How to Be a Safe Consultant Vascular Surgeon from Day One

This is a highly pragmatic and down-to-earth guide to the "real world" of vascular surgery, written to help trainees pass the FRCS (Vasc) Examination the first time around, hopefully with flying colours! Through clear and concise chapters, a review of relevant vascular surgery papers, a solid grounding in up-to-date and relevant UK and European guidelines, and mock examination questions, this book should give candidates a fighting chance at exam success.

Using his early experience, and insight gained from senior consultant vascular surgeons and mentors, author James Forsyth dispenses both facts and pearls of wisdom as he takes the prospective vascular surgeon through the core topics pertinent to a day one vascular consultant.

This guide specifically covers:

- "Building a strong foundation" with a focus on patient counselling, presentation skills, clear documentation, professionalism, and a foundational grasp of the key evidence base for vascular surgery
- "Core vascular surgery topics" from chronic limb-threatening ischaemia to aorto-iliac aneurysms to symptomatic carotid artery disease to chronic venous disease
- Pragmatic guide to the "bread & butter" vascular surgery operations
- Fifty mock SBA assessment questions and answers, and numerous mock FRCS short and long cases that are blended into reality-based discussions to draw out key learning points

This book is essential to any budding vascular surgeon intending to sit the FRCS (Vasc) examinations, and those who are about to start off as real day one consultant vascular surgeons. Indeed, the FRCS (Vasc) Examination is a bridge to becoming a true consultant vascular surgeon, and this book therefore is a "must-read" for anyone looking to cross that bridge.

James Michael Forsyth, MBBS MSc (HPE) FRCSEd (Vasc.Surg) is a Vascular Surgery Consultant at the Leeds Vascular Institute, United Kingdom. His special interests include diabetic foot disease, chronic limb-threatening ischaemia, vascular access, and major trauma.

HOW TO BE A SAFE CONSULTANT VASCULAR SURGEON FROM DAY ONE

The Unofficial Guide to Passing the FRCS (VASC)

James Michael Forsyth, MBBS MSc (HPE) FRCSEd (Vasc.Surg)

Vascular Surgery Consultant
Leeds Vascular Institute, UK

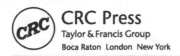

CRC Press
Taylor & Francis Group
Boca Raton London New York

CRC Press is an imprint of the
Taylor & Francis Group, an **informa** business

First edition published 2023
6000 Broken Sound Parkway NW, Suite 300, Boca Raton, FL 33487-2742

and by CRC Press
4 Park Square, Milton Park, Abingdon, Oxon, OX14 4RN

CRC Press is an imprint of Taylor & Francis Group, LLC

ISBN: 978-1-032-28585-6 (hbk)
ISBN: 978-1-032-28547-4 (pbk)
ISBN: 978-1-003-29754-3 (ebk)

DOI: 10.1201/b22951

Typeset in Times New Roman
by KnowledgeWorks Global Ltd.

My son, there is something else to watch out for. There is no end to the writing of books, and too much study will wear you out.

Ecclesiastes 12:12

I dedicate this book to my parents John and Linda.
Thanks for all your help and support over the years
I would not be here without you

Contents

INTRODUCTION   x

Section One   Strong Foundation

1 20 PAPERS FOR FRCS (PLUS A FEW MORE)   1

2 PATIENT COUNSELLING   38

3 CLEAR DOCUMENTATION   40

4 BE PROFESSIONAL   42

5 HOW TO PRESENT A VASCULAR PATIENT   45

Section Two   Core Vascular Surgery Topics

6 INTERMITTENT CLAUDICATION   51

7 DIABETIC FOOT DISEASE   54

8 CHRONIC LIMB-THREATENING ISCHAEMIA (CLTI)   68

9 ACUTE LIMB ISCHAEMIA   77

10 AORTOILIAC ANEURYSMS   103

11 THORACOABDOMINAL AORTIC ANEURYSM   131

12 POPLITEAL ANEURYSM   134

13 DESCENDING THORACIC AORTIC ANEURYSM   137

14 TYPE B AORTIC DISSECTION   145

15 SYMPTOMATIC CAROTID ARTERY DISEASE   150

16 VASCULAR ACCESS   163

17 THE IVDU GROIN   185

18 CHRONIC VENOUS DISEASE   189

19 LOWER LIMB VENOUS THROMBOEMBOLISM   199

20 MESENTERIC ARTERIAL DISEASE   211

21 VASCULAR TRAUMA   223

22 VASCULAR GRAFT AND ENDOGRAFT INFECTION   256

Section Three   "Bread & Butter" Vascular Surgery Operations

23 OPEN AAA REPAIR (ELECTIVE, INFRA-RENAL)   273

24 CAROTID ENDARTERECTOMY   278

25 COMMON FEMORAL ENDARTERECTOMY   282

26 FEMORAL ABOVE-KNEE POPLITEAL BYPASS: REVERSED IPSILATERAL GSV   284

27 FEMORAL BELOW-KNEE POPLITEAL BYPASS: REVERSED IPSILATERAL GSV   286

28 FEMORAL EMBOLECTOMY   289

29 POPLITEAL EMBOLECTOMY   291

30 BRACHIAL EMBOLECTOMY   293

31 LOWER-LIMB FASCIOTOMY   296

32 HALLUX AMPUTATION   298

33 FOOT DEBRIDEMENT   300

34 TRANSMETATARSAL AMPUTATION   302

35 ABOVE-KNEE AMPUTATION   304

36 BELOW-KNEE AMPUTATION   306

37 GUILLOTINE AMPUTATION (ABOVE ANKLE)   309

38 GSV ENDOVENOUS ABLATION   311

39 SAPHENOFEMORAL JUNCTION LIGATION, GREAT SAPHENOUS VEIN STRIPPING, AND MULTIPLE STAB AVULSIONS   313

40 TEMPORAL ARTERY BIOPSY   315

41 BRACHIOCEPHALIC FISTULA CREATION   317

42 PERITONEAL DIALYSIS TUBE INSERTION (OPEN)   320

43 PERITONEAL DIALYSIS TUBE REMOVAL   322

Section Four   Single Best Answer Assessment

44 QUESTIONS   325

45 ANSWERS   342

KEY REFERENCES FOR BOOK   345

INDEX   349

Introduction

If you have bought this book, it is highly likely that you are a senior vascular surgery trainee who is a few months away from sitting the FRCS Vascular Surgery Examination. It is also quite likely that if you are successful in passing this exam, the next challenge looming over the horizon is that of starting off as a day one consultant. Or perhaps, and less likely, you have been a Consultant Vascular Surgeon for a few years and want a "refresher" on all the stuff you learned to pass the FRCS exam, and that which you have now mostly forgotten! Whatever your justification for picking up this book, let's be honest with each other: nobody really likes studying and I don't think anyone who has gone through the FRCS Examination process has ever truly enjoyed it.

In terms of my own experience of the FRCS Examination, being honest, I did not really enjoy it. I spent months upon months reading through different books (massive ones, big ones, smaller ones), guidelines, journal papers, listening to audio podcasts, watching videos on the internet, doing mock MCQs online, seeing patients and presenting them to senior vascular surgeons who then grilled me, writing mock clinical scenarios out on pieces of paper and then filming myself explaining how I would manage such scenarios (e.g., ruptured AAA, ischaemic arm, major trauma), asking countless people for advice, and trying to get an idea of what was likely to come up …. To make matters worse, the COVID-19 pandemic struck in between my sitting FRCS Vascular Surgery Part A and Part B. This meant that my period of required revision was extended by 6 months. It is also meant I had to revise in a fairly isolated and restricted context. The examination was also conducted in what I can only describe as "weird" conditions. I had to sit the exam in a hotel in Glasgow wearing a facemask (*with my glasses continually fogging up*), in a massive room full of examiners and candidates sitting at big tables with no patients and only tablets being used to show pictures/clinical information. I don't know what your experience will be, but hopefully it will be a bit more "normal."

As I was approaching the end of my speciality training, I felt the "burden" of the FRCS Examination steadily looming over me. I knew it was coming, but for a couple of years, I didn't really have to think about it. And yet, once ST7 arrived, I knew it was inescapable. This is about the time when you are probably pretty confident in vascular surgery and will have a fairly good grasp of most of the core topics and probably think revising for the examination is unnecessary. It is also at this time when you will have already jumped through countless hoops, sat numerous examinations, been to various award ceremonies (e.g., MRCS, BSc, MBBS, PhD, MSc …). You will also probably feel tried, burned out, and fed up with training and just want to be free of examinations. You may also just want to focus on your family, settle down, chill out, and so on.

However, the truth is that you have to do the exam. Nobody ever said you had to like it. It is a pain, it is tedious, and I am sure you think you have better things to be doing. But guess what, you are not alone in feeling this. We all feel like this. So, it is alright to feel negative and frustrated at times. However, you must not let this negativity get the better of you. You have to put your game face on, pull your socks up, and go to work. This means being positive and facing the challenge like a true warrior.

I have witnessed first hand through my earlier years of training other senior vascular surgery trainees going for the examination. There are always a few candidates who do not pass it first time and have to re-sit it. I have also seen candidates fail the examination multiple times and have to instead go and sit the European examination. This does not mean these are bad vascular surgery trainees nor are they bad vascular surgeons. However, this is a reality which you have to accept → *this examination is a beast that either you will slay, or it will slay you*. You may have a chilled-out approach to life, be horrifically (*and falsely*) positive, and think you can "wing" this examination. Maybe you think you are gifted and examinations come easy to you. You may therefore adopt a minimalistic approach to sitting the FRCS Examination. If this is you, hey, you may be successful and I wish you good luck with this approach. However, I just do not recommend this approach. This is a serious, difficult, demanding, and challenging examination and the standards are set high. If you don't rise to the challenge, there is a very high likelihood that you will fail the examination. If you fail it, you just have to keep re-sitting it. Re-sitting it is not only demoralising, it is also time-consuming and expensive. I am very serious about this point. **This examination is not to be underestimated**. Imagine you are getting into a boxing ring with a ferocious world heavyweight champion boxer. If you think you can get away with doing 10 press-ups, 5 sit-ups, and hitting the heavy bag for 5 minutes, don't be surprised when you are knocked out in the first round.

I passed the FRCS Vascular Surgery examinations (Parts A and B) first time around. I also passed both of them under fairly challenging circumstances. If I can get through these examinations the first time, so can you. I am writing this book as an aid memoir, and hopefully it will be a relatively concise guide that gives you some high yield material that will increase your chances of success. I also hope it gives you some much-needed motivation and perhaps even a good kick up the rear to keep you moving forwards. However, I must emphasise that you must not rely upon this book alone. I prepared for this examination properly and that is why I passed it first time. I am not a genius and the reason I was successful is this: **HARD WORK**.

Finally, when I was approached by my publishing editor Miranda Bromage, the idea for this book was originally supposed to be just a revision guide for passing the FRCS Examination. However, this did not sit comfortably with me. I did not want this book to be a standard revision guide that sits amongst 10,000 other similar revision guides. No, this book is more than that. Let me remind you that you are not sitting the FRCS Vascular Surgery Examination in isolation. The FRCS Examination is an exit exam, and more than anything, it is a stepping stone to become a real day one consultant vascular surgeon. The examination is really a test to see whether or not you are competent and trustworthy to work as a day one consultant vascular surgeon. Therefore, I thought it would be better to focus the book on this domain. This means I will use my acquired knowledge, early experience as a consultant, and pearls of wisdom that I have picked up from senior vascular surgeons (*who have mentored me*) to help guide you. This book will therefore be "academic," but it will also be heavily pragmatic and "real world" at the same time.

I hope you find the book useful.

James Michael Forsyth

Cautionary Note

Every author selects what to include in their book, and what not to include. Every book is by design, every author has an agenda, and every author has their own biases. My agenda is to write a book that I hope will help shape a vascular surgery consultant who is down to earth, sensible, pragmatic, does the basics well, can do the "bread & butter" operations, is a decision-maker, assertive when necessary, and above all is safe. I also want to encourage adherence to guidelines and evidence-based medicine. In terms of bias, I consider myself to be a vascular surgeon as opposed to an endovascular surgeon. This agenda and biases are important to remember as you read this book.

This book is not an atlas of vascular surgery. It does not cover everything. It does not want to cover everything. It is big enough as it is without having covered everything! Therefore, don't be surprised if you don't find things like aortic arch pathology, thoracic outlet syndrome, hyperhidrosis, miscellaneous topics, statistics, etc. You will also not find a dedicated chapter on endovascular skills. Don't think though that I am ignorant of these other topics, nor should you think that you are not expected to have a grip on them. Hyperhidrosis did come in my Part B exam (*it was a rabbit in the headlights moment for me*), other candidates who were in my Part B Examination had thoracic outlet syndrome come up a few times, and in the Part A Examination there were a few miscellaneous topics and aortic arch pathology came up too. Henceforth, I do encourage you to do further self-directed learning beyond this book.

Finally, do please remember that this is **NOT** an official guide to passing the FRCS Examination. I have written my own book and it reflects my own character and my outlook on the world at this early stage of my career. Therefore, take what I say with a pinch of salt. If you find what I say useful and you think it is authoritative, please use it to your own advantage. However, if you think what I have said is wrong, feel free to ignore me.

CHAPTER 1

20 Papers for FRCS (Plus a Few More)

There are a lot of papers to cover. We could also spend an enormous amount of time on these papers. However, I don't really think this is necessary. For the examination, you need to be individually reading each of the recommended papers on your own, getting into the details, and having an idea in your own mind of the pros and cons of each paper. I am writing this chapter as if you are in a hotel room the night before your FRCS exam. You have already read all the papers a hundred times, and are running low on enthusiasm. You just want something to read that will give you the salient points. That is what I am trying to achieve here. I am putting some core papers and their key points / results / conclusions all in one place for convenience. This chapter will also be helpful in your day to day practice to summarise the key results that you can apply in your clinical decision-making.

I will also include other papers that I think are relevant for the FRCS examination and your real world practice. You don't have to focus on these too much, but I personally think they are useful. Also, your knowledge of them will give you something else to talk about in the exam and help you score the highest points

Risk of Major Amputation in Patients with Intermittent Claudication Undergoing Early Revascularisation

Background

- In the real world we know that loads of patients with intermittent claudication get treated with revascularisation.
- This is mainly in the form of endovascular intervention.
- This is despite the fact that most current clinical guidelines recommend supervised exercise programmes, smoking cessation, and best medical therapy for this cohort of patients.
- In this prospective study the incidence of major amputation was compared between cohorts of patients with intermittent claudication initially managed by revascularisation or conservative treatment during long term follow-up.
- This was a three centre, prospective study from Australia.
- The study ran from 2002 to 2016.
- Of the patients managed conservatively, this included—antiplatelet and statin, smoking cessation advice and support, identification of diabetes and referred to diabetologist/cardiologist as indicated, and advice to exercise regularly. No formal supervised exercise programme was available.
- Of the patients managed with intervention, this involved revascularisation within the first 6 months of initial assessment in addition to medical management and advice to undertake a home-based exercise programme.
- In general, endovascular management was first chosen for tight stenoses or occlusions affecting the iliac or superficial femoral arteries.
- Aorto-bifemoral bypass was preferred for widespread long occlusions of the common iliac and external iliac arteries, or occlusion of the infra-renal aorta.

DOI: 10.1201/b22951-1

1

- Femoropopliteal bypass grafts were considered for long flush occlusions of the superficial femoral artery where adequate long saphenous vein was available.
- The primary outcome of the study was major amputation, including above- and below-knee amputations.
- Secondary outcomes were the requirement for subsequent revascularisation and the incidence of myocardial infarction, stroke, and all-cause mortality.
- 456 patients diagnosed with PAD who presented with symptoms of intermittent claudication with follow-up of at least 1 year since recruitment were included in the study.
- Of these, 39% underwent early revascularisation and 61% had initial conservative management.
- Patients were followed up for a mean length of 5 years.

Results

- During this time, 12 patients (2.6%) required a major lower limb amputation, including five below-knee and seven above-knee amputations, at a mean of 4.75 years after recruitment.
- In univariable analysis, subsequent requirement for major amputation was associated with the prescription of fibrates (and therefore higher HDL-C), lower BMI, higher eGFR, and early revascularisation.
- Nine of the major amputations occurred in patients who had early revascularisation at a mean of 3.92 years after recruitment, and the other three were in patients initially treated conservatively at a mean of 7.23 years after recruitment (P = 0.010).
- Kaplan–Meier analysis showed that the estimated 5-year incidence of major amputation was 6.2 and 0.7% in patients undergoing early revascularisation and initial conservative treatment, respectively (P = 0.003).
- Unadjusted and adjusted Cox proportional hazard models indicated that early revascularisation was independently associated with subsequent requirement for major amputation.
- Of the nine patients who had early revascularisation and subsequently required a major amputation, the initial revascularisation procedure was an open operation alone in five patients, an endovascular procedure alone in three patients, and a combined endovascular and open procedure in one patient.
- Before major amputation, seven of the nine patients underwent multiple further revascularisation procedures.
- In Kaplan–Meier analysis, the estimated 5-year incidence of subsequent revascularisation was 49.1 and 31.5% in patients undergoing early revascularisation and initial conservative treatment, respectively (P < 0.001).
- The incidences of myocardial infarction, stroke, and death during follow-up were similar in the two groups.

Conclusions

- For patients with intermittent claudication, early revascularisation was associated with a greater risk of subsequent requirement for major amputation than initial conservative treatment.

- Both endovascular and open surgical revascularisation have limited long term durability, as illustrated by the higher rate of subsequent revascularisation in patients having early revascularisation than in those initially treated conservatively in the present study.
- The short term benefits of revascularisation, in terms of symptom relief, may potentially be offset by the longer-term hazards of major amputation.

Bypass versus Angioplasty in Severe Ischaemia of the Leg (BASIL): Multicentre Randomised Controlled Trial. BASIL Trial Participants

Background

- This trial was performed because of a stark lack of level 1 RCT evidence in regards to whether bypass or angioplasty was better for the treatment of patients with severe limb ischaemia related to infra-inguinal arterial disease.
- The BASIL trial compared the outcomes of a surgery-first strategy with an angioplasty-first strategy in patients with severe limb ischaemia.
- Severe limb ischaemia was defined as rest pain or tissue loss (ulcer or gangrene) of presumed arterial aetiology for more than 2 weeks, and who on diagnostic imaging had a pattern of disease which could equally well be treated by either infra-inguinal bypass surgery or balloon angioplasty.
- The study ran for 5 years from 1999 to 2004.
- 27 UK hospitals were involved.
- 452 patients were randomised.

Results

- 86% of 228 patients assigned to bypass surgery and 96% of 224 to balloon angioplasty underwent an attempt at their allocated intervention at a median of 6 days after randomisation.
- At the end of follow-up, 248 (55%) patients were alive without amputation (of trial leg), 38 (8%) were alive with amputation, 36 (8%) were dead after amputation, and 130 (29%) were dead without amputation.
- After 6 months, the two strategies did not differ significantly in amputation-free survival.
- There was no difference in health-related quality of life between the two strategies.
- For the first year the hospital costs associated with a surgery-first strategy were about one-third higher than those with an angioplasty-first strategy.
- There was a higher immediate failure and 12-month re-intervention rate in angioplasty than in surgery; however, morbidity associated with angioplasty was low and the hospital stay was short (thus the costs were lower).
- In the short term, a surgery-first strategy was associated with a significantly higher rate of morbidity, significantly greater length of hospital stay, and greater use of the high-dependency unit and intensive-therapy unit than that of an angioplasty-first strategy. Therefore, hospital costs of surgery for the first 12 months after randomisation were about a third higher than those after angioplasty. There was also a higher occurrence of cardiovascular, infective, and wound complications after surgery, and a small but clinically significant re-intervention rate for graft revision, thrombectomy, and evacuation of haematoma.
- However, in the long term, after 2 years, surgery seemed to be associated with a significantly reduced risk of future amputation, death, or both—i.e., if a patient was

alive with their leg intact at 2 years after randomisation, they seemed to be more likely to remain alive in the future with their leg intact if they had been assigned to receive surgery first than angioplasty first.

Conclusions

- Patients presenting with severe limb ischaemia due to infra-inguinal atherosclerosis and who seem technically suitable for both treatments can reasonably be treated with either method in the first instance.
- However, notwithstanding the high failure and re-intervention rate associated with angioplasty, patients who are expected to live for less than 1–2 years and have significant comorbidity should probably, when possible, be offered angioplasty first.
- By contrast, in patients expected to live more than 2 years and who are relatively fit, the apparent improved durability and reduced re-intervention rate of surgery could outweigh the short term considerations of increased morbidity and cost.

Bypass versus Angioplasty in Severe Ischaemia of the Leg (BASIL) Trial: Analysis of Amputation Free and Overall Survival by Treatment Received

This paper came out 5 years after the original BASIL trial results. Essentially, the authors followed all of the original trial patients to 3 years, with more than half beyond 5 years.

Key Recommendations

- "The overall recommendation from BASIL is that severe limb ischaemia patients predicted to live 2 years, and with a useable vein, should usually have bypass first. This is because the long term results of saphenous vein bypass are good, the rate of balloon angioplasty failure is high, and results of bypass after failed balloon angioplasty are significantly worse than for primary bypass. However, patients expected to live less than 2 years, and those without a useable vein, should usually have balloon angioplasty first because they will not survive to reap the longer-term benefits of surgery and the results of prosthetic bypass are poor."

Lower Limb Amputation in England: Prevalence, Regional Variation and Relationship with Revascularisation, Deprivation, and Risk Factors. A Retrospective Review of Hospital Data

Background

- This study's aim was to ascertain whether regional differences in the prevalence of major lower limb amputation exist in England and whether these are associated with reduced revascularisations, social deprivation, or different risk factor profiles of regional populations.
- The authors interrogated the Hospital Episode Statistics (HES) database which captures every hospital—patient encounter in England with approximately 52 million in-and outpatient episodes added each year.
- Information regarding patient demography, risk factors, diagnosis, and intervention was collected.
- From HES information was gathered on patients aged 50–84 years who underwent major lower limb amputation and revascularisation (both endovascular and surgical and including diagnostic angiograms).
- Social deprivation was measured using Indices of Multiple Deprivation 2010 (IMD) score.

Results

- There were approximately 90 million inpatient hospital episodes between 2003 and 2009.
- From this sampling frame, 25,312 major lower limb amputations and 136,215 revascularisations were extracted.
- The mean age of amputees was 70.6 years, 68.5% were men, and 28.6% were from the most deprived areas.
- The commonest disease risk factors were diabetes (44%), hypertension (39%), and coronary heart disease (23%).
- The overall age standardised prevalence rate of amputations and revascularisations in England for those aged 50–84 years was 26.3/100,000 and 141.6/100,000, respectively.
- Rates were double in men than women for both amputations and revascularisations.
- Regionally, the rates, per 100,000, of amputations and revascularisation were higher in Northern England—North 31.7 and 182.1; Midlands 26.0 and 121.3; and South 23.1 and 124.9.
- 7543 amputations (29.8%) were matched to a revascularisation.
- There were increased odds of having an amputation associated with a revascularisation with increasing age, male sex, and all risk factors except diabetes.
- Diabetics, however, were more likely to have an amputation with no revascularisation.

Conclusions

- The prevalence of major lower limb amputation and revascularisation in England is double in men than women and significantly higher in Northern England compared with the South.
- Amputees from Northern England had higher levels of social deprivation, coronary heart disease, and smoking but lower levels of diabetes, hypertension, and hypercholesterolaemia.
- The odds of having an amputation with a revascularisation were not significantly different between the Midlands and Southern England but were higher in the North even after controlling for demographic and disease risk factors.

Key Message from the Trial

- "We believe the challenge for PAD management is to reduce the inequality in major lower limb amputation rates across England. This should involve organising and delivering healthcare in a targeted manner and include the community as well as hospital care with particular focus on Northern England."

The Society for Vascular Surgery Lower Extremity Threatened Limb Classification System: Risk Stratification Based on Wound, Ischaemia, and Foot Infection (WIfI)

- I suggest you just read the original paper.
- If you get asked in the exam you may need to calculate the WIfI stage yourself ….
- As for me, in my real world practice, I just use the Society of Vascular Surgery mobile application.
    1. Firstly, determine the ulceration (no ulcer, small shallow ulcer, deep ulcer, or extensive and deep ulcer).

2. Secondly, determine the gangrene (none, limited to distal phalanx, gangrenous changes to digits, extensive gangrene).
3. Thirdly, determine the level of ischaemia (toe pressure or ankle systolic pressure).
4. Fourthly, determine the infection grade (uninfected, mild, moderate, severe).
- Whack in the numbers and you will be given a WIfI clinical stage! BOOM POW!

Shall We Do Some Examples?

1. Patient with a small shallow ulcer at the tip of 5th toe with surrounding dry gangrene, no infection, but with a toe pressure of 34 mmHg. WIfI stage is 2, meaning a low amputation risk and moderate potential benefit from revascularisation.
2. Patient with a deep ulcer of the hallux with exposed bone and MTP joint, gangrene of the hallux and adjacent toes, a toe pressure of 22 mmHg, and a nasty tracking infection in the forefoot with evidence of systemic upset. WIfI stage is 4, meaning high risk of amputation and high potential benefit of revascularisation.
3. Patient with a small ulcer over the plantar aspect of the fifth MTP. Pus coming from ulcer with MTP joint exposed. Forefoot is swollen and cellulitic. Patient is systemically well but WBC of 16 and CRP of 187. Toe pressure unrecordable. WIfI stage is 4, meaning again high amputation risk and high potential benefit from revascularisation.
4. Patient with rest pain in the left foot and minor dry gangrene to tip of left second toe. No signs of infection. Toe pressure of 49 mmHg. WIfI stage is 1, meaning very low risk of amputation and low potential benefit from revascularisation.

Six-Year Prospective Multicentre Randomised Comparison of Autologous Saphenous Vein and Expanded Polytetrafluoroethylene Grafts in Infrainguinal Arterial Reconstructions

Background

- This is an "old school" paper that I think is great.
- It is from 1986, by Frank Veith et al.
- Basically at the time of this study, you get the impression there was a big controversy about whether PTFE or autologous saphenous vein was better for infra-inguinal bypasses.
- This study, which started in 1978, was a randomised prospective multicentre comparison between PTFE and autologous vein grafts as infra-inguinal arterial bypass conduits in patients with atherosclerotic lower limb ischaemia.
- The three vascular centres were in New York, Chicago, and Milwaukee.
- Autologous vein and PTFE grafts were compared in 845 infra-inguinal bypass operations, 485 to the popliteal artery, and 360 to infra-popliteal arteries.

Results

- The primary patency for randomised PTFE grafts to the popliteal artery were similar to vein grafts for 2 years, and then became significantly different, with a 4-year patency rate of around 68% for vein versus 47% for PTFE.
- The 4-year patency differences for above-knee grafts were not statistically significant, but for below-knee grafts there were significant patency differences (vein patency around 76% and PTFE around 54%).

- The 4-year limb salvage rates for popliteal bypasses for critical ischaemia did not differ between the two different types of randomised grafts.
- The primary patency at 4 years for below-knee popliteal bypasses with randomised vein was significantly better than with randomised PTFE (around 49% for vein versus 12% for PTFE).

Conclusions

- Femoropopliteal bypasses performed with randomised PTFE grafts have patency rates inferior to those performed with randomised autologous saphenous vein grafts.
- This fact does not support the routine preferential use of PTFE grafts for femoropopliteal arterial reconstructions.
- The present study confirms the clear superiority of randomised autologous saphenous vein grafts over randomised PTFE grafts for arterial reconstructions to infra-popliteal arteries.
- PTFE may be used preferentially in selected poor-risk patients for femoropopliteal bypasses, particularly those that do not cross the knee.
- Although every effort should be made to use autologous saphenous vein for infra-popliteal bypasses, a PTFE distal bypass is a better option than a primary major amputation.

Risk of Death Following Application of Paclitaxel-Coated Balloons and Stents in the Femoropopliteal Artery of the Leg: A Systematic Review and Meta-Analysis of Randomised Controlled Trials

Background

- The authors of this paper highlighted that a couple of RCTs with longer-term follow-up have shown hints of increased late patient mortality with the use of paclitaxel DES or DCB, and in the absence of obvious causal links, these findings have been dismissed by expert review panels as statistical artefacts or anomalies, and both devices are currently under clinical use with extended on label indications.
- Henceforth, this study was an updated systematic review and quantitative meta-analysis of RCTs investigating paclitaxel-coated balloons and stents in the femoropopliteal artery, in order to analyse the early and late risk of death associated with these novel endovascular technologies that deliver paclitaxel to the vessel wall of the lower limbs.
- The literature search was last updated in August 2018.
- Trials were considered for inclusion in the present meta-analysis if they fulfilled the following inclusion criteria: (1) Randomised controlled study design, (2) investigation of a paclitaxel-coated/paclitaxel-eluting stent or balloon in the femoropopliteal artery, (3) patient population with peripheral arterial disease (PAD) of the femoral and/or popliteal artery and symptoms of intermittent claudication and/or critical limb ischaemia, and (4) clinical follow-up of at least 1 year available.
- 28 RCTs with 4663 patients were finally included in the present meta-analysis.
- Paclitaxel-coated balloons and stents were used primarily for the treatment of short-distance intermittent claudication (n = 4133 of 4663 subjects; 89%) in the majority of the study population and infrequently for a critical limb ischaemia indication (n = 530).

Results

- All-cause death at 1 year → there was good evidence that the pooled risk of death did not differ significantly between the active use of paclitaxel-coated balloons or stents versus the control arms.
- All-cause death at 2 years → there was good evidence that application of paclitaxel-coated devices in the femoropopliteal artery was related to significantly increased risk of death (significant 68% relative risk increase of all-cause death with a corresponding NNH of 29 patients).
- All-cause death up to 5 years → the risk of death increased further in the long term analysis with a 93% relative risk increase and an NNH of 14.

Conclusions

- There seems to be an increased long term risk of death beyond the first year following femoropopliteal application of paclitaxel-coated balloons and stents in the lower limbs.

JMF Reflections on the Paclitaxel Controversy

This is a big topic and it has had a large global effect on the endovascular community. It is advisable to have a good understanding not just of this paper but also the numerous other papers out there that either support its position or challenge its position. As far as I am concerned, I can see both sides of the equation. Generally speaking, however, my position is to remain cautious, and therefore my gut feeling is to say that there is no smoke without fire. However, at the same time (despite my feeling that there is something suspicious about paclitaxel), I have recently been to two London-based vascular surgery conferences where the majority of the audience seemed to think paclitaxel is beneficial for patients. In any case, you can draw your own conclusions. I guess time will ultimately tell what the answer is.

MRC/BHF Heart Protection Study of Cholesterol Lowering with Simvastatin in 20,536 High-Risk Individuals: A Randomised Placebo-Controlled Trial

Background

- 20,536 UK adults (aged 40–80 years) with coronary disease, other occlusive arterial disease, or diabetes were randomly allocated to receive 40 mg simvastatin daily or matching placebo.
- Analyses were of the first occurrence of particular events, and compare all simvastatin-allocated versus all placebo-allocated participants.
- This was an intention to treat analysis (85% compliance in statin cohort, 17% non-study statin use in the placebo cohort).
- Primary outcomes were mortality (for overall analyses) and fatal or non-fatal vascular events (for subcategory analyses), with subsidiary assessments of cancer and of other major morbidity.

Results

- All-cause mortality was significantly reduced among those allocated simvastatin versus placebo (12.9 versus 14.7%; $P = 0.0003$).

- This was due to a highly significant 18% proportional reduction in the coronary death rate (5.7 versus 6.9%; P = 0.0005).
- There was a marginally significant reduction in other vascular deaths (1.9 versus 2.2%; P = 0.07).
- There were highly significant reductions of about one-quarter in the first event rate for non-fatal myocardial infarction or coronary death (8.7 versus 11.8%; P < 0.0001), for non-fatal or fatal stroke 4.3 versus 5.7%, P < 0.0001), and for coronary or non-coronary revascularisation (9.1 versus 11.7%; P < 0.0001).
- For the first occurrence of any of these major vascular events, there was a definite 24% reduction in the event rate (19.8 versus 25.2%; P < 0.0001).
- During the first year the reduction in major vascular events was not significant, but subsequently it was highly significant during each separate year.
- The annual excess risk of myopathy with this regimen was about 0.01%.
- There were no significant adverse effects on cancer incidence or on hospitalisation for any other non-vascular cause.

Conclusion

- Lowering cholesterol with 40 mg simvastatin daily produces substantial reductions in the rates of major vascular events among a wide range of high-risk individuals irrespective of their initial cholesterol concentrations.

Effects of Statin Therapy and Dose on Cardiovascular and Limb Outcomes in Peripheral Arterial Disease: A Systematic Review and Meta-Analysis

Background

- According to the authors of this paper, the guidelines around statin prescribing in patients with PAD are inconsistent.
- Indeed, the authors highlighted that NICE recommends "high intensity statins" for patients with PAD, although the evidence for specific PAD patients is lacking.
- This meta-analysis aimed to collate, review, and analyse recent data on statin use and dose in patients with a diagnosis of PAD.
- 24 studies were included in this meta-analysis.
- 22 of the 24 studies were cohort studies, of which 9 were prospective and 13 retrospective.

Results

- Statin therapy was significantly protective for all-cause mortality and amputations.
- High doses of statins were significantly better protective against all-cause mortality but work less significantly for major adverse cardiovascular events (MACE).
- Amputations were less frequent in patients on high doses.

Conclusion

- Higher dosing of statins confers a significant improvement in patient outcomes, especially all-cause mortality and amputations, although the quality of the evidence was variable.

Collaborative Meta-Analysis of Randomised Trials of Antiplatelet Therapy for Prevention of Death, Myocardial Infarction, and Stroke in High Risk Patients. Antithrombotic Trialists' Collaboration

Background

- This big study aimed to determine the effects of antiplatelet therapy among patients at high risk of occlusive vascular events.
- It was a collaborative meta-analysis that included randomised trials of an antiplatelet regimen versus control or of one antiplatelet regimen versus another in high-risk patients.
- Studies reviewed 287 studies involving 135,000 patients in comparisons of antiplatelet therapy versus control and 77,000 in comparisons of different antiplatelet regimens.
- The main outcome measure was "serious vascular event": non-fatal myocardial infarction, non-fatal stroke, or vascular death.

Results

- Overall, among these high-risk patients, allocation to antiplatelet therapy reduced the combined outcome of any serious vascular event by about one-quarter; non-fatal myocardial infarction was reduced by one-third, non-fatal stroke by one-quarter, and vascular mortality by one-sixth.
- In each of these high-risk categories, the absolute benefits substantially outweighed the absolute risks of major extra-cranial bleeding.

Conclusion

- Aspirin (or another oral antiplatelet drug) is protective in most types of patients at increased risk of occlusive vascular events, including those with an acute myocardial infarction or ischaemic stroke, unstable or stable angina, previous myocardial infarction, stroke or cerebral ischaemia, and PAD.

A Randomised, Blinded, Trial of Clopidogrel versus Aspirin in Patients at Risk of Ischaemic Events (CAPRIE)

Background

- CAPRIE was a randomised, blinded, international trial designed to assess the relative efficacy of clopidogrel (75 mg once daily) and aspirin (325 mg once daily) in reducing the risk of a composite outcome cluster of ischaemic stroke, myocardial infarction, or vascular death.
- Their relative safety was also assessed.
- The population studied comprised subgroups of patients with atherosclerotic vascular disease manifested as either recent ischaemic stroke, recent myocardial infarction, or symptomatic PAD.
- 19,185 patients, with more than 6300 in each of the clinical subgroups, were recruited over 3 years, with a mean follow-up of 1.91 years.

Results

- An intention-to-treat analysis showed that patients treated with clopidogrel had an annual 5.32% risk of ischaemic stroke, myocardial infarction, or vascular death compared with 5.83% with aspirin.

- These rates reflect a statistically significant (P = 0.043) relative-risk reduction of 8.7% in favour of clopidogrel.
- On-treatment analysis yielded a relative-risk reduction of 9.4%.
- Reported severe bleeding was more common with aspirin, with the difference in severe gastrointestinal bleeding being statistically significant.

Conclusions

- Long term administration of clopidogrel to patients with atherosclerotic vascular disease is more effective than aspirin in reducing the combined risk of ischaemic stroke, myocardial infarction, or vascular death.
- The overall safety profile of clopidogrel is at least as good as that of medium-dose aspirin.

Rivaroxaban with or without Aspirin in Patients with Stable Peripheral or Carotid Artery Disease: An International, Randomised, Double-Blind, Placebo-Controlled Trial

Background

- Before this study the mainstay for treating patients with PAD was mainly single antiplatelet therapy.
- This was mainly focused on preventing MACE.
- Other antithrombotic regimens had been tested including vitamin K antagonists and newer antiplatelet agents used alone or in combination with aspirin, but none had been shown to be superior to antiplatelet therapy alone.
- This was multicentre, double-blind, randomised, placebo-controlled trial comparing low-dose rivaroxaban with aspirin or rivaroxaban alone (with aspirin placebo) versus aspirin alone (with rivaroxaban placebo) for prevention of cardiovascular death, myocardial infarction, and stroke in patients with coronary artery disease or peripheral artery disease.
- The trial ran from 2013 to 2016.
- It enrolled 7470 patients with peripheral artery disease from 558 centres.
- The median duration of treatment was 21 months.

Results

- The combination of rivaroxaban plus aspirin compared with aspirin alone reduced the composite endpoint of cardiovascular death, myocardial infarction, or stroke (5 versus 7%; hazard ratio [HR], 0.72; 95% CI, 0.57–0.90; P = 0.0047).
- Major adverse limb events including major amputation was reduced (1 versus 2%; HR, 0.54; 95% CI, 0.35–0.82; P = 0.0037).
- The use of the rivaroxaban plus aspirin combination increased major bleeding compared with the aspirin alone group (3 versus 2%; HR, 1.61; 95% CI, 1.12–2.31; P = 0.0089), which was mainly gastrointestinal.

Conclusion

- Low-dose rivaroxaban taken twice a day plus aspirin once a day reduced major adverse cardiovascular and limb events when compared with aspirin alone. Although major bleeding was increased, fatal or critical organ bleeding was not.

Rivaroxaban in Peripheral Artery Disease after Revascularisation (VOYAGER Trial)

Background

- This is the follow-up to the COMPASS trial.
- It was a double-blind randomised controlled trial.
- Eligible patients were at least 50 years old and had documented lower-extremity peripheral artery disease, including symptoms, anatomical evidence, and hemodynamic evidence.
- Patients were eligible after a successful revascularisation procedure performed within the previous 10 days for symptoms of peripheral artery disease.
- Patients were randomly assigned to receive rivaroxaban (2.5 mg twice daily) plus aspirin or placebo plus aspirin.
- Clopidogrel could be administered for up to 6 months after revascularisation at the discretion of the investigator.
- The primary efficacy outcome was a composite of acute limb ischaemia, major amputation for vascular causes, myocardial infarction, ischemic stroke, or death from cardiovascular causes.
- The principal safety outcome was major bleeding.
- A total of 6564 patients underwent randomisation from 2015 to 2018 at 542 sites in 34 countries.
- Overall, there were 14,752 patient-years of follow-up.
- 80% of patients were taking statin therapy and 63% were taking angiotensin-converting—enzyme inhibitors or angiotensin-receptor blockers; 51% were taking clopidogrel.
- Approximately two-thirds of patients were been treated with an endovascular procedure (65%), and one-third were treated surgically (35%).
- Around 76% of revascularisation procedures were performed for intermittent claudication, and around 23% of revascularisation procedures were performed for critical limb ischaemia.

Results

- The primary efficacy outcome occurred in 508 patients in the rivaroxaban group and in 584 in the placebo group; the Kaplan–Meier estimates of the incidence at 3 years were 17.3 and 19.9%, respectively (HR, 0.85; 95% CI, 0.76–0.96; $P = 0.009$).
- TIMI major bleeding occurred in 62 patients in the rivaroxaban group and in 44 patients in the placebo group (2.65 and 1.87%; HR, 1.43; 95% CI, 0.97–2.10; $P = 0.07$).
- ISTH major bleeding occurred in 140 patients in the rivaroxaban group, as compared with 100 patients in the placebo group (5.94 and 4.06%; HR, 1.42; 95% CI, 1.10–1.84; $P = 0.007$).

Conclusions

- The addition of rivaroxaban at a dose of 2.5 mg twice daily to aspirin in patients with symptomatic peripheral artery disease who had undergone lower-extremity revascularisation reduced the incidence of the composite outcome of acute limb ischaemia, amputation for vascular causes, myocardial infarction, ischemic stroke, or cardiovascular death.

- The incidence of the principal safety outcome of TIMI major bleeding was not significantly higher with rivaroxaban plus aspirin than with aspirin alone, but rivaroxaban plus aspirin was associated with a significantly higher incidence of the secondary safety outcome of ISTH major bleeding.

Efficacy of Oral Anticoagulants Compared with Aspirin after Infra-Inguinal Bypass Surgery (The Dutch Bypass Oral Anticoagulants or Aspirin Study): A Randomised Trial

Background

- This was a multicentre, randomised, open trial.
- 77 centres were involved between 1995 and 1998.
- 2690 patients who had undergone infra-inguinal grafting were randomly assigned oral anticoagulants (target international normalised ratio 3.0–4.5, n = 1339) or aspirin (80 mg daily, n = 1351).
- Patients were followed up for a mean of 21 months.
- The primary outcome was graft occlusion.

Results

- 308 graft occlusions occurred in the oral anticoagulants group compared with 322 in the aspirin group (HR, 0.95), which suggested no overall advantage for either treatment.
- Oral anticoagulants were beneficial in patients with vein grafts, whereas aspirin had better results for non-venous grafts.
- The composite outcome of vascular death, myocardial infarction, stroke, or amputation occurred 248 times in the oral anticoagulant group and 275 times in the aspirin group (0.89 [0.75–1.06]).
- Patients treated with oral anticoagulants had more major bleeding episodes than those treated with aspirin.

Conclusions

- Oral anticoagulation is the optimum treatment to prevent infra-inguinal vein graft occlusion, and is generally more effective in lowering the rate of ischaemic events, at an acceptable risk of haemorrhage.
- Aspirin is the first choice of treatment to prevent non-venous graft occlusion. Although it is associated with a higher risk of ischaemic stroke and myocardial infarction, the risk of haemorrhage is lower than that with oral anticoagulants.

Results of the Randomised, Placebo-Controlled Clopidogrel and Acetylsalicylic Acid in Bypass Surgery for Peripheral Arterial Disease (CASPAR) Trial

Background

- This was a prospective, multicentre, randomised, double-blind, placebo-controlled study of the efficacy and safety of clopidogrel plus aspirin as compared to aspirin alone in patients undergoing unilateral below-knee arterial bypass grafting.
- Patients were eligible for recruitment to the trial 2–4 days after bypass surgery.
- There was chronic background treatment with daily aspirin started at least 4 weeks before surgery.

- The pre-specified minimum duration of treatment and follow-up was 6 months and the maximum was 24 months.
- The primary endpoint was defined as the first occurrence, over the duration of follow-up, of the following cluster of events: occlusion of the index bypass graft. Any surgical or endovascular revascularisation procedure on the index bypass graft or para-anastomotic region or amputation above the ankle of the index limb or death.
- Secondary endpoints included the first occurrence of any individual component of the primary endpoint, and the first occurrence of the following during follow-up: CV death or myocardial infarction or stroke or any amputation above the ankle.
- The primary safety endpoint was severe bleeding.
- 851 patients were enrolled in 87 sites in 13 European countries and Australia, between 2004 and 2006.
- Of these, 425 were randomised to receive clopidogrel and aspirin (venous grafts, 297; prosthetic grafts, 128), and 426 to receive placebo plus aspirin (venous grafts, 301; prosthetic grafts, 125).
- Around 75% of bypasses were to the below-knee popliteal artery, 21% were to the crural vessels, and around 3% were to the pedal vessels.

Results

- In the overall population, the primary endpoint occurred in 149 of 425 patients in the clopidogrel group versus 151 of 426 patients in the placebo (plus ASA) group (HR, 0.98; 95% CI, 0.78–1.23).
- In a pre-specified subgroup analysis, the primary endpoint was significantly reduced by clopidogrel in prosthetic graft patients (HR, 0.65; 95% CI, 0.45–0.95; P = 0.025) but not in venous graft patients (HR, 1.25; 95% CI, 0.94–1.67, not significant).
- Although total bleeds were more frequent with clopidogrel, there was no significant difference between the rates of severe bleeding in the clopidogrel and placebo (plus ASA) groups (2.1 versus 1.2%).

Conclusions

- There was no significant benefit within the whole population from dual clopidogrel and aspirin therapy in terms of the primary endpoint.
- Patients receiving prosthetic grafts were analysed separately, and a statistically significant result was seen showing that clopidogrel reduced the composite primary endpoint, and the secondary endpoints of graft occlusion and amputation.

General Anaesthesia versus Local Anaesthesia for Carotid Surgery (GALA): A Multicentre, Randomised Controlled Trial

Background

- This was a parallel group, multicentre, randomised controlled trial.
- 3526 patients with symptomatic or asymptomatic carotid stenosis from 95 centres in 24 countries.
- Participants were randomly assigned to surgery under general (n = 1753) or local (n = 1773) anaesthesia between 1999 and 2007.

- The primary outcome was the proportion of patients with stroke (including retinal infarction), myocardial infarction, or death between randomisation and 30 days after surgery.
- Analysis was by intention to treat.

Results

- The primary outcome events were observed in 4.8% of GA patients, and 4.5% of LA patients.
- This difference was not statistically significant.
- Similarly, there were no differences between LA and GA for patients aged > or <75 years or for those considered at higher risk from surgery.
- However, there were differences in those patients with contralateral carotid occlusion. In 310 patients with contralateral carotid occlusion there were 23 primary outcome events (10%) in GA patients, versus 8 primary outcome events (5%) in LA patients.

Core Findings/Recommendations from GALA

- Both methods of anaesthesia are safe and that the anaesthetist and surgeon, in consultation with the patient, should probably determine the method of anaesthesia.
- However, for patients with a contralateral carotid occlusion LA may offer some added benefit.

European Carotid Surgery Trialist's Collaboration: Reanalysis of the Final Results of the European Carotid Surgery Trial

Background

- The original ECST and NASCET trials measured carotid stenoses in different ways.
- This disparity leads to inconsistent and slightly confusing clinical recommendations.
- This trial focused on re-measuring the ESCT patient in the same way as NASCET, such that both trials could be more easily compared (i.e. the original carotid angiograms were reassessed).
- 3018 patients from ECST were followed up for a mean of 73 months.

Results

- Surgery reduced the 5-year risk of any stroke or surgical death by 5.7% in patients with 50–69% stenosis and by 21.2% in patients with 70–99% stenosis without "near occlusion."
- These benefits were maintained at the 10-year follow-up.
- Surgery was of no benefit in patients with near occlusion.
- The effect of surgery in this group was highly significantly different from that in patients with 70–99% stenosis without near occlusion.
- Surgery was harmful in patients with 30% stenosis and of no benefit in patients with 30–49% stenosis.

Trial Conclusion

- Surgery was highly beneficial for 70–99% stenosis and moderately beneficial for 50–69% stenosis. Surgery was of little benefit in patients with carotid near occlusion.

Early Endarterectomy Carries a Lower Procedural Risk Than Early Stenting in Patients with Symptomatic Stenosis of the Internal Carotid Artery: Results from Four Randomised Controlled Trials

Background

- This paper looks at carotid endarterectomy versus carotid stenting for symptomatic carotid artery disease.
- It also takes into account the timing of intervention in relation to the risk/benefit profile.
- Four randomised controlled trials were included in the analysis; EVA-3S, SPACE, ICSS, and CREST.
- The pooled data set for all 4 trials included 4754 patients with symptomatic ICA stenosis. 2361 patients were randomised to CEA (49.7%) and 2393 patients to CAS.

Results

- The risk of any stroke or death within 30 days after treatment was higher for the CAS compared with the CEA group for the entire study population: 7.3% versus 3.3%.
- In the early period (0–7 days), CAS had the highest number and proportion of peri-procedural strokes and deaths (8.4%), compared with CEA (1.3%).
- Patients in the CAS group had a higher risk of any stroke or death in the crude and adjusted models.
- Compared with those treated within 7 days, patients treated after 7 days had fewer strokes and deaths in the CAS group (7.1%), whereas the risk of stroke and death in the CEA group slightly increased (3.6%).
- The relative risk for CAS compared with CEA was still higher in this later treatment group.
- Results were almost identical for the outcome analysis of any stroke.
- The analysis of fatal or disabling stroke outcome at 30 days also showed that the crude relative risk was higher for CAS than the CEA group within 7 days and after 7 days.

Paper's Conclusion

- CAS is not as safe as CEA in the treatment of patients with symptomatic stenosis of the ICA irrespective of the timing of treatment. The difference in safety between CAS and CEA is particularly potent in patients treated within 7 days of symptom onset. Therefore early CEA compared with early CAS after an initial neurological event offers the highest stroke prevention benefit for the patient at risk.

Cochrane Review: Carotid Endarterectomy for Symptomatic Carotid Stenosis

Background

- Three relevant randomised studies were included: ECST 1998, NASCET 1991, and VACSP 1991.
- Original carotid angiograms from the studies were re-analysed.

Results

- Carotid surgery is beneficial for people with a significant degree of carotid artery stenosis.

- The degree of stenosis above which surgery is beneficial is 50%, although benefit in patients with 70–99% stenosis is markedly more than in those with 50–69% stenosis.
- Patients with carotid near occlusion are different from patients with 70% or greater stenosis without near occlusion, and have a lower risk of stroke on medical treatment. The evidence indicates that benefit from carotid endarterectomy in patients with carotid near occlusion is marginal.
- Benefit from CEA is greater in men than women and in the elderly.
- Benefit from surgery decreases with increased time delay from last neurological symptom.
- Women had a lower risk of ipsilateral ischaemic stroke with medical treatment and a higher operative risk compared with men.
- Carotid endarterectomy is very clearly beneficial in women with 70–99% symptomatic stenosis, but not in women with 50–69% stenosis.

Conclusion from Paper

- Early and appropriate intervention will continue to be highly beneficial for symptomatic patients with high grade ipsilateral carotid artery stenosis.

Mid-Term Migration and Device Failure Following Endovascular Aneurysm Sealing with the Nellix Stent Graft System: A Single Centre Experience

Background

- The Achilles heel of endovascular aneurysm repair (EVAR) is long term durability.
- The Nellix device was specifically designed to eliminate or reduce the risk of all endoleaks after endovascular abdominal aortic aneurysm (AAA) repair.
- The system is based upon two balloon expandable stents attached to "endobags" that are filled in situ with a soluble polymer that "seals" the aneurysm.
- In the short term there appeared to be seemingly positive results.
- People had also been using this technology outside of IFU, and also in the context of using parallel stents (i.e. chimney endovascular aneurysm sealing—EVAS).
- Sounded like a great concept.
- However, over time there were increasing concerns in regards to long term durability and device failure.
- This was a single centre study from Cambridge that did quite a few Nellix device insertions. However, the Cambridge team noticed a higher than expected rate of device failures, and thus published this paper to alert other units.
- This was a retrospective review of all patients treated with the Nellix device at Cambridge University Hospital trust between February 2013 and August 2017.

Results

- Nellix stent grafts were implanted in 161 patients.
- This included both elective and emergency cases (emergency = 20).
- The median follow up was 4.4 years.
- In general, this cohort included patients with complex anatomy for EVAR.

- 29% of patients had anatomy outside the original Nellix IFU, 46% of patients were deemed suitable for conventional EVAR, and 25% of patients had no other endovascular option.
- In total, failure in 42 of 115 patients was identified. There were 12.2 failures per 100 person-years and device failure frequently occurred more than 2 years following implant.
- Device failure was higher when used outside the original IFU.
- Freedom from failure at 4 years was 42%.
- There were five failures within 1 year of the index procedure. Two of these were type 1b endoleaks and the remainder type 1a endoleaks.
- The mechanism for failure in most cases was caudal migration of the stents, separation of the endobags, and pressurisation of the sac, often in the absence of a visible endoleak on duplex or triple phase CT scan.

Author's Discussion

- Collectively, the early results were encouraging in both standard and challenging anatomies and it was felt that EVAS may have significant advantages over standard EVAR and was a potential game changer with regard to long term freedom from re-intervention.
- This has proved not to be the case and in retrospect the enthusiasm should have been tempered by the lack of long term durability data.
- Post-operative imaging of Nellix failure can be challenging, and sac pressurisation and rupture may occur in the absence of a visible endoleak.
- *Key message in the article:* Absence of a visible endoleak on duplex scanning does not rule out proximal device failure and there should be meticulous scrutiny of stent position, new thrombus formation, sac size increases, or evidence of stent separation. All of these features are concerning. Any inferior migration, even subtle, can be catastrophic as the endobag polymer cast no longer fits the aorta.
- As part of the ongoing concern about the durability of the Nellix devices in this patient cohort, "duty of candour" letters have been sent to all surviving patients and the patients have all been reviewed again in clinic to explain the findings and answer their questions.
- All surviving patients are now undergoing enhanced surveillance, with clinical assessment, six monthly duplex ultrasound, and plain abdominal X-ray, to identify device migration and endoleaks.

Author's Conclusion

- Poor outcomes for AAA patients treated with the Nellix endovascular sealing device beyond the first 2 years following implantation have been demonstrated. Of the patients surviving more than 3 years, approximately half of the grafts have shown signs of failure. Diagnosis and management of proximal graft failure is challenging and often requires graft explant. Nellix is no longer routinely used at CUH because of these problems.

Systematic Review and Meta-Analysis of Sex Differences in Outcomes after Endovascular Aneurysm Repair for Infrarenal Abdominal Aortic Aneurysm

Background

- Women face distinctive challenges when they receive EVAR treatment, and according to the previous studies, sex differences in outcomes after EVAR for infra-renal AAA remain controversial.

- This study aimed to compare the short term and long term outcomes between women and men after EVAR for infra-renal AAA.
- This was a comprehensive systematic review and meta-analysis of all available studies reporting sex differences after EVAR for infra-renal AAA.
- The time period of selected studies was from 2009 to 2018, and the publications were all in English.
- All the studies were retrospective cohorts from America and Europe.

Results

- The overall pooled odds ratio (OR) suggested that women were associated with a significantly increased risk of 30-day mortality than men (OR, 1.67; 95% CI, 1.50–1.87; $P < 0.001$).
- The pooled results from ten cohorts with 63,858 patients demonstrated that women had a significantly higher risk of in-hospital mortality (OR, 1.90; 95% CI, 1.43–2.53; $P < 0.001$), especially in patients with intact AAA (OR, 2.10; 95% CI, 1.79–2.48; $P < 0.001$).
- Women experienced significantly higher risk of limb ischaemia within 30 days after EVAR (OR, 2.44; 95% CI, 1.73-2.43; $P < 0.001$).
- The pooled result indicated a trend towards worse outcomes in women in regards to visceral/mesenteric ischaemia; however, it did not reach statistical significance.
- Women were associated with a higher risk of 30-day renal complications without significant heterogeneity (OR, 1.73; 95% CI, 1.12-2.67; $P = 0.028$).
- Women had a significantly increased risk of cardiac complications within 30 days of EVAR with a low level of heterogeneity (OR, 1.68; 95% CI, 1.01–2.80; $P = 0.046$).
- There was no significant sex difference in 30-day re-interventions.
- Women had a significantly higher risk of long term all-cause mortality than men (HR, 1.23; 95% CI, 1.09–1.38; $P = 0.01$).
- There was no significant difference between women and men in late endoleaks.
- There was no significant sex difference in late re-interventions.

Possible Explanations Given by Authors to Explain These Results

- Women tend to be older than men at the time of their intervention.
- Women have smaller access arteries, more hostile infra-renal necks.
- Women are perhaps susceptible to inferior medical treatment.
- Perhaps women have previously had their AAA intervened at too large a size i.e. 5.5 cm. The authors say that the threshold should be lowered to probably around 5.0 cm.

Conclusions

- Female sex was associated with a significantly increased risk of 30-day mortality, in-hospital mortality, limb ischaemia, renal complications, cardiac complications, and long term all-cause mortality. However, there was no evident difference in outcomes by sex for visceral/mesenteric ischaemia, 30-day re-interventions, late endoleaks, or late re-interventions.
- Women should be enrolled in a strict and regular long term surveillance after EVAR.

Meta-Analysis of Fenestrated Endovascular Aneurysm Repair versus Open Surgical Repair of Juxtarenal Abdominal Aortic Aneurysms over the Last 10 Years

Background

- The aim of this systematic review was to compare short- and long term outcomes of FEVAR and OSR for the management of juxtarenal aortic aneurysms.
- Prospective and retrospective cohort studies, as well as case series involving more than 20 patients, published from 2007 to 2017 were included.
- Owing to variance in definitions, the terms "juxta/para/suprarenal" were considered sufficient for inclusion; strict anatomical definitions were not mandated. TAAA were excluded, including Crawford type 4 aneurysms.
- Only elective repairs were included, thereby excluding ruptures.
- When considering FEVAR, only series describing custom-made fenestrated devices were included.
- This excluded "off the shelf" devices and physician-modified grafts.
- All other forms of endovascular repair, including chimney and snorkel repairs, and branched devices, were excluded.
- All forms of OSR were included, including transperitoneal and retroperitoneal approaches, and all variations of visceral vessel reconstruction.
- A total of 2975 patients were included, 1476 of whom underwent FEVAR and 1499 of whom had OSR.
- There were 14 series within retrospective cohort studies, one case—control study and a single prospective non-randomised trial.
- Patients undergoing FEVAR had more medical comorbidities. Pre-existing renal dysfunction was twice as high in the FEVAR cohort. These patients also displayed higher rates of ischaemic heart disease and pulmonary dysfunction.

Main Results

- The pooled rate of early post-operative mortality following FEVAR was 3.3% compared with 4.2% after OSR.
- Estimated long term survival was similar for FEVAR and OSR.
- After FEVAR, the pooled rate of post-operative renal insufficiency was 16.2% compared to 23.8% after OSR.
- Following FEVAR, the pooled major complication rate was 23.1% compared with 43.5% after OSR.
- The rate of cardiac complications was 3.9% after FEVAR and 13.4% after OSR.
- The overall rate of early re-intervention (at less than 30 days) after FEVAR was 6.1% compared with 7.4% after OSR.
- The rate of late re-intervention following FEVAR was higher than that after OSR: 11.1% and 2.0%, respectively.
- Overall, the incidence of type 1/3 endoleak was 4.9%.
- Target vessel preservation was high, with rates of occlusion during follow-up between 2% and 4%.

Conclusions

- No significant difference was noted in 30-day mortality; however, FEVAR was associated with significantly lower morbidity than OSR.
- Long term durability is a concern, with far higher re-intervention rates after FEVAR.
- Ideally, a randomised trial would be conducted to determine definitively which procedure patients should be offered as a first-line intervention.

Multicentre Aneurysm Screening Study (MASS): Cost Effectiveness Analysis of Screening for Abdominal Aortic Aneurysms Based on 4-Year Results from Randomised Controlled Trial

Background

- At the time of this study it was not clear whether screening for AAA was cost-effective/beneficial.
- The multicentre aneurysm screening study (MASS) assessed the benefit of screening on mortality related to AAAs in a randomised trial.
- The trial assessed the benefit of screening on AAA mortality, and also estimated the cost effectiveness of screening over the observed 4-year follow up period.

Methods

- During 1997–1999, 67,800 men aged 65–74 years from four centres in the United Kingdom were individually randomised to be invited for screening (intervention arm) or not (control arm).
- Those who attended for screening underwent ultrasonography of the abdominal aorta with a portable ultrasound machine in a primary care setting.
- Those found to have a normal aorta (<3 cm diameter) received no further clinical follow up.
- Those with an aortic diameter of 3.0–4.4 cm were allocated to annual scans in hospital.
- Those with an aortic diameter of 4.5–5.4 cm were allocated to scans every 3 months.
- Men with an aneurysm with an aortic diameter >5.5 cm, rapid expansion (>1 cm within 1 year), or symptoms attributable to the aneurysm were referred to a vascular consultant for assessment of suitability for surgery.
- Costs were determined for the screening process itself and surgery.

Results

- A cost-effectiveness analysis of data with follow-up over 4 years showed 47 fewer deaths and additional costs of £2.2 m in the group invited to screening.
- The adjusted net cost per patient was £63.39 and per life year gained was £28,400.
- The projected cost per life year gained after 10 years was £8000, which is substantially lower than the perceived NHS threshold value.

Conclusion

- The 4-year analysis shows a cost-effectiveness ratio already at the margin of acceptability and the projection shows that this will fall considerably even at 10 years. The clinical analysis and this economic analysis of the MASS trial together provide clear evidence to support the cost effectiveness of this particular form of screening in elderly men.

Final Follow-Up of the Multicentre Aneurysm Screening Study (MASS) Randomised Trial of Abdominal Aortic Aneurysm Screening

Key Findings

- The benefit of being invited to AAA screening continued to accumulate throughout the 13-year follow-up in the MASS trial.
- The risk of AAA-related mortality and AAA rupture was almost halved, and there was a small but convincing reduction in all-cause mortality.
- The number needed to be invited to screening to save one AAA-related death over 13 years was estimated to be 216 (which is better than breast cancer screening).
- For every 10,000 men screened, this would have saved 75 ruptured AAAs (58 fatal), leading to an extra 119 elective AAA procedures, with an associated 5 post-operative deaths, over 13 years.
- The overall balance of benefit to harm in terms of mortality was in favour of screening again.
- The mortality benefit was somewhat less in years 10–13 after screening than before year 10. This was at least partly due to ruptured AAA in men originally screened normal, with a steady increase in these ruptures from year 8 onwards; the large majority of these were fatal.
- About half of these ruptures were in men with an initial aortic diameter of 2.5–2.9 cm.
- The cost per life-year gained was estimated as £7600 at 10 years, and using health economic modelling as £2300 over the lifetime of men aged 65 years.
- These figures are both below the guideline threshold figure of around £20,000 per life-year gained for the acceptance of medical technologies by the National Institute for Health and Clinical Excellence in the United Kingdom.

Chief Conclusions

- Long term follow-up of the MASS trial has shown that it is possible to achieve almost a halving of the AAA-related mortality rate by screening men aged 65–74 years.
- Rescreening of all those originally screened normal is not justified, but consideration should be given in future to offering a further scan after about 5 years for the small proportion of men with an aortic diameter in the range 2.5–2.9 cm.

Final 12-Year Follow-Up of Surgery versus Surveillance in the UK Small Aneurysm Trial

Background

- This publication details the long term results of the original UK Small Aneurysm Trial.
- The aim was to compare long term survival and AAA treatment costs between surgery and surveillance, and to contrast survival of patients with a small AAA compared with the general population of similar age and sex.
- Between 1991 and 1995, the original trial recruited 1276 patients aged 60–76 years considered fit for elective surgery, with an asymptomatic (non-tender), infra-renal AAA between 4.0 and 5.5 cm in diameter identified.
- 1090 patients, in 93 different hospitals, were assigned randomly to receive treatment by either early elective open surgery or ultrasound surveillance.
- At randomisation, the mean age of the patients was 69.3 years, and 17.2% were women.

- Patients randomised to ultrasound surveillance with an AAA of 4.0–4.9 cm in diameter were reviewed at 6-monthly intervals, and those with an AAA of 5.0–5.5 cm in diameter were reviewed at 3-monthly intervals.
- When AAA diameter exceeded 5.5 cm, the growth rate exceeded 1 cm per year or the AAA became tender or symptomatic, elective repair was recommended to the patient.
- The direct health service costs of aneurysm surveillance and repair to the UK National Health Service (NHS) were estimated.
- The primary endpoint for the trial was all-cause mortality. Secondary outcomes included costs of the two treatments and a comparison with the death rate in the general population matched for age and sex.

Results

- After 12 years, mortality in the surgery and surveillance groups was 63.9 and 67.3%, respectively, and unadjusted HR 0.90 (P = 0.139).
- Three-quarters of the surveillance group eventually had aneurysm repair, with a 30-day elective mortality of 6.3% (versus 5.0% in the early surgery group, P = 0.366).
- Estimates suggested that the cost of treatment was 17% higher in the early surgery group, with a mean difference of £1326.
- The death rate in these patients was about twice that in the population matched for age and sex.
- About 60% of deaths were attributed to a cardiovascular cause.

Conclusions

- The trial did not find a late survival benefit for a policy of early elective surgery.
- Early surgery also does not appear to be cost-effective.
- Surveillance is a safe treatment option until the aneurysm reaches 5.5 cm in diameter or symptoms referable to the aneurysm develop.
- Patients with small screen-detected AAAs should be targeted for cardiovascular risk reduction.

Endovascular or Open Repair Strategy for Ruptured Abdominal Aortic Aneurysm: 30-Day Outcomes from IMPROVE Randomised Trial

Background

- At the time of this study it was suspected that emergency EVAR may be associated with a lower 30-day mortality rate compared to emergency open AAA repair.
- The *Immediate Management of Patients with Rupture: Open versus Endovascular Repair* (IMPROVE) trial aimed to answer this question and test the hypothesis that a strategy of endovascular repair, if anatomically feasible, reduced the 30 day mortality of patients with a clinical diagnosis of ruptured AAA, compared with treatment by open repair.
- It was a multicentre trial that randomised patients with a clinical diagnosis of ruptured AAA to either an endovascular strategy of immediate computed tomography and emergency EVAR, with open repair for patients anatomically unsuitable for EVAR (endovascular strategy group), or to the standard treatment of emergency open repair (open repair group).
- This trial was conducted in 29 eligible centres in the United Kingdom and one in Canada.

- The centres were chosen by their clinical credentials, including audited volumes of elective EVAR of more than 20 cases a year out of at least 50 cases of aortic surgery, evidence of good interdisciplinary team working, availability of the team for at least 66% of the week, rapid access to emergency computed tomography (target 20 minutes), and audited experience of emergency EVAR (minimum of five cases).
- All patients aged over 50 years with a clinical diagnosis of ruptured AAA or ruptured aortoiliac aneurysm, made by a senior trial hospital clinician (either in emergency medicine or vascular surgery), were recorded and were eligible for inclusion.
- The study took place between 2009 and 2013.
- 1275 patients (78% male) were admitted with a diagnosis of ruptured aortoiliac aneurysm across the trial centres, and 623 (49%) patients were randomly assigned to the two study groups.

Results

- Overall 30-day mortality was 35.4% in the endovascular strategy group and 37.4% in the open repair group (unadjusted OR, 0.92, 95% CI, 0.66–1.28; P = 0.62).
- After adjustment for age, sex, and Hardman index, no difference in 30-day mortality existed between the endovascular strategy and open repair groups (OR, 0.94; 0.67–1.33; P = 0.73).
- The endovascular strategy seemed to be more effective in women than in men (P = 0.02).
- For women, 30 day mortality was 37% in the endovascular strategy group and 57% in the open repair group, compared with 35 and 32% for men.
- 24-hour mortality was 22% in the endovascular strategy group and 19% in the open repair group.
- The number and type of re-interventions within 30 days was similar between the randomised groups.
- The average lengths of stay in critical care and in hospital were shorter in the endovascular strategy group.
- 94% of discharges within 30 days were directly to home in the endovascular strategy group compared with only 77% in the open repair group (P < 0.001).
- The average hospital costs within the first 30 days of randomisation were similar between the randomised groups overall.

Conclusions

- The endovascular strategy did not reduce either 30-day mortality or costs overall in comparison to emergency open AAA repair.
- However, patients were discharged earlier and more often to home, and women seem to have better survival with an endovascular strategy.

Comparative Clinical Effectiveness and Cost Effectiveness of Endovascular Strategy versus Open Repair for Ruptured Abdominal Aortic Aneurysm: 3-Year Results of the IMPROVE Randomised Trial

Key Findings

- After AAA rupture an endovascular strategy offers no significant reduction in operative mortality at 30 or 90 days.

- There is however an interim midterm survival advantage (3 months to 3 years).
- Together with the early gains in quality of life, this leads to a mid term gain in QALYs after 3 years.
- Re-interventions related to the aneurysm, particularly those for life threatening conditions, occurred at a similar rate in both groups.
- The cost differences observed at 30 days (non-significantly in favour of the endovascular strategy group) were not eroded by an increased burden of re-interventions in later follow-up, and therefore the endovascular strategy is cost effective.

The UK Endovascular Aneurysm Repair (EVAR) Randomised Controlled Trials: Long Term Follow-Up and Cost-Effectiveness Analysis

Background

- Before the advent of EVAR, open surgical repair was the only surgical treatment available for aortic aneurysms.
- In the spring of 1990, word came of a novel endovascular technique which was being used to treat AAAs. It was originally designed to be of use mainly in patients unfit for open AAA repair.
- By 1996, it was evident that commercial EVAR devices would become available shortly. The urge was to learn the new device method, but it would require comparison with open repair for those patients medically fit for open repair.
- The EVAR trials (EVAR trial 1 [EVAR-1] and EVAR trial 2 [EVAR-2]) were set up to meet the above need.
- EVAR-1 focused on comparing elective EVAR with elective open AAA repair for "fit" patients.
- EVAR-2 focused on patients who were unfit for open AAA repair, randomising such unfit patients to EVAR or observation.
- This paper describes the long term results of the EVAR-1 and EVAR-2 trials.

EVAR-1 Long Term Results

- From 1999 until 2004, 1252 patients were recruited to participate in this trial.
- The patients were equally, and randomly, assigned to the two treatment groups. There were no differences in baseline characteristics between the groups, mean age 74 years, 1135 men.
- Patients were followed until 2015.
- The most striking finding of these very long term results is that both aneurysm-related and total mortality rates are greater in late follow-up for patients who were randomised to EVAR than those randomised to open surgical repair.
- The significant late divergence of the survival curves in favour of OR can be partly explained through greater contribution to late mortality from aneurysm-related and cancer deaths in the EVAR group.
- Total and aneurysm-related mortality were lower in patients who received EVAR in the first 6 months, but increased after 6 months' follow-up, leading to a significantly higher rate after 8 years' follow-up in EVAR than in those who received open surgical repair.
- After the first 6 months, the increased aneurysm-related deaths in the EVAR group were predominantly from secondary sac rupture.

- Re-interventions occurred in both groups throughout follow-up, including those who were free from re-intervention after 2 or even 5 years.
- However, the rate of re-intervention was higher in the EVAR group at all time periods.
- These late re-interventions included those with high severity score, indicating that there was never a safe period to abandon follow-up for patients with EVAR.
- EVAR showed greater overall health benefit but higher costs than OR. The initial benefit after EVAR was attenuated by late mortality and re-interventions, which are associated with a decrement in health-related quality of life. Over the lifetime of the patient, these two factors outweigh the initial gain in operative mortality and faster recovery from surgery. Lifetime costs are greater for EVAR because of the price of the stent graft, the need for surveillance, and the need for re-interventions. The incremental cost-effectiveness ratio is >£200,000 per QALY, considerably above the threshold of £20,000–30,000 per QALY that conventionally applies in the United Kingdom.

Significance of Type 2 Endoleaks

- Type 2 endoleaks are a common complication after EVAR.
- There is no evidence of a substantial increase in either all-cause or aneurysm-related mortality following a detected type 2 endoleak within the first 3 years, or for individuals who survive beyond 3 years.
- However, type 2 endoleak as part of the "cluster" of complications is associated with secondary rupture. The 'cluster' included type 2 endoleak with sac expansion in its definition and it seems that sac expansion is the important measure here.

EVAR-2 Results

- From 1999 to 2004, 404 patients were recruited to participate in EVAR-2.
- A total of 197 patients were randomly assigned to the endovascular group and 207 were assigned to the no-intervention group.
- There were no significant differences between the two study groups with respect to baseline characteristics, mean age was 76.8 years and 347 (86%) were men.
- These patients were older and more physically frail than patients randomised to EVAR-1.
- Patients were followed for mortality until 2015.
- The benefit of EVAR in terms of aneurysm-related mortality persisted throughout follow-up.
- However, although some patients (<10%) survive to 12 years, either with or without aneurysm repair, the majority of EVAR-2 patients had a limited life expectancy, and hence at no time does aneurysm repair confer an overall survival benefit.
- Although longer follow-up shows benefits in terms of aneurysm-related mortality, primarily through prevention of late aneurysm rupture, patients in this trial had a limited life expectancy, regardless of whether the aneurysm was repaired or no intervention was performed.
- Life expectancy was estimated to be 4.2 years in both the EVAR and no-intervention groups.
- By 2009, only 98 patients had survived.
- By 2015, only 23 patients were still alive.

Conclusions

- EVAR has an early survival benefit but an inferior late survival benefit compared with open surgical repair, which needs to be addressed by lifelong surveillance of EVAR and re-intervention if necessary.
- EVAR does not prolong life in patients unfit for open repair.
- Type 2 endoleak alone is relatively benign, although type 2 endoleak with sac expansion is concerning given its association with secondary AAA rupture.

Meta-Analysis of Individual-Patient Data from EVAR-1, DREAM, OVER and ACE Trials Comparing Outcomes of Endovascular or Open Repair for Abdominal Aortic Aneurysm over 5 Years

Background

- EVAR-1 was not the only trial that compared elective EVAR to open surgical repair for infra-renal AAAs.
- There were three other trials—DREAM (Dutch study), ACE (French study), and OVER (American study).
- This is a meta-analysis of these four multicentre randomised trials of EVAR versus open repair.
- It reported on mortality, aneurysm-related mortality and re-intervention.
- The analysis included 2783 patients, with 14,245 person-years of follow-up (median 5.5 years).
- Between 0 and 6 months, mortality was lower for the EVAR groups, with 46 deaths versus 73 for open repair (HR, 0.61; 0.42–0.89) and no evidence of heterogeneity between the trials.
- The early survival advantage of EVAR in the first 6 months was largely attributable to the lower 30-day operative mortality for EVAR versus open repair.
- After this, the early advantage for the EVAR group was lost and the HRs moved (non-significantly) in the direction of open repair.
- By 5 years, the estimated survival rate was 73.6% in both the EVAR and open repair groups.
- The findings for aneurysm-related mortality were similar in direction, with relative benefit for the EVAR groups 0–6 months after randomisation.
- In later time periods, the results moved in the direction of open repair.
- For those who received aneurysm repair, analysis by time from repair showed a strong relative advantage for the EVAR group in the first 30 days; between 30 days and 3 years there was no difference between the groups, but after 3 years there was a significant relative advantage for the open repair group.
- The overall rates of re-intervention reported were higher in the EVAR group than in the open repair group for all trials.

Conclusions

- These four randomised trials, from Europe and the United States, provide the best evidence for the early survival advantage offered by EVAR rather than open repair.

- This survival advantage is lost within 3 years of randomisation, so that the life-years saved from EVAR over 5 years are minimal.
- Between 0 and 6 months after randomisation, total and aneurysm-related mortality rates were lower for the EVAR group, mainly because of the 2.5-fold lower 30-day operative mortality in this group.
- However, after this interval, the early EVAR group advantage was eroded progressively. By 3 years after aneurysm repair, aneurysm-related mortality was five times higher in the EVAR group (mainly due to secondary rupture or re-interventions) and this is likely to have contributed to the "catch-up" in mortality.
- The re-intervention rate was consistently higher in the EVAR groups.
- Surveillance must focus on reducing aneurysm-related deaths in the mid and longer term, particularly deaths resulting from re-interventions and secondary ruptures after EVAR.

Randomised Comparison of Strategies for Type B Dissection: The Investigation of Stent Grafts in Aortic Dissection (INSTEAD) Trial

Background

- This paper was published in 2009.
- At that stage TEVAR was already established as a life-saving treatment option for patients with acute complicated type B aortic dissection.
- However, its role in improving outcomes of uncomplicated type B aortic dissection was yet unknown.
- The traditional method of managing stable patients was medical treatment, however, long term outcomes were poor because of aneurysmal expansion of the false lumen and late complications.
- The authors of this study therefore wanted to test the hypothesis that endovascular stent reconstruction of the dissection might improve the long term prognosis in these patients.
- Consecutive patients at seven centres in Germany, Italy, and France who had uncomplicated type B aortic dissection between 2 and 52 weeks after onset were considered candidates for random assignment to TEVAR plus optimal medical therapy or to medical treatment alone between 2003 and 2005.
- 140 patients were enrolled.
- The primary end point was all-cause death at 2 years, whereas aorta-related death, progression (with need for conversion or additional endovascular or open surgery), and aortic remodelling were secondary end points.

Results

- There was no difference in all-cause deaths, with a 2-year cumulative survival rate of 95% with optimal medical therapy versus 89% with TEVAR ($P = 0.15$).
- The aorta-related death rate was not different ($P = 0.44$), and the risk for the combined end point of aorta-related death (rupture) and progression (including conversion or additional endovascular or open surgery) was similar ($P = 0.65$).
- Finally, aortic remodelling (with true-lumen recovery and thoracic false-lumen thrombosis) occurred in 91.3% of patients with TEVAR versus 19.4% of those who received medical treatment ($P = 0.001$), which suggests ongoing aortic remodelling.

Conclusions

- This trial justifies medical management for uncomplicated type B aortic dissection and corroborates excellent survival rate with tight blood pressure control and close surveillance.
- For patients who fail to respond to medical management and with progressive expansion or late malperfusion, deferred endovascular therapy is feasible and safe.

Endovascular Repair of Type B Aortic Dissection. Long Term Results of the Randomised Investigation of Stent Grafts in Aortic Dissection Trial (INSTEAD-XL Trial)

Key Points

- Basically, the INSTEAD trial was extended for a few more years.
- After 5 years, the all-cause mortality trended lower in patients randomised to TEVAR than with best medical therapy alone (11.1±3.7 versus 19.3±4.8%; P = 0.13).
- Kaplan–Meier curves demonstrated survival benefit with TEVAR seen between 2 and 5 years (100 versus 83.1±4.7%; P = 0.0003), but not yet within 2 years of follow-up (88.9±3.7 versus 97.9±2.0%; HR, 3.96; 95% CI, 0.84–18.6; P = 0.082).
- At 5 years, the aorta-specific mortality was 6.9±3.0% with TEVAR and 19.3±4.8% with best medical therapy alone (P = 0.045).
- Again, Kaplan–Meier curves diverged during late follow-up with landmark analysis demonstrating survival benefit of TEVAR compared with best medical therapy between 2 and 5 years (100 versus 83.1±4.7%; P = 0.0005) rather than during the initial 2 years (93.1±3.0 versus 97.1±2.0%, HR, 2.46, 95% CI, 0.48–12.7; P = 0.283).
- At 5 years of follow-up cumulative freedom from disease progression and aorta-specific events was 53.9±6.1% with OMT alone and 73.0±5.3% with TEVAR.
- There was also ongoing evidence of improved aortic remodelling following TEVAR compared to best medical therapy alone.
- Complete false lumen thrombosis was confirmed in 90.6% at thoracic level with morphological evidence of remodelling in 79.2% at 5 years after TEVAR.
- Conversely, best medical therapy alone failed to demonstrate significant true lumen recovery or false lumen shrinkage, but was associated with expansion of maximum aortic diameter from 43.6±9.2 to 56.4±6.8 mm (P < 0.0001).

Conclusions

- TEVAR in the subacute (stable) phase of distal aortic dissection induces aortic remodelling and reduces aorta-related mortality >5 years as compared with controlled medical management with optional crossover to TEVAR or open repair when complications emerge.
- Early hazard with TEVAR is likely counterbalanced by prevention of late complications and (mostly emergent) crossover procedures.
- A reduction of aorta-specific mortality becomes evident after 24 months of follow-up.
- Although pre-emptive TEVAR was associated with an excess early mortality (attributable to peri-procedural hazards), the procedure turned beneficial at 5 years of follow-up with the number needed to treat as 13.
- Thus, INSTEAD-XL corroborates recent observational evidence, suggesting long term beneficial results of TEVAR in subacute and chronic dissection.

Endovascular Repair of Acute Uncomplicated Aortic Type B Dissection Promotes Aortic Remodelling: 1-Year Results of the ADSORB Trial

Background

- This trial looked at TEVAR in the setting of uncomplicated acute type B aortic dissection (i.e. within 14 days).
- The aim of this prospective randomised trial was to compare best medical treatment (BMT) with BMT and Gore TAG stent graft in patients with uncomplicated AD.
- The primary endpoint was a combination of incomplete/no false lumen thrombosis, aortic dilatation, or aortic rupture at 1 year.
- 31 patients were randomised to the BMT group and 30 to the BMT plus TEVAR group.
- The mean age was 63 years for both groups.
- The left subclavian artery was completely covered in 47% and in part in 17% of the cases.

Results

- Incomplete false lumen thrombosis was found in 13 (43%) of the TEVAR plus BMT group and 30 (97%) of the BMT group ($P < 0.001$).
- Aortic dilatation was found in 11 (37%) of the TEVAR plus BMT patients and 14 (45%) of the BMT patients.
- The maximum false lumen diameter decreased in the BMT plus TEVAR group by 7.0 mm compared to an increase of 4.3 mm in the BMT group ($P < 0.001$).
- The maximum true lumen diameter increased in the BMT plus TEVAR group by 8.4 mm compared to 1.9 mm for BMT ($P = 0.022$).
- There were no deaths within 30 days.
- No aortic ruptures were reported within 365 days of randomisation in either treatment group.

Conclusions

- Uncomplicated acute type B aortic dissection can be safely treated with the Gore TAG device.
- Remodelling with thrombosis of the false lumen and reduction of its diameter is induced by the stent graft, but long term results are needed.

A Randomised Trial Comparing Treatments for Varicose Veins (Class Trial)

Background

- This trial investigated the outcomes following endovenous laser, surgery, and foam sclerotherapy for patients with unilateral or bilateral primary symptomatic varicose veins (grade C2 or higher according to the CEAP classification system).
- Outcomes were assessed at baseline and at 6 weeks and 6 months after treatment.
- The primary outcome measures were patient-reported disease, specific quality of life, and generic quality of life.
- The secondary outcomes were as follows: clinical success at 6 weeks and 6 months (as measured by the proportion of patients with residual varicose veins), venous clinical severity score, and ablation rates of the main trunks of the saphenous vein according to duplex ultrasonography at 6 weeks and 6 months.

- 785 patients participated in the trial.
- 11 UK centres were involved.
- The trial ran from 2008 to 2012.

Results

- The mean disease-specific quality of life was slightly worse after treatment with foam than after surgery (P = 0.006) but was similar in the laser and surgery groups.
- There were no significant differences between the surgery group and the foam or the laser group in measures of generic quality of life.
- The frequency of procedural complications was similar in the foam group (6%) and the surgery group (7%) but was lower in the laser group (1%) than in the surgery group (P < 0.001).
- The frequency of serious adverse events (approximately 3%) was similar among the groups.
- Measures of clinical success were similar among the groups, but successful ablation of the main trunks of the saphenous vein was less common in the foam group than in the surgery group (P < 0.001).

Conclusions

- This trial showed no clinically substantial between-group differences in quality of life.
- Moderate differences in disease-specific quality of life favoured surgery over treatment with foam.
- Moderate differences in generic quality of life favoured laser treatment over foam.
- All treatments had similar clinical efficacy, but there were fewer complications after laser treatment, and ablation rates were lower after treatment with foam.

Five-Year Outcomes of a Randomised Trial of Treatments for Varicose Veins (Class Trial)

Key Findings

- Disease-specific quality of life 5 years after treatment was better after laser ablation or surgery than after foam sclerotherapy.
- The majority of the probabilistic cost-effectiveness model iterations favoured laser ablation at a willingness-to-pay ratio of £20,000 per QALY.

Long Term Results of Compression Therapy Alone versus Compression Plus Surgery in Chronic Venous Ulceration (ESCHAR): Randomised Controlled Trial

Background

- This trial was done before the endovenous revolution took place.
- It investigated whether recurrence of leg ulcers may be prevented by surgical correction of superficial venous reflux in addition to compression.
- By surgical correction we are talking about traditional open venous surgery.
- The ESCHAR study started recruiting in 1999 and finished in 2002.
- It took place in the South West of England.
- 500 patients (500 legs) with open or recently healed leg ulcers and superficial venous reflux were recruited.

- Patients with both superficial and deep venous reflux were included.
- Patients were randomly allocated to treatment with multilayered compression therapy alone or compression plus superficial venous surgery.
- Patients with open ulceration were treated weekly with multilayered compression bandaging aiming for 40 mmHg of pressure at the ankle graduated to 17–20 mmHg at the upper calf.
- Patients with healed legs were prescribed class 2 elastic stockings and advised to wear these during the day.
- All patients were given standard written and verbal advice to elevate the affected leg and to exercise.
- Patients randomised to compression plus surgery were offered superficial venous surgery guided by findings on duplex scans. Patients with reflux at the saphenofemoral junction or long saphenous vein were offered saphenofemoral junction disconnection, stripping of the long saphenous vein to below the knee, and calf varicosity avulsions.
- Venous reflux in the short saphenous vein was treated with saphenopopliteal junction disconnection and calf varicosity avulsions.

Results

- Overall ulcer healing rates at 3 years were 89% in the compression group and 93% in the compression plus surgery group ($P = 0.737$).
- Ulcer recurrence rates at 4 years were significantly lower in the compression plus surgery group compared with the compression group (31 versus 56%; $P < 0.001$).
- For patients with isolated superficial reflux, recurrence rates at 4 years were 27% in the compression group and 51% in the compression plus surgery group ($P < 0.001$).
- For patients with superficial plus segmental deep reflux, recurrence rates at 3 years were 24% in the compression plus surgery group and 52% in the compression group ($P = 0.044$).
- For patients with superficial plus total deep reflux, recurrence rates at 3 years were 24% in the compression plus surgery group and 46% in the compression group, although this was not a statistically significant finding ($P = 0.23$).
- Cox regression analysis confirmed that randomisation to surgery significantly reduced ulcer recurrence ($P < 0.001$; HR, 2.926, 95% CI, 1.723–4.133).
- Patients randomised to compression plus surgery experienced significantly longer absolute (100 versus 85 weeks; $P = 0.013$) and proportional (78 versus 71%; $P = 0.007$) ulcer free time up to 3 years than those randomised to compression.

Conclusions

- Superficial venous surgery in addition to compression therapy for chronic venous leg ulceration reduced ulcer recurrence and improved ulcer-free time when compared with compression alone.
- The clinical benefit seemed greatest for patients with isolated superficial reflux but was also present for patients with coexistent segmental deep reflux.
- Although the improvement in ulcer recurrence rates was less impressive in the groups with segmental and total deep reflux, the subgroups were smaller and the actual benefit of surgery may have been underestimated.

A Randomised Trial of Early Endovenous Ablation (EVRA) in Venous Ulceration

Background

- At the time of this trial there was a lack of robust evidence that endovenous treatments helped venous ulcer healing.
- The Early Venous Reflux Ablation (EVRA) trial was performed to evaluate the role of early endovenous treatment of superficial venous reflux as an adjunct to compression therapy in patients with venous leg ulcers.
- It was a multicentre, parallel-group, randomised, controlled trial.
- 450 consented to participate in the trial and underwent randomisation.
- It ran from 2013 to 2016.
- There were 20 participating UK centres.
- Patients older than 18 years of age were eligible for inclusion if they had an open venous leg ulcer that had been present for a period of between 6 weeks and 6 months, an ankle—brachial index of 0.8 or higher, and primary or recurrent superficial venous reflux that was deemed by the treating clinician to be clinically significant.
- Deep venous reflux was recorded but was not an exclusion criterion.
- Compression therapy was administered by trained community and hospital-based nursing teams (multilayer elastic compression with two to four layers, short-stretch compression, and compression hosiery were all deemed to be acceptable.
- Patients assigned to the early intervention group were planned for superficial venous ablation within 2 weeks after randomisation.
- Patients in the deferred-intervention group were planned for ablation after the ulcer had healed or at least 6 months after randomisation if the ulcer had not healed.
- Endovenous laser or radiofrequency ablation, ultrasound-guided foam sclerotherapy, or non-thermal, non-tumescent methods of treatment (such as cyanoacrylate glue or mechanochemical ablation) were performed either alone or in combination.
- For all interventions, treating clinicians were asked to ablate the main refluxing truncal vein, treat to the lowest point of reflux where possible, and continue compression therapy immediately after endovenous treatment.
- Among the patients in the early-intervention group, duplex ultrasonography was to be performed 6 weeks after the intervention.
- The primary outcome measure was the time to ulcer healing from the date of randomisation through 12 months.
- Secondary outcomes included rate of ulcer healing at 24 weeks, rate of ulcer recurrence, ulcer-free time during the first year after randomisation, and patient-reported health-related quality of life.

Results

- 90% of patients in the early intervention group were treated within 2 weeks.
- 45.6% of patients in the deferred group were treated between 4 weeks and 6 months, followed by 29% treated past 6 months (and 24% never having intervention).
- 31.7% of patients in the early intervention group received endothermal ablation online, compared to 23.9% in the deferred intervention group.

- 49.6% of patients in the early intervention group received foam sclerotherapy alone, compared to 44% of patients in the deferred group.
- 12.1% of patients in the early intervention group received endothermal ablation and foam sclerotherapy, compared to 7.1% in the deferred group.
- The time to ulcer healing was shorter in the early-intervention group than in the deferred-intervention group.
- More patients had healed ulcers with early intervention (HR for ulcer healing, 1.38; 95% CI, 1.13–1.68; P = 0.001).
- The median time to ulcer healing was 56 days (95% CI, 49–66) in the early-intervention group and 82 days (95% CI, 69–92) in the deferred-intervention group.
- The rate of ulcer healing at 24 weeks was 85.6% in the early-intervention group and 76.3% in the deferred-intervention group.
- The median ulcer-free time during the first year after trial enrolment was 306 days (interquartile range, 240–328) in the early-intervention group and 278 days (interquartile range, 175–324) in the deferred-intervention group (P = 0.002).
- The most common procedural complications of endovenous ablation were pain and deep-vein thrombosis.

Conclusions

- Early endovenous ablation of superficial venous reflux as an adjunct to compression therapy was associated with a significantly shorter time to healing of venous leg ulcers than compression therapy alone.
- Patients assigned to the early-intervention group also had longer ulcer-free time during the first year after randomisation.

Long Term Clinical and Cost-Effectiveness of Early Endovenous Ablation in Venous Ulceration (Long Term Results from EVRA)

Key Findings

- Early endovenous ablation of superficial venous reflux was highly likely to be cost-effective over a 3-year horizon compared with deferred intervention.
- Early intervention accelerated the healing of venous leg ulcers and reduced the overall incidence of ulcer recurrence.

Pharmacomechanical Catheter-Directed Thrombolysis for Deep-Vein Thrombosis. ATTRACT Trial Investigators

Background

- Despite the use of anticoagulant therapy, the post-thrombotic syndrome (PTS) develops within 2 years in approximately half of patients with proximal deep vein thrombosis.
- The PTS commonly causes chronic limb pain and swelling and can progress to cause major disability, leg ulcers, and impaired quality of life.
- Pharmacomechanical catheter-directed thrombolysis (CDT) is the delivery of a fibrinolytic drug into the thrombus with concomitant thrombus aspiration or maceration.
- This trial investigated whether this approach prevents PTS in patients with proximal DVT.

- This was a phase 3, multicentre, randomised, open-label, assessor-blinded, controlled clinical trial.
- The trial ran from 2009 to 2014 in 56 clinical centres across the United States.
- 692 patients with acute proximal deep-vein thrombosis were randomised to receive either anticoagulation alone (control group) or anticoagulation plus pharmacomechanical thrombolysis (catheter-mediated or device-mediated intrathrombus delivery of recombinant tissue plasminogen activator [tPA] and thrombus aspiration or maceration, with or without stenting).
- Patients with symptomatic proximal deep-vein thrombosis involving the femoral, common femoral, or iliac vein (with or without other involved ipsilateral veins) were included.
- *This trial included not just ileo-femoral DVT but also fem-pop DVT—this is important to recognise.*
- The primary outcome was development of the PTS between 6 and 24 months of follow-up.
- Secondary outcomes included severity of PTS and patient-reported quality of life.
- Safety outcomes included bleeding, recurrent venous thromboembolism, and death, which were reported throughout follow-up and summarised through 10 days and 24 months.

Results

- In the primary analysis, the PTS developed over the 24-month period in 47% of patients assigned to the pharmacomechanical-thrombolysis group and in 48% of patients assigned to the control group (risk ratio, 0.96; 95% CI, 0.82–1.11; $P = 0.56$).
- There was no significant between-group difference in the percentage of patients who had major non-PTS treatment failure or overall treatment failure.
- Moderate-to-severe PTS (Villalta score, ≥10) occurred in 18% of the patients in the pharmacomechanical thrombolysis group and 24% of those in the control group (risk ratio, 0.73; 95% CI, 0.54–0.98; $P = 0.04$).
- The severity of the PTS, as assessed by the mean Villalta score and mean Venous Clinical Severity Score, was significantly lower in the pharmacomechanical-thrombolysis group than in the control group at all visits between 6 and 24 months.
- Over the 24-month period, there was no significant between-group difference in the change in venous disease—specific quality of life ($P = 0.08$) or general quality of life ($P = 0.37$).
- Major bleeding within 10 days occurred in 6 patients (1.7%) assigned to the pharmacomechanical-thrombolysis group, as compared with 1 patient (0.3%) assigned to the control group ($P = 0.049$).
- There was no significant difference in recurrent venous thromboembolism over the 24-month follow-up period (12% in the pharmacomechanical-thrombolysis group and 8% in the control group, $P = 0.09$).

Conclusion

- Among patients with acute proximal deep-vein thrombosis, the addition of pharmaco-mechanical CDT to anticoagulation did not result in a lower risk of the PTS but did result in a higher risk of major bleeding.

Endovascular Thrombus Removal for Acute Iliofemoral Deep Vein Thrombosis. Analysis from a Stratified Multicenter Randomised Trial

Basically this took the ATTRACT trial results, and just focused on patients with ileo-femoral DVT (i.e. we are *not* looking at femoral-popliteal DVT now).

Key Points

- 391 patients with acute deep vein thrombosis involving the iliac or common femoral veins were randomised to PCDT with anticoagulation versus anticoagulation alone (No-PCDT) and were followed for 24 months to compare short term and long term outcomes.
- In patients with acute iliofemoral deep vein thrombosis, PCDT did not influence the occurrence of PTS or recurrent venous thromboembolism.
- However, PCDT significantly reduced early leg symptoms and, over 24 months, reduced PTS severity scores, reduced the proportion of patients who developed moderate-or-severe PTS, and resulted in greater improvement in venous disease-specific quality of life.
- There was still an increased bleeding risk however with PCDT.

Conclusion of Trial Authors

- "The findings support early use of PCDT in patients with acute iliofemoral DVT who have severe symptoms, low bleeding risk, and who attach greater importance to a reduction in early and late symptoms than to the risks, costs, and inconvenience of PCDT."

Thrombolytic Strategies versus Standard Anticoagulation for Acute Deep Vein Thrombosis of the Lower Limb (Cochrane Systematic Review)

Background

- There have been quite a few trials now that looked at thrombolytic strategies for proximal DVT.
- This is a recent paper (from 2021).
- It included all randomised controlled trials of thrombolysis (with or without adjunctive clot removal strategies) and anticoagulation versus anticoagulation alone, for acute lower limb DVT.
- It included trials with the use of any thrombolytic agent, the principal ones being streptokinase, urokinase, and tPA; other agents were included if used for the treatment of acute DVT.
- All routes of drug lysis administration were considered, as were different dosing regimens of lytic agents. These included systemic and CDT methods.
- As combinations of clot removal strategies are now frequently used in clinical practice, it also included studies where adjunctive thrombus removal techniques such as thrombectomy, balloon maceration, balloon venoplasty, aspiration, stenting etc., were used in combination with thrombolysis, provided they were compared to standard anticoagulation alone.
- Primary outcomes → complete clot lysis, bleeding complications, and PTS.
- Secondary outcomes → any improvement in venous patency, stroke, venous ulceration rates, mortality, recurrent DVT, PE, quality of life, and cost.
- In total 19 trials were included with 1943 participants.

Results

- Complete clot lysis was more likely following thrombolysis at both early (RR, 4.75; 95% CI, 1.83–12.33) and intermediate time points (RR, 2.42; 95% CI, 1.42–4.12; moderate-certainty evidence).

- This benefit is offset by the increased incidence of major bleeding (RR, 2.45; 95% CI, 1.58–3.78; moderate-certainty evidence).

- Pooling all types of thrombolysis, the results showed a slight reduction in the risk of PTS with use of thrombolysis at the intermediate time point (RR, 0.78; 95% CI, 0.66–0.93; moderate-certainty evidence) and at late follow-up (RR, 0.56; 95% CI, 0.43–0.73; moderate-certainty evidence).

Author's Conclusions

- "Complete clot lysis occurred more frequently after thrombolysis (with or without additional clot removal strategies) and the proportion of patients with chronic disabling leg symptoms from post-thrombotic syndrome (PTS) was slightly reduced up to five years from treatment. There was an increased risk of bleeding after thrombolysis, but this risk has decreased over time with the use of stricter exclusion criteria of studies. Results from systemic thrombolysis and catheter-directed thrombolysis (CDT) appear similar. Using GRADE methods, we judged the evidence to be of moderate-certainty, due to many trials having small numbers of participants."

CHAPTER 2

Patient Counselling

Background

- Paternalism in surgery is dead.
- Patients have autonomy and it needs to be respected.
- Vascular surgery is a risky and invasive speciality, and what we do can bring significant benefit and harm to patients.
- The decisions that we make in vascular surgery can also significantly affect the families and friends of patients.
- It is not just about what the evidence recommends, what the MDT recommends, or what NICE and the various vascular society guidelines recommend ....
- Patients need to be fully informed of what they are signing up for, because ultimately the decision is really theirs alone, and what they think and feel is what definitively matters.
- It is the patient (and the family) who has to live with the consequences of such decisions, and therefore it is our job to help them make the best decision possible.
- This does not mean making everything sound wonderful, rattling off some risks and saying most of the time everything goes well, and then saying "please sign here."

How to Do It

- Full verbal explanation of what is being proposed.
- Try not to rush this.
- Avoid using medical jargon; speak so that the patient can understand what you are talking about.
- Ideally involve family members in important discussions/decisions.
- Explain the procedure and what is involved.
- Explain what the benefits are.
- Highlight the relevant risks.
- Discuss the realistic alternatives.
- If you honestly think that the risks outweigh the benefits, then tell the patient.
- If you are aware of any relevant evidence, guidelines, MDT recommendations, etc., then also include these in the discussions.
- Use diagrams to illustrate your points.
- Provide information leaflets.
- Allow the patient and/or family members to ask you questions.
- Give the patient sufficient time to make a decision if this is pragmatic.
- Ensure the patient actually has capacity (i.e. can they weigh up the information and effectively communicate a reasoned and meaningful decision to you).

DOI: 10.1201/b22951-2

- If the patient is signing a consent form, make sure your handwriting is legible, give the patient their copy of the consent form, and tick that the patient received their copy of the consent form.
- In the medical notes, I strongly suggest you clearly document all of the above.

JMF Reflections

All of this may seem like overkill, and you may question the relevance of this in regard to the FRCS examination. However, I must emphasise that this section represents the cornerstone of good surgical practice. In the FRCS examination if you apply such principles, you will demonstrate that you are interested in informed consent, respect patient autonomy, are able to build up a decent rapport with patients and their families, are capable of being professional and mature, and ultimately a responsible consultant-level decision maker. This is really good, and the examiners will recognise pretty quickly that you are a credible candidate. You are also scored on professionalism in the examination, so I would not skimp on patient counselling. I would also emphasise to you that in my FRCS Part B Examination, I was asked to counsel a patient on two occasions. Therefore, do be aware that something like this may come up, so take it seriously.

Also, in the context of your real world practice, if you genuinely do what I have described above, you will find yourself in a far stronger position when it comes to clinical governance. You will have a better relationship with patients and their families and almost certainly have fewer complaints. Even if complaints or coroner's inquests or complications come your way, you will be in a much more authoritative position to defend your practice and decision-making. I think patient counselling is a winner all round.

CHAPTER 3

Clear Documentation

I am not going to make a massive deal out of this because I think you already know the importance of documentation. However, what I will say is that, for me, vascular surgery can be a bit like writing a wonderful award-winning book with invisible ink. We all try our hardest and endeavour to do a good job. Despite this, our hard work and good results generally seem to go unnoticed. Nobody seems to really care if we have done a bypass that worked perfectly well. Nobody seems to notice when you consistently turn up to work early. Nobody seems to care that you never take a sick day off work. Nobody seems eager to pay you extra for staying a couple of extra hours to ensure important jobs get done.

However, you can bet that if there is a complication, this draws attention. The focus seems to be more on the bad things than the good things in surgery. This is a bit depressing to talk about, but I think it is a sad reality we have to confront and accept. I accepted this reality a few years ago, and I now embrace it.

There are countless benefits from clear documentation, such as clear lines of communication, seamless handover, and consolidating your professionalism. It is also vitally important for high-quality patient care and ensuring patient safety. However, in my eyes, the importance also lies within the realm of clinical governance. For me, I want my case notes to be robust and detailed because I want them to reflect the hard work and effort I have put in to try and uphold high standards and quality in my clinical care. I don't want to put an enormous amount of effort in, only to find that the case notes do not reflect this at all.

A few years back, a senior vascular surgeon told me this: "If it isn't documented in the medical notes, it didn't happen." This is a true statement. I suggest you always keep it in the back of your mind.

These are my recommendations / principles

1. If it is important or significant, document it.
2. If you spent a lot of time and effort doing it, document it.
3. Ensure that what you document actually reflects the truth of what took place.
4. Don't rush your documentation process.
5. Try to document things with your "retrospective" hat on, and imagine how a third party might interpret what you have written at a later date.
6. Remember that what you document in the casenotes will carry authority and be taken seriously, so be careful what you write and take things seriously.
7. Remember that the medical casenotes can either be your greatest friend or your worst enemy.

Very brief example: Imagine that you spend 2 hours doing a common femoral endarterectomy. It is a patient with a deep "high-risk groin". You do a good job, however. You washed your hands 3 times and used the scrubber on your finger nails. The patient is given prophylactic antibiotics. You prepped the groin with betadine twice (double-prep). You used Ioban drapes. You deliberately use a GSV patch instead of a bovine patch. You used a PICO dressing

DOI: 10.1201/b22951-3

post-operatively. You prescribed post-operative antibiotics. However, the operation note does not reflect any of these efforts to reduce the risk of infection *which genuinely took place*. The patient gets a wound infection that requires a trip back to theatre. The case is discussed in the clinical governance meeting 6 weeks later. You are not present in this governance meeting. Somebody who was not present in the operation is reviewing your operation notes. He / she remarks that the patient was not given antibiotics. Somebody else assumes you used a bovine patch, and says you should have used a vein patch. Somebody else comments on whether the department needs to do a handwashing audit. Someone else comments that they routinely use Ioban drapes in theatre, and ask whether this was used? Somebody else says a PICO dressing might have reduced the risk of infection.

On the contrary, imagine that you did clearly document all of your efforts to reduce the risk of surgical site infection. The case is discussed in the governance meeting. Again you are not present. However, the operation note clearly outlines all the efforts you made to reduce the risk of infection. Clearly you used a vein patch, gave antibiotics, prepped the groin properly, washed your hands properly, used a special negative pressure dressing etc. The audience concludes that every effort was made to reduce the infection risk, but this was a high-risk groin anyways so it was unfortunate but arguably unavoidable. You don't even need to be present in the meeting to justify your practice.

CHAPTER 4

Be Professional

I am going to start off with the absolute basics, that is, Good Medical Practice and Good Surgical Practice. After this, I will give you my own interpretation of what constitutes being a professional. If you are ever in a tight spot and don't know what to do, just come back to these core principles. Remember what I am about to describe to you is really "the law" in the field of medicine and surgery. Never forget these points, and never think that you will ever reach a position where you are "above the law." I encourage you to actually read the full guidance from Good Medical Practice and Good Surgical Practice. I am not including all of the points here, but, generally speaking, I have tried to apply these principles and others across this book and in my own practice.

Good Medical Practice—Overarching Principles

- Make the care of your patient your first concern.
- Be competent and keep your professional knowledge and skills up to date.
- Take prompt action if you think patient safety is being compromised.
- Establish and maintain good partnerships with your patients and colleagues.
- Maintain trust in you and the profession by being open, honest, and acting with integrity.

Good Surgical Practice—Some Points That Stand Out to Me for the FRCS Exam and Being a New Consultant

- Be respectful towards patients and their family members.
- Take full responsibility for patient management, leading the surgical team to provide the best care. Responsibility should encompass pre-operative optimisation and post-operative recovery.
- When providing elective care for patients with non-urgent conditions, carry out procedures that lie within the limits of your competence and the range of your routine practice, and refer where necessary.
- Carry out surgical procedures in a timely, safe, and competent manner, and ensure that you follow current clinical guidelines in your field.
- Use the skills and knowledge of other clinicians. When the complexity of the procedure is an issue, you should consider shared decision-making and shared operating with another expert consultant colleague.
- When appropriate, you should transfer the patient to another colleague or unit where the required resources and skills are available.
- Taking into account the patient's best interest ensure that, in an emergency, you only perform unfamiliar operative procedures if there is no safe clinical alternative, if there is no colleague available who is more experienced, or if, after consultation with the nearest specialist unit, transfer is considered a greater risk to the patient.
- Engage with the WHO surgical safety checklist.
- Take part regularly in morbidity and mortality and audit meetings.

DOI: 10.1201/b22951-4

- Do not work when your health is adversely influenced by fatigue, disease, drugs, or alcohol.
- Listen to and respect the views of other members of the team involved in the patient's care, and respond to any concerns they may have.
- Communicate effectively with colleagues within and outside your team.
- Attend multidisciplinary team meetings.
- Work effectively and amicably with colleagues in the multidisciplinary team, arrive at meetings on time, share decision-making, develop common management protocols where possible, and discuss problems with colleagues.
- Inform patients promptly and openly of any significant harm that occurs during their care, whether or not the information has been requested and whether or not a complaint has been made.
- Act immediately when patients have suffered harm, promptly apologise, and, where appropriate, offer reassurance that similar incidents will not reoccur.
- Report all incidents where significant harm has occurred through the relevant governance processes of your organisation.
- Reflect on any unanticipated events in a patient's care that you have been directly involved in and present them for discussion at appraisal.
- Treat complaints from patients or their supporters with courtesy and respect, and recognise the value of complaints for monitoring and improving care quality.
- You should respond to complaints promptly, openly and honestly, and cooperate fully with local complaints procedures, acknowledging harm and offering redress where appropriate.
- Participate fully, openly, and promptly to any investigations relating to the occurrence of significant harm, following local guidelines.
- If you appear to the Coroner's Court, you should provide prompt and complete evidence, including comprehensive and truthful reports.

JMF's Opinion on What It Is to Be Professional

- Be punctual.
- Be reliable.
- Take responsibility.
- Look like a professional.
- Don't use foul language or tell inappropriate jokes.
- Communicate clearly.
- Help your colleagues out when they are in trouble.
- Take the job seriously.
- Maintain a high standard.
- Do the basics properly (i.e. don't forget stuff like hand washing).
- Be humble.

How Does This Apply in the FRCS Exam?

- Turn up on time.
- Be prepared.

- Dress smart.
- Be polite.
- Be respectful.
- Speak clearly.
- Speak confidently.
- Adopt a posture that makes you look like a consultant vascular surgeon.
- Don't be arrogant.
- Be serious—don't try and crack jokes with the examiners as they are not your friends.
- Act like you are sensible and safe (don't say anything that makes you sound like a maverick).

CHAPTER 5

How to Present a Vascular Patient

I cannot give you a strict algorithm on how to present a vascular patient. However, what I am going to do is give you some general principles and provide you with some case examples. I am going to present cases incorrectly, and then correctly, so that you can contrast them and draw out the learning points. Hope you find this helpful.

General Principles

- Get to the point
- Have some form of logical structure
- Highlight the relevant issues
- Don't miss out the important stuff
- Construct your case selectively (you don't have to include everything!)
- Say what your plan is
- Try and justify your plan (evidence/guidelines/pragmatism/strength of argument)
- *When time is short and it is time for action, speak less, so that you can do more*
- *Avoid "war and peace" if there are no major issues*

In the FRCS examination, you are being deliberately tested on your presentation skills, so put your game face on and set out to impress your examiner. However, be pragmatic when you are in the real workplace. If you are handing over to a consultant colleague, and you have 30 patients to handover, try to wrap things up more succinctly. As for me, a lesson I try to always remember is this: ***Presentations should not go past 15 minutes***. Beyond 15 minutes, your audience stops absorbing information.

Another useful point for real world practice is to let your audience know what is expected from them immediately. This is particularly relevant for telephonic conversations. For example, if required, start off your conversation with something like this:

- Don't worry. I don't need you to come in. I just want to discuss something with you.
- Don't worry. This is not urgent. If you are busy, we can discuss this another time.
- I have a big problem here. I need your help urgently, you need to come in ….
- This patient needs an operation ….
- This patient is really sick ….
- It's *Top Knife* time matey. I need your help!
- Mate. I have a horrific liver trauma going to theatre. Are you in town?

These types of introductory statements "set the scene," and the person you are talking to can respond accordingly very quickly. In contrast to this, if you start off your presentation by presenting the history and examination, the CT results, talk about something else, and then finally say that the patient is about to die and you need help, well you have just wasted 5 minutes waffling on about stuff that is probably irrelevant now. The person on the phone will know you are a senior vascular surgeon, and if you say you need them to come in immediately, you likely won't need to provide a massive explanation to justify this.

In summary then, there is a time to do a big and impressive presentation, and there is a time not to.

Presenting Patient to Consultant Colleague on ICU Ward Round

This is a patient post-op following an aneurysm repair. He is on ICU doing well. He is probably at the stage where we can consider stepping him down to the ward.

This is Mr Smith. He is a 65-year-old gentleman 2 days post-op following an elective open infra-renal AAA repair with a tube graft. He is doing well. He is extubated, not requiring any oxygen, and not requiring any cardiovascular or renal support. He is passing good volumes of urine. He is eating and drinking, and his bowels are working. He is not in any pain. On examination his abdomen is soft and non-tender, and he has a full complement of lower limb pulses, although his popliteals feel bigger than normal. His post-op blood tests are reassuring with haemoglobin above 100, and a normal creatinine. I am pleased with his progress so far. His urinary catheter needs removing, he needs to sit out, he needs to work with the physiotherapists, and he can be stepped down to the ward. I think we should also get an ultrasound to make sure he does not have popliteal aneurysms.

Handing over to Night Consultant about Urgent Case for Theatre

This is a patient with an acutely ischaemic right leg. I have commenced the patient on intravenous heparin, requested an urgent CT angiogram, and provisionally consented the patient for theatre. I think the patient will require a femoral embolectomy

This is a 57-year-old gentleman with Rutherford 2B acute right leg embolic ischaemia. This is a delayed presentation, and the limb is barely salvageable. The patient has atrial fibrillation, but this is a new diagnosis. His symptoms started over 24 hours ago but he did not present to A&E initially because he thought it was nothing significant. The patient is otherwise fit and well and works as a carpenter. He has no pulses in the right leg, severely reduced power and sensation in the right foot and ankle, and he has a very tender calf. His upper and contralateral limb pulses are normal. There is some skin mottling up to the mid shin, but this is not fixed mottling. The CTA shows what looks like acute occlusion of the right iliac system. I have commenced him on intravenous heparin and gained consent from him for an urgent femoral/iliac embolectomy and fasciotomy. I have warned the patient that he may require a major amputation if this revascularisation attempt is unsuccessful. I have also spoken to ICU, and he will have a post-op bed there afterwards.

FRCS Long Case

This is a 45-year-old patient with rest pain, night pain, and tissue loss of the right foot. The patient has a right femoral pulse and nil distally. The arterial duplex shows an SFA occlusion. I think the patient is suitable for an endovascular approach. The patient is on best medical therapy.

This is a 45-year-old woman with chronic limb-threatening ischaemia of the right leg, with rest pain, night pain, and tissue loss. This woman has all the risk factors for atherosclerosis: Smoker, diabetic, hypertensive, and raised cholesterol. She is comorbid with significant background of ischaemic heart disease and severe COPD. She has a very poor exercise tolerance mainly because of her COPD. She is also very frail and physiologically is much older than 45. On examination she only has a right femoral pulse. In the right groin, there is current evidence of a fungal infection. She has dry gangrene of the right hallux, with no infection in the foot. She has weak monophasic foot signals with an ABPI of 0.37 and a toe pressure of 29 mmHg. Her WIfI stage is 3. She has had an arterial duplex which shows a short occlusion of the mid SFA. She has had a vein map that shows she has a good ipsilateral GSV. As per the BASIL trial, one could argue in favour of bypass for this woman. However, I do not consider her to be an ideal surgical candidate, and would support an endovascular-first approach in this case. I have recommended that she stops smoking, and commenced her on best medical therapy (aspirin 75 mg OD and atorvastatin 80 mg OD).

FRCS Long Case

This is a 78-year-old woman who has been referred by her GP with leg pain and an ulcer around her ankle. The patient says she has been getting pain around her ankle for years, and this ulcer developed around 3 weeks ago after hitting it on a door. The patient has a background of COPD, myocardial infarction, gout, diabetes, hypertension, hypothyroidism, and atrial fibrillation. She is currently on a statin, thyroxine, and allopurinol. She lives at home with her husband. On examination, she has an obvious venous leg ulcer around the medial malleolus. She also has GSV pattern varicosities. I think the patient will benefit from endovenous ablation and multiple stab avulsions.

This is a 78-year-old woman with mixed arteriovenous right leg ulceration. This is primarily a venous ulcer affecting the medial malleolus that developed around 3 weeks ago following trauma. I would classify this as CEAP C6 disease. She is describing general heaviness of the right leg and some minor varicose veins around her medial calf. She has not had any previous DVT, lower limb fractures, or varicose vein treatments. There is however a strong family history of varicose veins. She is not reporting classic rest pain, night pain, or intermittent claudication, and she sleeps with her legs flat in bed. However, she is an ex-smoker, diabetic, and hypertensive. She is also comorbid with an additional background of ischaemic heart disease, multiple myocardial infarctions, advanced COPD, and atrial fibrillation on warfarin. On examination, she looks frail. She has minor GSV pattern varicosities and has a small and superficial venous leg ulcer affecting the medial gaiter area. She only has a femoral pulse with an ABPI of 0.77 and an ankle pressure of 84 mmHg. My plan is to put this patient in reduced compression, and arrange for an urgent outpatient arterial and venous duplex. As per the EVRA trial and the up-to-date ESVS guidelines on chronic venous disease, this patient would ideally be treated with early endovenous ablation in addition to compression to encourage faster ulcer healing. I would avoid intervening on her arteries at this stage, but if this was required, I would prefer an endovascular-first approach. As per the ESVS guidelines, I would avoid interruption of her anticoagulation if I were to proceed with endovenous ablation.

Major Trauma Case

Hi mate. How are you doing? Are you at home? Yeah I am ok. I have a patient I would like to discuss with you. Is that alright? This is a 24-year-old woman who presented 40 minutes ago as a major trauma call. She was in a high speed RTA. When she came, her airway was patent, and she was speaking in full sentences. Her chest revealed some reduced air entry at the left base. Her abdomen revealed tenderness in the left upper quadrant with some peritoneal irritation. Her GCS was 15/15. Exposure revealed no other injuries. However, she was pretty stable initially. She went for a CT scan, and it has shown no major head or chest injuries. It has been reported by the radiology registrar. There does appear to be a pretty significant splenic injury. There is blood in the abdomen and active contrast extravasation. I discuss with interventional radiology consultant on-call about embolising the patient, and he is on his way in; however, she has deteriorated rapidly. She now has a systolic blood pressure of 80/40 mmHg and a heart rate of 110. I am taking her for a laparotomy. I have not done many open splenectomy operations before, can you come and help me?

Hi mate. Sorry to call you at this time but I need your help urgently. I have a 24-year-old female who is been in a high-speed RTA. Essentially, she has a grade 5 splenic rupture with a belly full of blood. She is in grade 4 haemorragic shock. I'm taking here to theatre now to do an emergency laparotomy and a splenectomy. I'm not that confident with emergency splenectomies, can you come and help me?

Busy Ward Round

This is a 78-year-old patient who is 3 weeks post-op following a left 2nd toe amputation for neuroischamic diabetic foot sepsis. The toe was removed and following this the patient had a successful crural angioplasty. After this the patient had a chest infection and also had issues with renal failure. He was seen by the care of the elderly team who adjusted his medications. He had a few nephrotoxic medications stopped including naproxen, ramipril, and his furosemide was reduced. He also had a renal tract ultrasound and renal review. He has also got some home issues and his wife is not so keen to take him back home. He currently has no medical issues. He has been medically fit for discharge for over one week now. The occupational health team are currently sorting out some stuff for his home, and we are trying to organise a package of care.

This patient is 3 weeks post-op following a left 2nd toe amputation and crural angioplasty for diabetic foot sepsis. He is on a 6 week course of oral co-amoxiclav as per the clean bone culture results. He has no medical issues. He is simply waiting for a package of care to be sorted which is taking forever. On discharge, we will follow him up in the diabetic foot clinic.

Discussing Angio Request with Consultant Interventional Radiologist

I have a patient who needs a crural angioplasty for CLTI. He has had an MRA.

Hi. How are you? Can I discuss a crural angioplasty request with you please? This is an 86-year-old gentleman with right-leg neuroischaemic ulceration/CLTI. He has tissue loss and exposed bone affecting his right 5th toe. He has a femoral and popliteal pulse, nil distally. He has monophasic foot signals and a toe pressure of 36 mmHg.

His medical history includes:

> ESRF on dialysis, T2DM on insulin, and peripheral vascular disease. We know he has crural vessel disease on an MRA from 9 months ago

> He does not look like a good surgical candidate, and he does not have suitable vein for a bypass option. His WIfI stage is 3, and his Rockwood frailty score is 7. As per the WIfI scoring, I think he is at moderate risk of amputation and high potential benefit of revascularisation.

> He is currently on best medical therapy and is not smoking. He dialyses on Tuesday, Thursday, and Saturday. Would you be happy to do an urgent angiogram with a view to likely crural angioplasty please? I have already counselled the patient on the angio procedure, discussed the potential risks, and given him an information leaflet. He is happy to proceed …

Seeking a Second Consultant Opinion for a Complex Case

Hi. Can you give me your second opinion on this patient? Here is the NHS number, he is upstairs on the vascular ward. I am not sure whether we should do a bypass on this gentleman, or just debride his foot and see how it does.

Hi. How are you? Can I ask for a favour? Can you give me your expert opinion please on this complex patient? I am not sure whether to do a bypass on him. He is Mr Smith, a comorbid 75-year-old gentleman with right leg CLTI and tissue loss. He is 4 days post-op following a radical foot debridement for quite nasty neuroischaemic diabetic foot sepsis. I looked at the wound this morning, and it is looking fairly reasonable, although it is a big wound. There are some areas of healthy granulation, but there is also some exposed bone at the base of the wound, and at this site, the tissues do not look as healthy. I think he will require further debridement. The patient has an ipsilateral femoral pulse only. His toe pressure is 29 mmHg and his WIfI stage is 4. As such he is at high risk of major amputation and has a high potential benefit from revascularisation. His MRA shows he has severe CFA disease and long SFA occlusion with a decent below-knee popliteal artery and two vessel run-off to the ankle. He also has a decent ipsilateral GSV. As such he is eminently suitable for a right CFA endarterectomy and femoral below-knee popliteal bypass using ipsilateral GSV.

However, he has quite a few comorbidities including emphysema and heart failure with an ejection fraction of 40%. He has previously been seen by an anaesthetist and deemed high operative risk-quoted mortality 10% and morbidity 75%. I'm not sure if I should just further debride this wound and hope it heals on its own, or take him for a full bypass and debride the wound in the same sitting. The other option is a primary below-knee amputation. There is no endovascular option. Would you mind giving me a second opinion? My gut feeling is to proceed with a bypass, acknowledging that it would be high risk and ideally be a two-consultant case.

CHAPTER 6

Intermittent Claudication

History

- Classically calf pain on exercise if SFA disease.
- Buttock/thigh pain on exercise if iliac disease.
- Worse on incline (stairs/going up a hill).
- Clarify the distance the patient can walk before they have to stop.
- Is the patient able to walk through the pain?
- Confirm no rest pain/night pain.
- Confirm patient sleeps with their legs flat in bed.
- Confirm patient has not noticed any ulcers/gangrene/tissue loss.
- *Rapid-fire assessment of risk factors*: "Do you smoke? Do you have high blood pressure? Do you have raised cholesterol? Are you a diabetic?"
- *Rapid-fire assessment of comorbidities*: "Do you have heart disease? Do you have chronic lung disease/COPD? Do you have chronic kidney disease? Have you had a stroke? Do you have pain in your abdomen after eating (i.e. chronic mesenteric disease)?"
- *Vascular history*: "Have you had any vascular surgery interventions before e.g. stents or bypass operations for your legs?"
- Clarify if there is a family history of vascular disease.
- *Best medical therapy*: "Are you on aspirin or clopidogrel? Are you on a statin to lower your cholesterol?"
- *Quality of life assessment*: "How badly are these symptoms affecting your quality of life? Mild, moderate or severe?"

Examination

- *Look around the bed for clues*: Walking stick, cigarette box, diabetic medication, etc.
- *Hands → face → chest → abdomen → legs*: Check the radial pulse, look in the eyes for signs of raised cholesterol/anaemia, look at the chest for signs of previous coronary artery bypass grafting (*theoretically you are supposed to auscultate the chest and listen for murmurs as well*), feel abdomen for a palpable aortic pulse and/or AAA, check groin pulses, then all lower limb pulses, check temperature/capillary refill time of feet, is there any tissue loss (check in between toes and under heel), is there muscle wasting, reduced hair growth.
- Use the handheld Doppler and determine the signals in the AT/DP/PT (i.e., monophasic, biphasic, or triphasic).
- Seriously, definitely, absolutely in the exam (*and in real world practice you should always ...*) say you will check the ankle brachial pressure index (ABPI).

Management Plan—*For the Exam → This is from NICE Guidelines 2021*

- Offer all people with peripheral arterial disease oral and written information about their condition (i.e., explain the diagnosis and give them an information leaflet).
- Strongly advise smoking cessation (and offer support).
- Dietary and weight management advice.
- Optimise management of hypertension and diabetes.
- *Best medical therapy (2× options here*: Antiplatelet and statin therapy, or the COMPASS regime).
- Offer a supervised exercise programme to all people with intermittent claudication.
- Offer duplex ultrasound as first-line imaging to all people with peripheral arterial disease *for whom revascularisation is being considered.*
- Offer contrast-enhanced magnetic resonance angiography to people with peripheral arterial disease who need further imaging (after duplex ultrasound) before considering revascularisation.
- Offer computed tomography angiography to people with peripheral arterial disease who need further imaging (after duplex ultrasound) if contrast-enhanced magnetic resonance angiography is contraindicated or not tolerated.

Revascularisation for Patients with Intermittent Claudication

- Offer angioplasty for treating people with intermittent claudication only when:
  1. Advice on the benefits of modifying risk factors has been reinforced.
  2. A supervised exercise programme has not led to a satisfactory improvement in symptoms.
  3. Imaging has confirmed that angioplasty is suitable for the person.
- Do not offer primary stent placement for treating people with intermittent claudication caused by aorto-iliac disease (except complete occlusion) or femoro-popliteal disease.
- Consider primary stent placement for treating people with intermittent claudication caused by complete aorto-iliac occlusion (rather than stenosis).
- Use bare metal stents when stenting is used for treating people with intermittent claudication.
- Offer bypass surgery for treating people with severe lifestyle-limiting intermittent claudication only when:
  1. Angioplasty has been unsuccessful or is unsuitable.
  2. Imaging has confirmed that bypass surgery is appropriate for the person.
  3. Use an autologous vein whenever possible for people with intermittent claudication having infrainguinal bypass surgery.

JMF's Management Plan for the Real World

- Patient gets lectured about why smoking is bad for them, and if they continue, they are at high risk of an MI, stroke, or losing their leg.
- *Use this analogy*: "The main motorway in your leg is blocked. If you continue to exercise your body will hopefully open up B roads that navigate around the blockage and in time your leg symptoms should improve as the blood supply gets better."

- I encourage patients to exercise as much as possible and try to push through the pain barrier.
- In principle I would refer to a supervised exercise programme, but actually I don't currently have one to offer.
- *Explain that vascular surgical interventions to improve the blood supply to their leg carry major risks including*: Bleeding, infection, nerve damage, worsening limb ischaemia, limb loss, stent/bypass infection, need for emergency surgery for groin complications, kidney failure ....
- I now routinely commence patients on the COMPASS regime (i.e., aspirin 75 mg OD plus rivaroxaban 2.5 mg BD) plus high-dose statin, i.e., atorvastatin 80 mg OD.
- *I would also check their bloods*: FBC, U&Es, lipid screen, HBA1c.
- I ask in letter to GP for hypertension/diabetic control to be optimised.
- I am generally reluctant to offer endovascular or open surgical intervention for patients with intermittent claudication. If asked to give a reason for this, I could spend about 1 hour giving examples of patients with intermittent claudication who went for an angioplasty or stent or bypass who had a nasty complication or ended up losing their leg ....

CHAPTER 7

Diabetic Foot Disease

This is a massive area and I cannot cover every possible avenue of diabetic foot disease in this book chapter alone. However, I do think that as complex and varied as diabetic foot disease can be, we can also visualise it in a fairly simple and pragmatic manner. Let's be honest, the diabetic foot problem will be neuroischaemic, neuropathic, Charcot, diabetic foot sepsis, or a combination of the above. I think the best way to do this chapter is to use some real life case scenarios, walk through their management, and draw out the core principles. Indeed, this is what I encountered in my FRCS VASC Part B Examination. The diabetic foot problem I was presented with was a fairly standard diabetic foot problem that I had dealt with in everyday life countless times before. Hence, I will present real life cases from my own practice but insert them into FRCS Part B Long/Short Case Scenarios.

CASE 7.1: Neuroischaemia

This is a new referral to the diabetic foot clinic.

History

- This is a 49-year-old gentleman with type 2 diabetes who has a discoloured right hallux.
- The toe started to become black at the tip about 1 week ago, and his general practitioner referred him urgently to the foot clinic.
- The patient is not complaining of any pain, and he confirms the sensation in his foot is poor (he is known to have neuropathy).
- He does not recall injuring his toe.
- He is not reporting classical rest pain or night pain, nor short distance claudication.
- *Rapid assessment of risk factors:* Does not smoke, does have high blood pressure, is on treatment for raised cholesterol, and we already know he has type 2 diabetes.
- *Rapid assessment of comorbidities:* No previous heart attacks, no angina, and no chronic lung disease, but is known to have mild chronic kidney disease.
- *Previous vascular history:* Tells you he has had a bypass on his left leg and a left forefoot amputation last year.
- *Medication history:* He says he is on clopidogrel, atorvastatin, amlodipine, ramipril, and metformin.
- *Social history:* Works as a lorry driver, but is currently having to take time off from his work because of his foot. Never smoked, drinks a minimal amount of alcohol. Lives at home alone, otherwise independent, exercise tolerance reported as being able to walk at least the length of a football field (mainly limited by trouble because of his left forefoot amputation which makes long-distance walking challenging).

Examination

- *End of the bed test:* This patient looks like a surgical candidate.
- Patient has a regular radial pulse.

DOI: 10.1201/b22951-7

- Abdomen soft and non-tender, no palpable AAA.
- Can feel right femoral and popliteal pulse, no foot pulses.
- Dry gangrenous changes developing at the tip of the right hallux.
- Neuropathy present around ankle level.
- No infection in the foot (clinically).
- Left leg full complement of pulses. Scars in below-knee popliteal region and medial malleolar region. Left forefoot amputation fully healed.

FRCS Question Time

What investigations would you do now?

- "As per the ESVS guidelines on chronic limb-threatening ischaemia, I would check the patient's toe pressure (right hallux). As per NICE guidelines on the management of patients with critical limb ischaemia I would first start off with a lower limb arterial duplex. After this if necessary I would request an MRA. As per NICE and ESVS guidelines I would also request a vein mapping ultrasound to assess the quality of the ipsilateral GSV."

You seem very versed with the NICE and ESVS guidelines. You don't need to labour the point. Just tell us what your plans are.

- "OK, sorry."

The patient's toe pressure is 28 mmHg, how would you determine the patient's WIfI stage?

- "Based upon my examination findings, this is how I would calculate the patient's WIfI score. He has no ulceration, gangrene limited to the top of the distal phalanx, a severely reduced toe pressure, and no signs of infection. As such I deem that this patient will have a WIfI stage of 3. This means his amputation risk is moderate and the potential benefit of revascularisation is high."

Would you not do an ABPI or ankle pressure?

- "In diabetic patients I find the ankle pressure and ABPI is often falsely elevated. Therefore I routinely focus on toe pressures to calculate the WIfI stage. However, in non-diabetics I would routinely check the ankle pressure and ABPI in addition to the toe pressure."

Can you interpret these duplex findings please?

You are shown a verbal report. The report says that the right CFA, SFA, AK popliteal, and BK popliteal all display triphasic flow with no significant disease. The AT appears to be occluded down to the ankle. The TPT is heavily diseased and there is diffuse disease of the PT and peroneal arteries all the way down to the ankle. You are then shown a scout MRA image. The inflow down to the BK popliteal looks intact. There is diffuse stenotic/occlusive disease of all three crural vessels. You are given a vein mapping report. It says that the ipsilateral GSV from groin down to mid calf is consistently > 0.3 cm.

- "These investigations demonstrate severe infra-popliteal disease that is common in diabetic patients. This is same disease pattern that the patient no doubt had in his contralateral limb that necessitated his previous pop-pedal bypass and forefoot amputation. Given his WIfI stage of 3, relative youth, lack of major comorbidities, and availability of ipsilateral autologous vein, my initial thoughts are this patient is heading for a pop-pedal bypass. However, I am not satisfied with the quality of the foot views on the MRA so I would at this stage request a formal diagnostic angiogram with dedicated foot views to see if I have a target in the foot for a bypass."

Now the examiner hands you another image of exactly what you have asked for. It is a lateral view of the right foot which shows a pretty decent right common plantar artery which appears to be feeding a decent right medial plantar artery. This vessel is passing forwards in the direction of the hallux. There appears to be a partial foot arch. You say to the examiners that this patient appears suitable for a BK popliteal to medial plantar artery bypass using ipsilateral GSV. The examiner asks if you are happy with one foot alone. You say you would prefer 2 foot views, and ask if there is an AP foot view. He seems happy with this and does not actually have another foot view to show you and you move on ….

What would you do now then?

- "I would ensure the patient is on best medical therapy. He is already on clopidogrel 75 mg OD as per the CAPRIE trial which I am happy with, and I would make sure he is on atorvastatin 80mg OD. I would also check the patient's lipid screen and ensure his LDL is < 1.4. I would work collaboratively with the diabetologist in the foot clinic, getting their expert help in ensuring the patient's hypertension is optimised (aiming for < 140/90 mmHg) and aiming for an HBA1c of ≤ 53. I would also discuss the case in the CLTI MDT and get expert opinions from my vascular surgery and interventional radiologists before I committed myself to a plan for bypass. If the CLTI MDT agreed with my plan I would counsel the patient on the proposed operation, discuss the indication, risks, benefits, and alternatives."

Would you not consider the COMPASS regimen in this patient?

- "Definitely. However, as I am planning a bypass, I would not start this yet, as I would likely only have to stop the low-dose rivaroxaban prior to surgery anyway. I would leave the patient on clopidogrel, and then after the bypass switch to the VOYAGER regimen."

What are the alternatives to a bypass?

- "The alternatives are conservative management alone, endovascular intervention, primary below-knee amputation, hallux amputation, forefoot amputation, or palliation."

Do you really think primary amputation and palliation are appropriate here?

- "No I don't think they are appropriate here at all but you just asked me what the possible alternatives are and so I told you."

Why wouldn't you consider endovascular intervention?

- "I would and I am. In fact that is one of the reasons I would put the case through the CLTI MDT. However, based upon the original BASIL trial, if patients are younger and fitter with a life expectancy beyond 2 years, then the original trial suggested that bypass was a more durable option. I personally am I favour of bypass in this patient."

Did the original BASIL trial specifically investigate this patient cohort?

- "No. The original BASIL trial was mainly focused on patients with infra-inguinal femoropopliteal disease, and any bypasses in the original trial were mainly from the common femoral artery. The below-knee territory was not the specific focus. Indeed, BASIL-2 and the BEST-CLTI trials will hopefully shed more light on this area."

If the patient did not have a suitable vein, would you consider a pop-pedal bypass using a prosthetic graft?

- "Not a chance."

What would you do about the ischemic toe?

- "Oh yes of course. I would have requested a foot X-ray to exclude underlying osteomyelitis. If the toe remained dry with no signs of infection I would be tempted to leave it alone. Ideally it would auto-amputate, and leave his metatarsal head intact which provides better foot biomechanics for mobilising. On the other hand, if there were signs of infection and spreading ischaemia I would probably do a hallux amputation at the same time as the bypass."

What if the patient had a severe hallux infection and was septic?

- "In that case I would do a hallux amputation +/− foot debridement before the bypass."

Relevant ESVS Guideline Recommendations

- Use objective hemodynamic tests to determine the presence and quantify the severity of ischaemia in all patients with suspected CLTI.
- Use a lower extremity threatened limb classification staging system (e.g., SVS's WIfI classification system) that grades wound extent, degree of ischaemia, and severity of infection to guide clinical management in all patients with suspected CLTI.
- Perform a detailed history to determine symptoms, past medical history, and cardiovascular risk factors in all patients with suspected CLTI.
- Perform a complete cardiovascular physical examination of all patients with suspected CLTI.
- Perform a complete examination of the foot, including an assessment of neuropathy and a probe-to-bone test of any open ulcer, in all patients with pedal tissue loss and suspected CLTI.
- Measure AP and ABI as the first-line non-invasive test in all patients with suspected CLTI.
- Measure TP and TBI in all patients with suspected CLTI and tissue loss.
- Consider DUS imaging as the first arterial imaging modality in patients with suspected CLTI.
- Consider non-invasive vascular imaging modalities (DUS, CTA, MRA) when available before invasive catheter angiography in patients with suspected CLTI who are candidates for revascularization.
- Obtain high-quality angiographic imaging of the lower limb (with modalities and techniques to be determined by local available facilities and expertise). This should

include the ankle and foot in all patients with suspected CLTI who are considered potential candidates for revascularization.

- Evaluate cardiovascular risk factors in all patients with suspected CLTI.
- Manage all modifiable risk factors to recommended levels in all patients with suspected CLTI.
- Treat all patients with CLTI with an antiplatelet agent.
- Consider clopidogrel as the single antiplatelet agent of choice in patients with CLTI.
- Consider low-dose aspirin and rivaroxaban, 2.5 mg twice daily, to reduce adverse cardiovascular events and lower extremity ischemic events in patients with CLTI.
- Do not use systemic vitamin K antagonists for the treatment of lower extremity atherosclerosis in patients with CLTI.
- Use moderate- or high-intensity statin therapy to reduce all-cause and cardiovascular mortality in patients with CLTI.
- Control hypertension to target levels of <140 mmHg systolic and <90 mmHg diastolic in patients with CLTI.
- Consider control of type 2 DM in CLTI patients to achieve a haemoglobin A1c of <7% (53 mmol/mol [International Federation of Clinical Chemistry]).
- Refer all patients with suspected CLTI to a vascular specialist for consideration of limb salvage, unless major amputation is considered medically urgent.
- Offer primary amputation or palliation to patients with limited life expectancy, poor functional status (e.g., non-ambulatory), or an unsalvageable limb after shared decision-making.
- Offer revascularization to all average-risk patients with advanced limb-threatening conditions (e.g., WIfI stage 4) and significant perfusion deficits (e.g., WIfI ischaemia grades 2 and 3).
- Obtain high-quality angiographic imaging with dedicated views of ankle and foot arteries to permit anatomic staging and procedural planning in all CLTI patients who are candidates for revascularization.
- Perform ultrasound vein mapping when available in all CLTI patients who are candidates for surgical bypass.
- Use autologous vein as the preferred conduit for infra-inguinal bypass surgery in CLTI.
- Avoid using a non-autologous conduit for bypass unless there is no endovascular option and no adequate autologous vein.

JMF Reflections

I did have a short case on a diabetic neuroischaemic problem in the FRCS Part B Exam. It was very fast and I didn't have much time to think. Most of the history and examination questions were fairly standard and I had to rattle through these to pick up the easy points. Things tend to get more and more challenging as you progress ....

Mentioning guidelines (such as NICE and ESVS) is a good thing and I would encourage you to do this to support any points you are making. However, don't labour the point. Mentioning toe pressures and WIfI stage is also a good thing. Getting in some good stuff about the best medical therapy, diabetic and blood pressure optimisation, etc., is also a good thing. Smash in something about using the MDT, getting second opinions from your expert colleagues, working collaboratively, and counselling the patient is all good as it demonstrates you are a safe and sensible clinician.

Quoting relevant randomised controlled trials is also a very good thing (e.g., BASIL, CAPRIE). However, just be careful here. As soon as you start mentioning 20 papers, evidence, and relevant studies like BASIL, etc., you have to be prepared to justify your use of the trials and to be questioned on them. The answer I have given above where I included BASIL is not a true answer that I gave in the exam. I use it to illustrate how using evidence can potentially backfire on you. Don't get me wrong; you do have to use the evidence in your answers to get the high marks (i.e. be a "high flyer"). However, using the evidence is a bit like walking around carrying a loaded gun. The fact that you have a loaded gun means you can theoretically use it to your advantage. However, you can just as easily shoot yourself in the foot with it or have it taken out of your hands and used on you by an opponent. My advice is: don't quote evidence or papers unless you genuinely know what you are talking about!

Finally, be aware of the fact that the examiners in front of you may not agree with your plan. For example, the examiners may not think much of the BASIL trial, and they may be massive endovascular enthusiasts. In fact, in their own practice, they may think the patient will be better served by primary attempt at endovascular intervention for this patient's infra-popliteal disease. Just be considerate of this possibility. This means don't make sweeping statements. It is perfectly acceptable to have **YOUR PLAN** but don't make the mistake of thinking that everybody else is obliged to agree with your plan.

CASE 7.2: Neuropathy 1

This is a new referral to the diabetic foot clinic.

History

- A 64-year-old female presents with an ulcer over her left first metatarsophalangeal joint (plantar aspect).
- This has been present for around 2 weeks.
- She is not reporting any pain, but the ulcer is smelly and her left hallux has swollen up over the past 48 hours.
- She has been feeling hot and sweaty.
- She is not reporting classical rest pain or night pain, nor intermittent claudication.
- *Rapid assessment of risk factors:* Does not smoke, does not have high blood pressure, is on treatment for raised cholesterol, and has type 2 diabetes.
- How good is your diabetes control? She says, "not very good …."
- *Rapid assessment of comorbidities:* No previous heart attacks, no angina, no chronic lung disease, and no chronic kidney disease. Patient says she has hypothyroidism and gastro-oesophageal reflux, and has had her gallbladder removed.
- No previous vascular surgery history.
- *Medication history:* She is on thyroxine, metformin, insulin, and lansoprazole.
- *Social history:* She is a retired secondary school teacher, and lives at home with her husband. Otherwise fit, well, and independent and has unlimited exercise tolerance.

Examination

- *End of the bed test:* Patient is systemically well, with slightly raised body mass index.
- Full complement of lower limb pulses.
- Left foot shows prominence of the metatarsal heads and clawing of the toes.

- Left hallux has a sausage appearance.
- 2-cm ulcer plantar aspect of first MTP.
- Bone is palpable at base of the wound.
- Foul smelling.
- A small amount of pus seeps out of ulcer when you squeeze it/probe it (you suspect it is going down to MTP joint).
- Cellulitis affecting hallux and forefoot.
- Adjacent toes do not appear to be involved.
- No obvious tracking sepsis/fluctuance/collection in plantar aspect of foot.
- Patient has reduced sensation around toes/forefoot.

FRCS Question Time

What is your diagnosis?

- "This is a 64-year-old poorly controlled type 2 diabetic with neuropathic diabetic foot sepsis. She has a sausage left hallux with ulceration and exposed bone at the 1st metatarsal head. There is purulent fluid coming from the 1st MTP joint so I suspect she has a septic arthritis of the 1st MTP as well."

What would be your initial investigations?

- "First of all, I would like to know her observations ...."

The examiner hands you a piece of laminated white paper.

> *Heart rate: 98*
> *Blood pressure: 150/90 mmHg*
> *Respiratory rate: 16*
> *Temperature: 37.9 degrees Celsius*
> *Blood sugar: 19*

- "This woman is not horrifically unwell at the moment. Based upon these readings I would not classify this as septic shock. However, her raised blood sugars suggest she is mounting a systemic inflammatory response which concerns me. Her relative tachycardia is also concerning, again suggesting she is starting to mount a systemic inflammatory response. Finally, she may not be officially pyrexial, but she almost is ...."

What other investigations do you want?

- "I would insert a large-bore intravenous cannula and send off bloods: FBC, U&Es, HBA1c, lipid screen, clotting, and group and save. I would request an urgent left foot X-ray to see if there was any evidence of osteomyelitis or gas in the tissues. I would also do an arterial blood gas to check her pH and lactate, and check her ketones to make sure she is not in diabetic ketoacidosis"

What is your management plan?

- "I would make the patient nil by mouth. I would give intravenous antibiotics for the treatment of severe diabetic foot sepsis as per local trust guidelines. I would elevate the patient's leg to reduce any swelling. Depending upon the results of the blood tests and the foot X-ray, I would counsel the patient for an urgent foot debridement +/− left hallux amputation."

The examiner hands you another white laminated piece of paper with some blood results.

- "The patient has a CRP of 240, and a WBC of 22. This shows that she has an active severe inflammatory/infective process. Her renal function is normal and her arterial blood gas reveals a normal pH and a normal lactate. This is reassuring because it suggests she has evidence of sepsis, but at the moment she is not in the range of organ failure. Her HBA1c is 95. This confirms she has poor long term blood glucose control. Her lipid screen reveals an LDL of 3.7, which means she has hypercholesterolemia that needs treating with a view to aiming for an LDL of <1.4. Her clotting is normal, her platelet count is normal, and her haemoglobin is 135, which means I do not have any surgical bleeding concerns at the moment"

The examiner hands you another white laminated piece of paper. There is an image of this patient's left foot X-ray.

- "There is advanced osteomyelitic destruction of the left 1st metatarsal head, and there is some gas in the tissues around the 1st MTP joint. The left hallux soft tissues are visibly swollen even on the X-ray. This X-ray confirms that this patient has a severe infection of the left hallux, and in my opinion confirms that she requires an urgent foot debridement and hallux amputation. I would explain this result to the patient, and counsel her for the proposed operation."

How would you counsel the patient? Talk to me as if I am the patient ….

- "I am sorry to be the bearer of bad news, but you have a very severe infection of your left big toe. There is purulent fluid coming out of the joint, the bone is exposed and infected, and your blood tests indicate that it is making you unwell. You are not dangerously unwell at the moment, but if we don't tackle this infection now, it could get much worse and put both your leg and your life at risk. We do need to put you on intravenous antibiotics and elevate your leg to get the swelling down, but I do not think this on its own is enough to stop the spread of infection. I think the most appropriate thing at this stage is to take you to theatre and drain the infection. There are two approaches here. One is to remove the joint at the base of the big toe and try and leave the toe itself intact. The other option is to remove the whole toe. I personally think that given the severity of the infection, and how your whole toe appears, I think it is safer to remove the whole toe at once to try and remove all the infection. I would only intend to remove the big toe, but I must mention that there is a risk that the adjacent toes may be involved in the infective process, and if that were the case I think it would be better to remove them at the same time. Also, if the infection was much worse at the time of surgery, I may need to carry out a more radical debridement."

What would be your surgical approach in this instance?

- "I would do the case preferably under a block, such as an ankle block or a popliteal block. I would prep the whole foot up to the lower calf. I would use a marker pen and draw an incision line around the base of the hallux and extend it proximally down the metatarsal shaft (tennis racket). I would use my knife and make a confident incision around the whole toe and remove it at the joint quickly to minimise blood loss. I would use a periosteal elevator to clear the metatarsal head and then use a powersaw to divide the metatarsal head at 45 degrees, ensuring I don't leave any proud bone. I would then wash out the wound, change my gloves, and use clean bone nibblers to send off clean bone samples for histology and microbiology. I would achieve haemostasis, pack the wound, and leave it open."

What would your post-operative plan be?

- "I would continue intravenous antibiotics for 24–72 hours depending upon the clinical condition of the patient, and whilst awaiting the clean bone sample results. I would review the wound at 48 hours. I would consider a VAC dressing at this point. If the clean bone samples were positive I would aim for 6 weeks of treatment for osteomyelitis. I would work closely with microbiology to ensure the antibiotics prescribed were appropriate. I would also ensure the patient was seen by either a diabetic specialist nurse or a diabetologist because her diabetic control is poor. I would also ensure she was on a high-dose statin. I would give the patient an information leaflet on diabetic foot care. I would also refer the patient to orthotics for special offloading footwear. I would follow the patient up in the diabetic foot clinic."

Would you not consider treating this patient with intravenous antibiotics for 24–48 hours, first of all, and try to avoid taking her to theatre? Shouldn't you try to preserve her toe?

- "No. I take diabetic foot sepsis very seriously. As far as I am concerned, pus coming from a diabetic foot means theatre. I have seen lots of cases of diabetic foot sepsis being managed conservatively, and I have seen quite a few of such cases where the infection has spread very rapidly, and this has led to the patient requiring a very radical foot debridement a few days later. I was told by one of my old bosses that I should never let the sun go down on a patient with diabetic foot sepsis …. This does not mean I think every diabetic foot infection needs to go to theatre. Not at all. But in my eyes if there is an amalgamation of systemic upset, pus, osteomyelitis, a sausage toe, spreading infection, necrosis/fluctuance/abscess/tracking sepsis …. these cases need to go to theatre urgently. I have an aggressive approach to diabetic foot sepsis. I would rather clear the infection and have a big wound, than be conservative with a tiny (or no wound) and a patient who is sick as a dog."

JMF Reflections

- This is a fairly straightforward case and does represent the "bread & butter" of vascular surgery. However, in an exam setting, it can still be challenging. Don't forget that you are presenting your management plan as you perceive the world to be. In my eyes, a patient with a big red stinking hallux with a massive ulcer pouring out pus with exposed bone needs to go to theatre to have that toe removed …. I think this is a no-brainer. But when you are asked about it you may start to doubt yourself. In fact, even as I write this now, I am slightly hesitant …. Surely other people agree with me in taking this patient to theatre to have the toe removed right …?

- But this is the nature of the beast, and this is what it is like being a consultant. You have to assess a patient, make sense of what is happening, come up with a plan, counsel the patient, and then execute that plan. This is what these questions are about. The examiners want to put you under pressure and see what you are made of. The examiner wants to know if you are safe and sensible. If the examiner is telling you that the patient is unwell, that pus is coming out of the foot, if the X-ray shows gas in the tissues, if the CRP is sky-high .... Seriously, we all know what the safe answer is. You are a vascular surgeon → the patient needs to go to theatre for source control! If on the other hand the patient is completely well, there is a tiny ulcer, there is no bone exposed, and the X-ray suggests early osteomyelitis, then I would not be diving in and doing a radical foot debridement in that setting. Again, it is just about making common sense decisions and coming across as a reasonable and safe vascular surgeon. Hope this helps anyways.

CASE 7.3: Neuroischaemia 2

This is a new referral to the diabetic foot clinic.

History

- A 59-year-old gentleman presents to diabetic foot clinic with a deep right heel ulcer.
- This ulcer has been present for about 3 weeks and has progressively got worse.
- The patient is not describing classical rest pain or night pain.
- His mobility is very poor and as such he is not describing intermittent claudication.
- The patient says he spends a lot of his time in bed at home and mobilises very little.
- He is well in himself and not reporting fevers/sweats/shakes or systemic upset.
- *Rapid assessment of risk factors:* Ex-smoker, does have high blood pressure, is on treatment for raised cholesterol, and has poorly controlled type 2 diabetes.
- *Rapid assessment of comorbidities:* Previous heart attack 2 months ago (had coronary stents), heart failure, chronic obstructive pulmonary disease, and stage 3 chronic kidney disease.
- *Previous vascular history:* Tells you he has had an angioplasty to his right leg 4 months ago.
- *Medication history:* He says he is on aspirin, ticagrelor, atorvastatin, furosemide, ramipril, amlodipine, metformin, and insulin.
- *Social history:* Unemployed, lives at home with his wife who is the main carer, practically housebound, uses wheelchair when leaves house.

Examination

- Patient is systemically well.
- Raised BMI.
- Right femoral and popliteal pulse palpable, no foot pulses palpable.
- Foot is reasonably warm, capillary refill time 2 seconds.
- Deep 4 × 5 cm ulceration to posterolateral heel, exposed bone and Achilles tendon.
- Macerated and sloughy tissues.
- No gross spreading infection, no pus from heel ulcer.
- DP and PT signals are weakly monophasic.
- Toe pressure = 37 mmHg.

FRCS Question Time

What is your diagnosis?

- "This is a poorly controlled diabetic with neuroischaemic heel ulceration. I suspect he has recurrent crural vessel disease and probably calcaneal bone osteomyelitis."

What initial investigations would you request?

- "I would first request routine blood tests: FBC, U&Es, LFTs, CRP, HBA1c, lipid screen, and a coagulation profile. I would also request a right heel X-ray and an arterial duplex to assess his crural vessel run-off as per NICE/ESVS guidelines +/− an MRA."

Please interpret these investigations.

- "His blood tests show a slightly raised WBC and CRP in-keeping with low grade sepsis. His LFTs show a low albumin indicating poor nutrition. His renal function is poor, as expected, with an eGFR of 28. His X-ray shows calcaneal osteomyelitis but no gas in the tissues. His duplex indicates severe crural vessel disease. All this indicates to me that this is a frail comorbid patient with a nasty neuroischaemic ulcer and secondary calcaneal osteomyelitis. The heel ulcer requires debridement, but as he is currently not septic, I would try to revascularise him first of all by way of an endovascular attempt. Given all the information I have so far, I do not think he is a suitable candidate for open surgical revascularisation."

What do you make of this MRA? (*examiner hands you a laminated paper with a scout MRA image*)

- "He has diffuse disease affecting all 3 crural vessels. The AT is stenosed at the origin and then diffusely diseased in the mid shin. It occludes at the ankle. The peroneal artery is occluded. The PT shows again diffuse stenotic disease along its length but it does appear to cross the ankle and it appears to be the vessel one would target from an endovascular perspective to improve perfusion to the heel. As such I would consider a right CFA antegrade approach with a view to mainly PT angioplasty."

The patient has a successful PT angioplasty with a good radiological result. What would you do now?

- "I would counsel the patient for a right heel debridement, with a view to Achilles tendon debridement and calcaneal shaving. If the patient agreed with this, this is what I would do next."

Post-operatively the patient continues to ooze from the right heel, and he continues to drop his haemoglobin. How would you manage this?

- "First of all, I would have tried to be meticulous with haemostasis at the time of surgery to prevent this. However, given the fact that the patient is on dual antiplatelets, this bleeding is not entirely unpredictable. I would liaise with cardiology, but in my experience I don't think we can stop the ticagrelor so soon after an acute coronary event. I may consider a pressure dressing, withholding any prophylactic enoxaparin, limb elevation, and possibly using local anaesthetic with adrenaline to under-run any bleeding points with 2-0 vicryl. If these attempts were unsuccessful I would consider formally taking the patient back to theatre for haemorrhage control."

How else would you manage this heel wound post-surgery?

- "I would consider a VAC dressing if there were no bleeding issues. I would also focus on offloading the heel to prevent further pressure damage. I would refer the patient to orthotics for appropriate footwear. I would also give the patient an information leaflet on diabetic foot care, and refer the patient to the diabetes team for optimisation of his blood sugar control. Finally, I would work closely with microbiology and if there were positive bone cultures from my clean bone samples that I took at the time of surgery, I would treat the patient with targeted antibiotics for 6 weeks. My routine practice would also be to closely monitor such a patient up in the diabetic foot clinic afterwards to ensure the heel wound was healing."

CASE 7.4: Fulminant Diabetic Foot Sepsis

This is an acute admission to A&E.

History

- This is a 68-year-old gentleman who has presented with a nasty left foot infection.
- The patient said he has had foot surgery in the past and is awaiting further foot surgery by podiatry in the next few weeks.
- He does not have much sensation in his foot and thinks he may have stood on a piece of glass in the kitchen a few days ago.
- His foot has swollen massively and there is a foul-smelling discharge from his sole.
- He feels unwell in himself, and last night, he was having hot and cold sweats and shakes in bed.
- *Rapid assessment of risk factors:* Smoker, poorly controlled type 2 diabetic, hypertension, and raised cholesterol.
- *Rapid assessment of comorbidities:* Atrial fibrillation, chronic kidney disease (eGFR 56).
- *Previous vascular history:* Not known to have problems with his leg arteries.
- *Medication history:* He says he is on apixaban, metformin, amlodipine, and simvastatin.
- *Social history:* Retired gardener, lives at home alone, mobilises with a walking stick, otherwise independent.

Examination

- Patient looks flushed from the end of the bed.
- His hands are warm and venodilated.
- His radial pulse is >100 bpm.
- There is a foul smell coming from the right foot.
- He has a full complement of right leg pulses.
- There is evidence of previous right foot surgery → the fourth toe has been amputated and there is a vertical scar from the fourth toe amputation site running along the plantar aspect of the foot (Loeffler—Ballard incision).
- This incision is dehisced and the tissues in the plantar aspect of the foot are boggy, blistered, and macerated.
- Purulent fluid is seeping from the wound.
- When you squeeze the foot pus pours out.
- This inflammatory/infective process has spread to the midfoot.
- The whole forefoot is oedematous and cellulitic.
- The patient has reduced sensation in the entire foot.

FRCS Question Time

What is your diagnosis?

- "This patient has limb and arguably life-threatening neuropathic diabetic foot sepsis. His right foot is grossly infected, and my clinical assessment suggests this patient is systemically unwell given the fevers, sweats, tachycardia, and vasodilatation."

What is your management plan?

- "This is a vascular surgery emergency. The patient will definitely require a radical right foot debridement +/− a guillotine amputation above the ankle. This is for source control. In terms of basics however, I would manage the patient according the sepsis 6 algorithm: High flow oxygen, blood cultures, intravenous antibiotics, intravenous fluids, check his blood lactate level, urinary catheter and careful fluid balance. I would keep the patient nil by mouth and alert the emergency theatre team and emergency anaesthetist. I would also alert intensive care in case the patient requires cardiovascular support post-operatively. Finally, I would speak to haematology about reversing his apixaban in preparation for theatre."

What would help you determine if you needed to do a guillotine amputation?

- "It depends upon my clinical findings, and to a certain degree this is a subjective assessment. In my practice, if I think the foot is salvageable I will proceed to a radical debridement. However, if the infection is tracking up towards the proximal midfoot/hindfoot/malleoli, the patient is systemically unwell, and I don't think the foot is realistically salvageable, then I would do a guillotine amputation."

Why not do a below-knee amputation if you think the foot is not salvageable?

- "If I am contemplating a guillotine amputation it is very likely that the patient is going to be extremely unwell. As such the lower limb tissues would likely be inflamed, infected and oedematous. The patient, if septic, may also require vasoconstrictor support. As such, I think in this context that a primary below-knee amputation would be at risk of wound breakdown and infection. I would rather do a guillotine amputation, rapidly clear the sepsis, get the patient fully recovered from this illness, and then do a formal below-knee amputation when they are better (with a better chance of healing)."

How do you do a guillotine amputation?

- "I would prefer the patient to be under a general anaesthetic, and if they are neuropathic with foot pulses I would use a tourniquet to minimise blood loss. The leg is draped as if I might need to do a below-knee amputation (i.e. prepare for the worst-case scenario). A knife is used to make a rapid circumferential incision around the lower tibia/fibula (just above the malleoli). The following vessels are ligated as they are encountered: GSV, SSV, anterior tibial artery, posterior tibial artery. A periosteal elevator is used to liberate the distal tibia and fibula at the level of bone transaction. A power saw is used to rapidly remove the whole foot. At this point, the peroneal artery is identified (often hiding medial to the divided fibula). This is ligated. The tourniquet is now released and haemostasis confirmed. Mepitel, blue gauze, wool and crepe are applied to the stump. The whole operation is ideally done in less than 10 minutes. Of note, if there is residual sepsis at the level of amputation the amputation can be made more proximal, or a vertical slit can be made in the skin and soft tissues and any proximal tracking sepsis can be decompressed and drained."

JMF Reflections

This was a real case. However, I never did a guillotine amputation. I did a radical foot debridement and cleared the sepsis. Over the next few months, the patient showed excellent wound healing with VAC therapy, and he kept a functional foot with an intact heel and ankle. However, this case demonstrates that you need to effectively counsel patients in this clinical context. You need to be discussing with patients about radical foot debridement +/− guillotine amputation/primary amputation when you have a case of horrific life-threatening diabetic foot sepsis like this. Diabetic foot sepsis is not pretty, and it is dealt with by vascular surgeons for a specific reason. We are there to drain the sepsis and save the patient's life. Limb salvage in these contexts is ideal and what we would prefer, but if it is a choice between life and limb, then life comes first.

CHAPTER 8

Chronic Limb-Threatening Ischaemia (CLTI)

CLTI is a massive topic. It also has a massive crossover with diabetic foot disease, which we have just covered. As such, I am going to cover some familiar territory but not labour the point with the ESVS guideline recommendations as I have already described in the diabetic foot chapter. We will review the history and examination of the patient cohort, the basic management principles, and then cover a few fairly standard case examples in FRCS Part B Examination settings.

History

- Ischaemic rest/night pain affecting the forefoot/toes.
- Made worse with recumbency (i.e. patient cannot sleep with legs flat in bed, often has to hang leg down or sleep in a chair).
- Ulceration or gangrene.
- Symptoms/signs present for >2 weeks.
- Will likely be complaining of short-distance claudication as well.
- *Rapid-fire assessment of risk factors:* "Do you smoke? Do you have high blood pressure? Do you have raised cholesterol? Are you a diabetic?"
- *Rapid-fire assessment of co-morbidities:* "Do you have heart disease? Do you have chronic lung disease/COPD? Do you have chronic kidney disease? Have you had a stroke? Do you have pain in your abdomen after eating (i.e. chronic mesenteric disease)?"
- *Vascular history:* "Have you had any vascular surgery interventions before e.g. stents or bypass operations for your legs?"
- Clarify if there is a family history of vascular disease.
- *Best medical therapy:* "Are you on aspirin or clopidogrel? Are you on a statin to lower your cholesterol?"
- *Quality of life assessment:* "How badly are these symptoms affecting your quality of life? Mild, moderate or severe?"
- *Social history:* "Where do you live? Who do you live with? Are you independent? Who does the cooking/cleaning/shopping? How active are you normally?"

Examination

- End of the bed test. This is subjective but trust your instincts. I ask myself 5× questions whenever I first eyeball a vascular patient with CLTI: Is this patient for conservative management, endovascular intervention, open revascularisation, major amputation, or palliation? This is just an impression, and the board is not set. However, remember that if you are going for the FRCS examination, you are already very experienced in vascular surgery and your subconscious mind can process vast amounts of information very quickly and draw very sensible conclusions. If you look at a patient and your "instinct" tells you they are an open surgical candidate, you are probably right.
- *Look around the bed for clues:* Walking stick, cigarette box, diabetic medication, etc.

DOI: 10.1201/b22951-8

- *Hands → face → chest → abdomen → legs:* Check the radial pulse, look in the eyes for signs of raised cholesterol/anaemia, look at the chest for signs of previous coronary artery bypass grafting (*theoretically you are supposed to auscultate the chest and listen for murmurs as well*), feel abdomen for a palpable aortic pulse and/or AAA, check groin pulses, then all lower limb pulses, check temperature/capillary refill time of feet, is there any tissue loss (check in between toes and under heel), is there muscle wasting, reduced hair growth ....
- Is there a sunset foot? Perform Buerger's test.
- *Describe any areas of ulceration:* Location, size, depth, margin, base of ulcer, are there signs of infection, is there tendon/bone exposed, is the joint involved, etc.
- *Describe any areas of gangrene:* Dry, wet, are there progressive ischaemic or infective changes in the dorsal or plantar aspect of the foot?
- Always check the heel and look in between the toes.
- Use the handheld Doppler and determine the signals in the AT/DP/PT (i.e. monophasic, biphasic, or triphasic).
- Say you would check the ABPI / ankle pressure.
- Also say you would check the toe pressure.
- Also visually inspect the leg to see if the patient has an obviously decent ipsilateral GSV.

Relevant Summary of ESVS and NICE Guideline Recommendations

- Calculate patient's WIfI stage.
- WIfI stage 1 → wound care, surveillance for deterioration.
- WIfI stage ≥2 and candidate for revascularisation → obtain further imaging.
- Duplex arterial ultrasound is first-line investigation.
- CTA/MRA second line.
- Request vein mapping ultrasound to confirm suitable autologous vein for bypass (*if patient is a surgical candidate*).
- Ensure patient on best medical therapy.
- Strongly advise smoking cessation, and offer support.
- Optimise analgesia (paracetamol in combination with opioids).
- Consider referral to pain team.
- Use an integrated, limb-based anatomic staging system (such as GLASS) to define complexity of a preferred target arterial pathway (TAP) to facilitate evidence-based revascularisation (EBR) in CLTI patients.
- High-risk patient → perform endovascular intervention if possible.
- If standard risk patient and suitable vein conduit available → revascularise using preferred strategy (endovascular or open).
- In addition to above, perform urgent surgical drainage and debridement (including minor amputation if needed) and commence antibiotic treatment in all patients with suspected CLTI who present with deep space foot infection or wet gangrene.
- If there is no option for revascularisation and/or patient is not a candidate for limb salvage, options are either primary amputation or palliation/wound care.
- As per NICE, avoid offering major amputation to patients with CLTI unless all other options for revascularisation have been explored and considered by the vascular MDT.

- Make sure patient (and ideally family) is fully involved in any decision-making (*shared decision-making*).
- Patients with CLTI should be managed by the vascular multi-disciplinary team.

CASE 8.1: Severe Aortoiliac Occlusive Disease

- A 50-year-old gentleman presents with bilateral rest pain/night pain in his feet with short-distance calf claudication.
- He has no pulses in either leg.
- He has no tissue loss.
- He has very poor monophasic foot signals.
- He has toe pressures of 30 mmHg on the left and 36 mmHg on the right.
- He is a heavy smoker and has chronic obstructive pulmonary disease.

Your FRCS Short Case Begins

What is your diagnosis?

- "This is a heavy smoker with what sounds like severe aortoiliac occlusive disease causing bilateral chronic limb-threatening ischaemia. I would estimate his WIfI stage to be 2, giving him a low amputation risk and a moderate potential benefit from revascularisation."

What is your management plan?

- "Immediate smoking cessation. Best medical therapy, in this case clopidogrel 75 mg OD and atorvastatin 80 mg OD. I would arrange for an urgent CT angiogram, echocardiogram and pulmonary function tests. I would discuss the case in the CLTI MDT when the above results were available."

Why not request an arterial duplex as per the NICE/ESVS guidelines?

- "I suspect the primary issue that needs investigating and treating here is an inflow issue, i.e. the aortoiliac segment. In my opinion CT is the best imaging modality for this pattern of disease to help diagnose and plan intervention."

Can you please interpret this CT angiogram?

- "This CT angiogram reveals severe bilateral common femoral artery disease, and severe external iliac artery disease bilaterally. The common iliac arteries are slightly diseased, but the infra-renal aorta appears disease free. Both the internal iliac arteries appear occluded. The superficial femoral arteries are patent and there is three-vessel run off below the knee."

What are your definitive management options then?

- "Conservative management is always an option. Indeed, it may be the best option here. The patient can be advised to stop smoking, continue best medical therapy, and try to exercise as much as possible to encourage collaterals to develop. The other options are an aortobifemoral bypass (with bilateral common femoral endarterectomies), or bilateral common femoral endarterectomies and iliac stenting, or an axillobifemoral bypass with bilateral common femoral endarterectomies."

What would be your preferred option?

- "I think that the "best" option with the "best" durability would be an aortobifemoral bypass. However, this is risky invasive surgery, and the patient does not sound like he has great lungs. If I were contemplating this I would first want to know the results of the patient's lung function tests, and I would also ask for a review by a consultant vascular anaesthetist. I would also counsel the patient on the risks of surgery, and try to balance them with the benefits."

The lung function tests reveal he has an obstructive lung disease pattern. The vascular anaesthetist advises that aortic surgery is possible, but it would be high risk. The patient himself would rather avoid major open surgery if at all possible, but he does not think he can cope with his symptoms at the moment and does not feel conservative management is appropriate because he can barely walk 20 m before his claudication forces him to stop and rest ....

- "In this case then I think bilateral common femoral endarterectomies with iliac stents is a suitable compromise. I would consider dual consultant operating (one for each groin) to make the operation faster. I would also work collaboratively with the anaesthetist, and perhaps a spinal/epidural approach would be better given his bad chest. If this were the plan I would also stop the patient's clopidogrel and switch him to aspirin to allow the spinal approach."

Your FRCS Short Case Ends

CASE 8.2: Multi-Level SFA Disease with Tissue Loss

- A 78-year-old patient presents with right foot rest pain, night pain, and fifth toe gangrene.
- He also has cellulitis in the forefoot.
- He is systemically well.
- He is an ex-smoker, type 2 diabetic, hypertensive, and has raised cholesterol.
- He has chronic kidney disease (eGFR 48), has had a previous myocardial infarction, and a left below-knee amputation (for a failed left femoral-popliteal bypass).
- He lives at home alone and has carers twice a day.
- He is frail.
- He has bilateral femoral pulses, nil distally.
- He has weak monophasic foot signals and a toe pressure of 16 mmHg.

Your FRCS Short Case Begins

What is your working diagnosis?

- "This is a frail, comorbid gentleman with chronic limb-threatening ischaemic with tissue loss of the right leg. As he only has a femoral pulse, I suspect he has right SFA disease +/− crural disease."

What is your immediate management plan?

- "I would send off urgent bloods for: FBC, U&Es, clotting, HBA1c, lipid screen, and group and save. I would request a right foot X-ray to exclude osteomyelitis and gas in the soft tissues. I would also request an urgent right leg arterial duplex and do a vein mapping request. The patient needs to be on best medical therapy (i.e. ensure he is on a suitable antiplatelet and high-dose statin therapy). Finally, he needs intravenous antibiotics for is right foot infection."

Would you take him to theatre to debride his right foot now, or after revascularisation?

- "It depends. If he was systemically well and this was mainly a case of forefoot cellulitis, ideally one would simply manage this with antibiotics, and then take him to theatre after revascularisation. If this was a really nasty foot infection however and the patient was systemically unwell, I would do an urgent debridement before revascularisation."

The patient does not actually go for an arterial duplex. He goes for an MRA instead. Can you interpret the images please?

- "The patient has severe diffuse stenotic disease of his right SFA. There is also a short occlusion in the adductor canal. The below-knee popliteal artery appears disease free, and there is three vessel run-off to the ankle. Theoretically this is suitable for either an endovascular recannalisation or a femoral below-knee popliteal artery bypass, depending upon the availability of vein."

Here is the vein mapping report. Your opinion?

- "The ipsilateral great saphenous vein is consistently above 0.3 cm in diameter from groin down to the lower calf. This is therefore suitable for a below-knee bypass."

So what would be your revascularisation approach?

- "According to the original BASIL trial, in patients with a life expectancy beyond 2 years, bypass affords greater durability and is probably better for the patient in the long term. In this case therefore there is an argument to support a bypass as I think this patient has a life expectancy beyond 2 years. However, one can also make the argument that he is not the fittest surgical candidate, and perhaps this pattern of disease is more suited to an endovascular-first approach. My gut feeling in this case would be to go for an endovascular-first strategy. However, I would counsel the patient in regards to the options, and also discuss the case in the CLTI MDT."

The patient and the CLTI MDT support an endovascular-first strategy. Angioplasty achieves a poor result so the whole length of the SFA is stented. There is a good radiological and clinical result. What would you do now?

- "I would take the patient to theatre for right foot debridement +/− 5th ray amputation. I would also make sure the patient was on dual antiplatelet therapy for his stent."

What if the endovascular approach had been unsuccessful and the below-knee popliteal artery has been dissected?

- "I would consider a femoral-distal bypass using ipsilateral GSV."

What if endovascular intervention has been unsuccessful in crossing the short SFA occlusion, and the patient had no suitable vein for a bypass?

- "I would consider a prosthetic bypass to the below-knee popliteal artery using a venous cuff."

Your FRCS Short Case Ends

JMF Reflections

This was a real case. I accepted the patient from another hospital with the results of the vein mapping and MRA already available. The patient was accepted provisionally on the basis of doing a bypass. However, the patient was not a great surgical candidate, and the MRA images made one salivate at the notion of endovascular treatment. The patient, when offered the options between bypass and endovascular, said he was "no spring chicken" and wanted to get out of hospital as soon as possible. Henceforth, despite BASIL, the patient went for an endovascular-first strategy. He did require a long SFA stent, but there was a good result. I do not think, however, if we had done a bypass, it would have been the wrong answer. Indeed, in the FRCS examination, if you had said bypass and justified your position, I don't think anyone would really have a problem with this.

CASE 8.3: Chronic Limb-Threatening Ischaemic Right Leg with Tissue Loss, Failed Previous SFA Angioplasty

- A 64-year-old female patient presents with right fifth toe dry gangrene with rest pain/ night pain.
- She had a right SFA angioplasty 6 months previously for rest pain.
- 1 month ago her rest/night pain suddenly returned and her fifth toe has deteriorated since then.
- She is a smoker, type 2 diabetic, hypertensive.
- She has a right femoral pulse, nil distally.
- The right foot power and sensation are normal.
- She has weak monophasic foot signals with a right toe pressure of 29 mmHg.
- There is minor dry gangrene to the tip of the fifth toe with no signs of infection.
- She lives at home with her husband and says she is otherwise independent.

Your FRCS Short Case Begins

What is your working diagnosis?

- "This is a 64-year-old woman with chronic limb-threatening ischaemia of the right leg with minor tissue loss. I suspect her continued smoking has resulted in the previous SFA angioplasty site occluding 4 weeks ago. I would estimate her WIfI stage to be 3, putting her at moderate risk of amputation, and high potential benefit from revascularisation."

What is your immediate management plan?

- "Ensure she is on best medical therapy i.e. antiplatelet and high-dose statin. I would strongly recommend immediate smoking cessation, and would also provide support to help her achieve this. As per the NICE/ESVS guidelines I would request an urgent right leg arterial duplex, and a vein map to assess if she has suitable vein for an autologous bypass. I would request blood tests: FBC, U&Es, lipid screen, HBA1c, clotting, and group and save. I would also request a right foot X-ray."

The arterial duplex confirms that the SFA is occluded from the upper thigh to the lower thigh. The below-knee popliteal artery appears to be patent and the crural vessels are all patent but demonstrate reduced monophasic flow. The right leg vein map shows that the ipsilateral great saphenous vein is very small (<0.25 cm from groin to ankle). What would you do now?

- "I would request an urgent MRA, and also vein mapping of the contralateral leg and both upper limbs."

Please interpret these scans.

- "The MRA shows that the right CFA and profunda are patent. There is an SFA occlusion that is about 10 cm long. There is reconstitution of the above-knee popliteal artery. The below-knee popliteal artery is also relatively disease-free, and there is three vessel run-off down to the ankle. The contralateral leg vein map again shows that the great saphenous vein is unsuitable. Both upper limb vein maps suggest the cephalic veins are suitable on both sides. Essentially, these scans suggest that the patient is theoretically suitable for a right femoral above-knee popliteal artery bypass using arm vein."

Would you not consider a repeat endovascular attempt?

- "This is of course possible. However, the first endovascular attempt was not durable, henceforth I don't think a second attempt would be durable either. As per the BASIL trial, I think this patient has a predicted life-expectancy beyond 2 years, therefore I think a bypass would be the best option for her now in terms of durability."

Which arm would you use for the bypass?

- "I would preferentially choose the non-dominant arm. I would alert the vascular team to this likelihood in advance and deter people from taking blood or cannulating the non-dominant arm to protect the cephalic vein."

OK. You take the patient to theatre for a bypass using arm vein. However during the arm vein harvest, you find that the vein is quite poor quality. There are segments that are sclerotic and occluded, mainly around the antecubital fossa. The other arm has not been prepped. What would you do now?

- "Firstly I would not have found myself in this situation because I would have scanned the arm vein in the anaesthetic room to confirm the vein was of decent quality. In any case, in this situation I would likely make a pragmatic decision and do the bypass using PTFE with a venous cuff."

You complete the bypass and use some proximal great saphenous vein to create a Miller cuff. The patient goes into recovery. After 15 minutes you are called urgently because there is a massive haematoma in the right groin. The patient is peri-arrest. What would you do now?

- "I would press on the right groin to achieve proximal control. The differential diagnosis here is that the proximal anastomosis is bleeding, or the saphenofemoral junction is bleeding from the vein harvest site. I would take the patient straight back to theatre and ensure the patient was being simultaneously resuscitated with blood."

You reopen the groin and there is a large amount of dark blood gushing upwards at you. What is the diagnosis?

- "The sapheno-femoral junction ligation tie has likely slipped off. Essentially this is a large bleed from the common femoral vein. I would manage this by asking my assistant to press above and below the saphenofemoral junction, then I would simply pick up the junction with my forceps and transfix it properly using 2-0 vicryl."

Your FRCS Short Case Ends

CASE 8.4: Acute-on-Chronic Right Leg Ischaemia Following Iliac Angioplasty

- A 66-year-old gentleman has acute right foot rest pain and night pain after a right iliac/CFA angioplasty performed yesterday.
- This patient is seen on a ward round in a district general hospital that is 20 minutes from your main tertiary arterial centre.
- This patient was having issues with tissue loss affecting the right foot and short-distance claudication.
- The patient went for a right iliac angioplasty (retrograde approach via left groin). This was successful. The interventional radiologist crossed the CFA with the wire and then did an angioplasty here. Unfortunately, the right CFA then occluded.
- The patient now has rest pain and night pain, and slept last night with his leg hanging out of the bed.

Your FRCS Short Case Begins

How would you first assess this patient?

- "First of all I would introduce myself to the patient. I would assess him from the end of the bed to gauge whether I thought he was an open surgical candidate. I would take a thorough history and examine him. In particular I am interested in the Rutherford status of the right limb. I would also want to clarify exactly what procedure was done, and if there was any pre-operative imaging."

The patient can move and feel his right foot. His right calf is soft and non-tender. There are no pulses in the right leg. He has minor tissue loss around the toes. Would you like to interpret his MRA?

- "With the information you have given me, this patient currently has a viable limb. It is Rutherford 1 acute-on-chronic ischaemia. His prior MRA showed a severe right external iliac artery stenosis. He also had significant right common femoral and profunda artery origin disease. He had a full length SFA occlusion. The below-knee popliteal artery was diseased. He had single vessel run-off to the ankle via the peroneal artery. The patient had multi-level peripheral arterial disease causing CLTI, and this attempted CFA angioplasty has resulted in acute thrombosis of his inflow. This has now left him with worsening ischaemia that is causing rest pain and night pain."

What would your management plan be in this context?

- "I would first counsel the patient on the diagnosis, and potential therapeutic options. On the one hand we could manage this conservatively with just anticoagulation. However,

I suspect this would carry a high risk of limb loss. Another option is a complex hybrid operation involving a right common femoral endarterectomy and profundaplasty, iliac angioplasty/stenting +/− a femoral to peroneal artery bypass. I would highlight that there is no guarantee this operation would be successful, and we would need to find suitable autologous vein to do the bypass. I would mention there is a risk of major limb loss, and he may ultimately require an amputation. After this, I would ensure the patient was on best medical therapy (i.e. antiplatelet and high-dose statin), commence him on intravenous heparin, make him nil by mouth, and arrange for immediate transfer to the tertiary vascular centre after discussion with the vascular consultant on-call."

The patient has his vein map and it shows he has a decent ipsilateral great saphenous vein from groin to ankle. Unfortunately, he starts spiking temperatures over the next 24 hours and develops a productive cough. A chest X-ray shows a right basal pneumonia. What would you do now?

- "I would continue to assess the Rutherford status of the right limb. On the assumption that it remained viable, I would prefer to treat this presumed chest infection first of all before taking him to theatre."

His chest infection improves and you aim to take him to theatre the following day. Are you still intending to do a femoral-peroneal bypass, or is there another option?

- "Actually I would re-discuss the case in the vascular MDT, and reappraise the original MRA. The below-knee popliteal artery was reported as diseased on the original MRA report, but this may still be a potential target."

It is interesting that you should say that. The vascular MDT recommended exploring the below-knee popliteal artery at the time of operation and/or doing an on-table angiogram. Indeed the popliteal artery was suitable for a bypass and he had a successful femoral below-knee popliteal artery bypass using reversed ipsilateral great saphenous vein. What would be your post-operative plan for this patient?

- "I would commence the patient on the VOYAGER regimen after counselling the patient. I would ensure he was on a high-dose statin. I would also request routine vein graft ultrasound surveillance. I would ensure the patient received post-operative chest physiotherapy."

What is the VOYAGER regimen?

- "Aspirin 75 mg OD plus rivaroxaban 2.5 mg BD. This regimen has been demonstrated in a large randomised controlled trial to improve MALE and MACE outcomes in patients following lower limb revascularisation. There is a theoretical increased risk of mainly non-fatal GI bleeding. I would routinely start patients on this regimen 48 hours post-surgery as long as there were no bleeding concerns."

Your FRCS Short Case Ends

CHAPTER 9

Acute Limb Ischaemia

This is a very big topic. I have chosen to focus on the core principles, highlight the core ESVS guideline recommendations, and then try to bring everything together with some interesting case examples. Hope you find it helpful for both the examination and your clinical practice. Note that the answers I provide in these cases are designed to stimulate your thinking and prepare you for what you may encounter. I encourage you to think of your own answers to the questions as well, after all with acute limb ischaemic there is often "more than one way to skin a cat."

Acute Limb Ischaemia (Lower Limb)

History

- Patient presents with acute onset pain and/or sensorimotor disturbance in lower limb.
- Alternatively, may present with new short distance claudication.
- When did these symptoms begin? How have the symptoms progressed?
- Prior claudication symptoms?
- Possibly, a history of palpitations/chest discomfort prior to this.
- Any drug abuse (*ask this question carefully and in the right context*)?
- Any fevers/sweats/shakes?
- Any instrumentation in groins recently, e.g., coronary angiogram?
- *Rapid-fire assessment of risk factors:* "Do you smoke? Do you have high blood pressure? Do you have raised cholesterol? Are you a diabetic?"
- *Rapid-fire assessment of comorbidities:* "Do you have heart disease? Do you have chronic lung disease/COPD? Do you have chronic kidney disease? Have you had a stroke? Do you have pain in your abdomen after eating (i.e. chronic mesenteric disease)? Any previous vascular surgery procedures?"
- Clarify if there is a family history of vascular disease, atrial fibrillation, thyroid disease, and aneurysms.

Examination

- End of the bed test
- Does patient have a regular pulse?
- Neck examination for signs of thyroid gland enlargement
- Auscultate the chest for murmurs
- Palpate the abdomen for an aortic pulse/AAA
- Palpate lower limb pulses (check both sides)
- Palpate upper limb pulses as well (*don't get caught out by aortic dissection*)
- Handheld Doppler assessment
- Determine Rutherford status of limb

DOI: 10.1201/b22951-9

Relevant ESVS Guideline Recommendations

- For patients presenting with acute limb ischaemia, the Rutherford classification for acute limb ischaemia is recommended for clinical evaluation.
- For patients presenting with acute limb ischaemia, diagnostic imaging is recommended to guide treatment, provided it does not delay treatment, or if the need for primary amputation is obvious.
- For patients presenting with acute limb ischaemia, computed tomography angiography is recommended as the first-line modality for anatomical imaging.
- For patients presenting with acute limb ischaemia, duplex ultrasound or contrast-enhanced magnetic resonance angiography may be considered for alternative imaging before starting treatment, depending on availability and clinical assessment.
- For patients presenting with acute limb ischaemia, it is not recommended to use results of myoglobin and creatine kinase on admission to base the decision to offer revascularisation or primary amputation.
- For patients with acute limb ischaemia awaiting revascularisation, heparin is recommended.
- For patients with acute limb ischaemia awaiting revascularisation, supplemental oxygen is recommended.
- For patients with acute limb ischaemia awaiting revascularisation, adequate analgesia and intravenous rehydration are recommended.
- It is recommended that patients diagnosed with acute limb ischaemia in a non-vascular centre be transferred to a vascular centre that offers the full range of open and endovascular interventions with an urgency that depends on the severity of the ischaemia.
- It is recommended that patients with acute limb ischaemia should have access to treatment in a hybrid theatre, or operating theatre with C arm equipment, and by a clinical team able to offer a full range of open or endovascular interventions during a single procedure.
- For patients requiring surgical thrombo-embolectomy for acute limb ischaemia, regional or local anaesthesia may be considered, but always with an anaesthetist present.
- For patients requiring surgical thrombo-embolectomy for acute limb ischaemia, the use of over the wire embolectomy catheters under fluoroscopic control should be considered.
- For patients requiring an infra-inguinal bypass procedure for acute limb ischaemia, the preferential use of a vein graft should be considered.
- For patients undergoing open and endovascular surgery for acute limb ischaemia, completion angiography is recommended.
- For patients with residual thrombus after open surgery for acute limb ischaemia, intra-operative local thrombolysis may be considered.
- For patients with acute limb ischaemia caused by graft occlusion, identification and treatment of the cause of graft occlusion are recommended.
- After open revascularisation for acute limb ischaemia, simultaneous endovascular treatment addressing inflow or outflow stenosis should be considered.
- For patients with acute limb ischaemia, intravenous thrombolysis is not recommended.
- For patients with acute onset claudication (Rutherford grade 1) that does not threaten the limb, (percutaneous) catheter-directed thrombolysis is not recommended.

- For patients with Rutherford grade 2a acute limb ischaemia, it is recommended that (percutaneous) catheter-directed thrombolysis is considered an alternative to surgery.
- For patients with Rutherford grade 2b acute limb ischaemia, (percutaneous) catheter-directed thrombolysis may be considered, if initiated promptly, and may be combined with percutaneous aspiration or thrombectomy.
- For patients with acute limb ischaemia undergoing thrombolysis, it is recommended that recombinant tissue plasminogen activator or urokinase is used.
- For patients undergoing thrombolytic therapy for acute limb ischaemia, routine monitoring of plasma fibrinogen is not recommended.
- For patients undergoing thrombolysis for acute limb ischaemia, continuous systemic therapeutic heparinisation is not recommended.
- It is recommended that patients undergoing thrombolytic treatment for acute limb ischaemia should be monitored for vital signs, access site complications, and the condition of the limb.
- For patients treated for acute limb ischaemia, it is recommended that thrombolysis be stopped if major bleeding occurs during treatment.
- For patients treated for acute limb ischaemia who have minor bleeding during thrombolysis, continued treatment should be considered, after evaluation of the risk and benefit of stopping or continuing.
- For patients with acute limb ischaemia, aspiration and mechanical thrombectomy should be considered.
- For patients with acute limb ischaemia secondary to thrombosis of a popliteal artery aneurysm, repair of the aneurysm with a saphenous vein bypass should be considered.
- For patients with acute limb ischaemia secondary to popliteal artery aneurysm, pre-operative or intra-operative thrombolysis to improve runoff should be considered.
- For patients with acute limb ischaemia secondary to popliteal artery aneurysm, stent grafting is not recommended as first-line treatment.
- For patients revascularised for acute limb ischaemia of embolic origin, it is recommended that, whenever possible, the source of the embolus be investigated, to prevent recurrence.
- After revascularisation for acute limb ischaemia caused by an embolus secondary to atrial fibrillation or intracardiac thrombus, long term anticoagulation is recommended.
- Antiplatelet therapy or anticoagulation and statins are recommended long term to reduce cardiovascular events following acute limb ischaemia revascularisation caused by native artery thrombosis, thrombosis of a popliteal artery aneurysm, or failure of previous revascularisation.
- For patients with acute limb ischaemia secondary to acute aortic occlusion, it is recommended that revascularisation is performed urgently.
- For patients who have undergone revascularisation for acute limb ischaemia secondary to acute aortic occlusion, close collaboration is recommended with anaesthetists and intensivists to reduce the complications of ischaemia reperfusion injury.
- For patients with acute limb ischaemia, it is recommended that the best interests of the patient are considered before deciding on treatment; to obtain informed consent to management if at all possible; and to record decisions clearly.
- For patients with acute limb ischaemia and underlying malignant disease, active revascularisation in selected patients should be considered, as the immediate post-operative outcome is comparable to patients without malignancy.

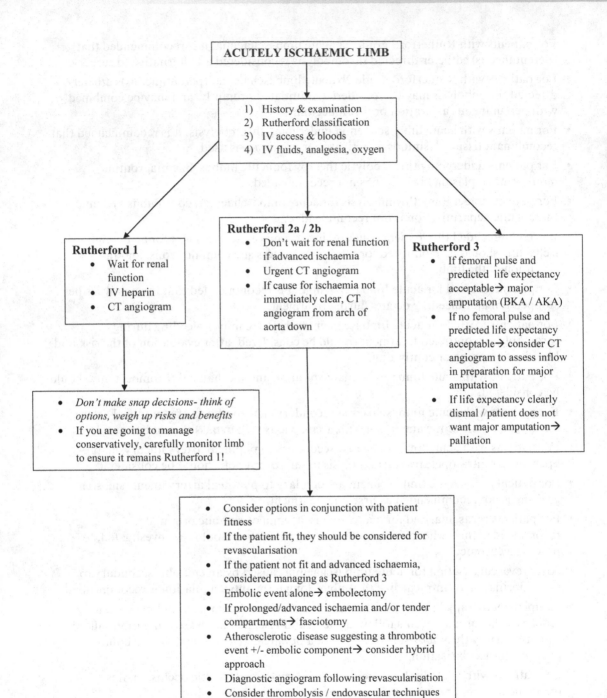

ACUTELY ISCHAEMIC LIMB

1) History & examination
2) Rutherford classification
3) IV access & bloods
4) IV fluids, analgesia, oxygen

Rutherford 1
- Wait for renal function
- IV heparin
- CT angiogram

Rutherford 2a / 2b
- Don't wait for renal function if advanced ischaemia
- Urgent CT angiogram
- If cause for ischaemia not immediately clear, CT angiogram from arch of aorta down

Rutherford 3
- If femoral pulse and predicted life expectancy acceptable→ major amputation (BKA / AKA)
- If no femoral pulse and predicted life expectancy acceptable→ consider CT angiogram to assess inflow in preparation for major amputation
- If life expectancy clearly dismal / patient does not want major amputation→ palliation

- *Don't make snap decisions- think of options, weigh up risks and benefits*
- If you are going to manage conservatively, carefully monitor limb to ensure it remains Rutherford 1!

- Consider options in conjunction with patient fitness
- If the patient fit, they should be considered for revascularisation
- If the patient not fit and advanced ischaemia, considered managing as Rutherford 3
- Embolic event alone→ embolectomy
- If prolonged/advanced ischaemia and/or tender compartments→ fasciotomy
- Atherosclerotic disease suggesting a thrombotic event +/- embolic component→ consider hybrid approach
- Diagnostic angiogram following revascularisation
- Consider thrombolysis / endovascular techniques

Acute Limb Ischaemia (Upper Limb)

We are not going to labour the same points as we have just covered with acute lower limb ischaemia. Let's focus on the important stuff.

Diagnosis and Immediate Work-Up

- Upper limb acute ischaemia is more likely to be embolic than thrombotic.
- Cardiac embolism is the usual culprit (i.e. often atrial fibrillation).
- It is less likely to be limb threatening.
- *Acute treatment is going to be much the same:* Systemic anticoagulation, intravenous fluids, oxygen, and analgesia.
- You can usually detect where the embolus is by pulse identification.
- If you strongly suspected this was an embolic event, the hand is immediately threatened, and there is an axillary pulse, you might proceed straight to brachial embolectomy.
- However, if this was an atypical case, you would be very wise to get further imaging before rushing in (fools rush in where angels fear to tread). Atypical cases may include young patients where thoracic outlet syndrome or a cervical rib is suspected, thrombosis associated with radiotherapy, subclavian aneurysm or aortic dissection.
- If in doubt get some imaging, you can either go with an arterial duplex or CT angiogram. For me, if I was planning intervention, I would routinely go for a CT angiogram as it is faster and gives me more information on the proximal vessels.
- If the axillary pulse was not palpable and I was contemplating intervention, I would definitely get a CT angiogram first. Doing a blind embolectomy in this setting may not improve the blood flow to the hand and may simply make the ischaemia worse.
- If you are anticipating difficulties, consider requesting a vein map before going to theatre (i.e. of arm/leg veins).
- Prophylactic fasciotomy is often not required.
- However, if the limb were profoundly ischaemic, and the ischaemic time were for many hours, it is worth considering.
- If you are going to do an upper limb fasciotomy, I would recommend asking for plastic surgical assistance.

Relevant ESVS Guideline Recommendations

- For patients with acute ischaemia of the upper limb, preoperative imaging is recommended, unless embolic occlusion is obvious, the limb is immediately threatened, and axillary or proximal brachial pulses are palpable.
- For a patient with acute ischaemia of the upper limb, conservative treatment with anticoagulation alone is not recommended if the arm is threatened, or if limb function is important to quality of life.

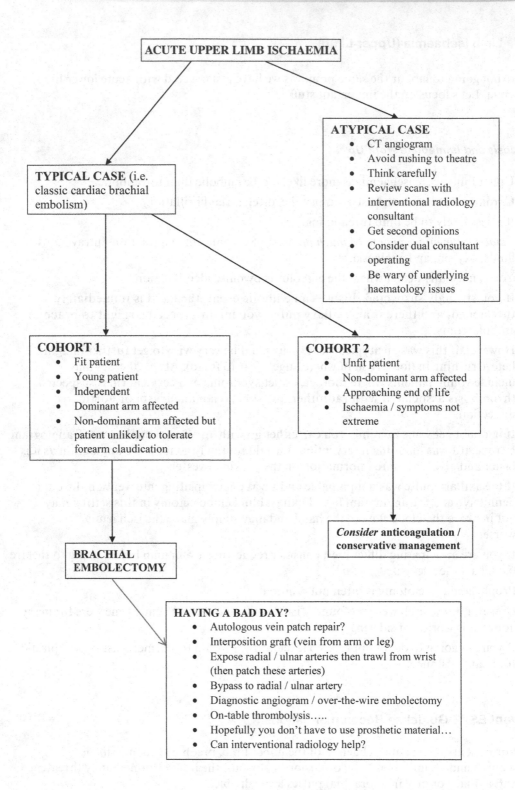

ACUTE UPPER LIMB ISCHAEMIA

ATYPICAL CASE
- CT angiogram
- Avoid rushing to theatre
- Think carefully
- Review scans with interventional radiology consultant
- Get second opinions
- Consider dual consultant operating
- Be wary of underlying haematology issues

TYPICAL CASE (i.e. classic cardiac brachial embolism)

COHORT 1
- Fit patient
- Young patient
- Independent
- Dominant arm affected
- Non-dominant arm affected but patient unlikely to tolerate forearm claudication

COHORT 2
- Unfit patient
- Non-dominant arm affected
- Approaching end of life
- Ischaemia / symptoms not extreme

Consider anticoagulation / conservative management

BRACHIAL EMBOLECTOMY

HAVING A BAD DAY?
- Autologous vein patch repair?
- Interposition graft (vein from arm or leg)
- Expose radial / ulnar arteries then trawl from wrist (then patch these arteries)
- Bypass to radial / ulnar artery
- Diagnostic angiogram / over-the-wire embolectomy
- On-table thrombolysis.....
- Hopefully you don't have to use prosthetic material...
- Can interventional radiology help?

Compartment Syndrome (Lower Limb)

History

- Patient post-op following revascularisation for limb ischaemia.
- Anticoagulated patient who has fallen on leg and developed painful swelling.
- Patient who has been abroad and think they may have been bitten by an insect/spider.
- Patient post-op following lower limb fracture fixation.
- Severe pain in leg.
- Swelling of muscle compartment(s) of leg.
- Patient has noticed sensory/motor disturbance.
- Increasing analgesia requirements reported by nursing staff (not controlling pain).
- Severe buttock pain (perhaps after iliac artery revascularisation).

Examination

- Tender muscle bellies on palpation (buttock/thigh/calf/shin).
- Sensory disturbance (e.g., loss of sensation in 1st webspace demonstrating deep peroneal nerve compression, inability to extend knee with femoral nerve compression in thigh compartment syndrome).
- Motor disturbance e.g., cannot move toes, foot drop.
- The patient may not have any pain at all (*I have seen genuine cases of compartment syndrome where the patient did not have pain but presented with foot drop following a revascularisation procedure 8 hours beforehand*).
- Leg may be tense and swollen.
- Severe pain elicited on passive movement.

Relevant ESVS Guideline Recommendations

- For patients who have had revascularisation for acute limb ischaemia, clinical examination is recommended to diagnose post-reperfusion compartment syndrome.
- Compartment pressure measurement may be considered to diagnose post-reperfusion compartment syndrome, when the clinical diagnosis is uncertain.
- For patients who have had revascularisation for acute limb ischaemia, routine prophylactic fasciotomy is not recommended, as it is associated with prolonged hospital stay, local infection, and development of late deep venous insufficiency.
- Prophylactic four compartment fasciotomy should be considered if ischaemia before revascularisation has been profound or prolonged.
- Emergency four compartment fasciotomy is recommended to treat post-ischaemic compartment syndrome.
- When post-ischaemic compartment syndrome is diagnosed, fasciotomy should be considered as soon as possible, and always within 2 hours.
- When post-ischaemic compartment syndrome of the lower limb is diagnosed, delaying fasciotomy by more than 6 hours is not recommended.

CASE 9.1: Patient with Rutherford 2A Left Arm Ischaemia. Brachial Pulse Palpable. No Wrist Pulses

- 85-year-old gentleman who is 2 days post-op following a right below-knee amputation for chronic limb-threatening ischaemia.
- He is heavily comorbid and frail.
- He is known to have atrial fibrillation.
- His normal warfarin had recently been stopped because of issues with upper GI bleeding, and for him to have his amputation.
- He has also only just recovered from hospital-acquired pneumonia.
- The patient is right handed (i.e. it is his non-dominant arm that is ischaemic).
- The patient has reduced sensation to the tips of his fingers.

The power in his hand and wrist is 5/5. He is not in significant pain.

Your FRCS Short Case Begins

What is your management approach now?

- "Given the patient's age, comorbidities, frailty, and that this is his non-dominant arm affected, and that this is arguably Rutherford 1/2a ischaemia, I would be veering on a conservative management approach at this point. There is an argument to say that this may well be a terminal event, and palliation may even be an option if he were to deteriorate."

So do you think that all frail elderly people with ischaemic arms should be palliated?

- "Oh no, not at all. I was providing an overall holistic opinion on this patient taking into account his age, frailty, comorbidities, and the fact that he is having multiple medical and surgical issues. As ischaemic leg that has required a major amputation, gastrointestinal bleeding, pneumonia, and now an ischaemic arm …. I am not saying that conservative management or palliation is the only option, but it should be considered."

What other options are available for this patient?

- "The other surgical options include a brachial embolectomy (+/− bypass) and primary amputation. Endovascular treatments such as percutaneous thrombectomy, aspiration thrombectomy, or catheter-directed thrombolysis may also be considered."

Would you do thrombolysis on this patient given he is only 2 days post-op following a major amputation, and in the context of recent upper GI bleeding?

- "No I would not."

Then why did you mention catheter-directed thrombolysis?

- "Well, you did ask me what the other potential options for this patient are. I am not saying I would advocate all the options I mentioned, but they are worth considering."

Let's say that you do manage the patient conservatively with intravenous heparin for 48 hours, but his hand deteriorates. He is now complaining of reduced power in his hand, and he is struggling to sleep because of pain. The patient is actually systemically well, his amputation stump is healing nicely, and he is engaging with the physiotherapists. He has not had any further GI bleeding. His chest infection has been treated ....

- "In this context I would re-consider revascularisation. However, I would want to do some further imaging first. As he has a brachial pulse and no wrist pulses I suspect any embolic material has showered down his forearm vessels. As such I think an arterial duplex would be ideal here. At the same time I would also ask for a vein map of his ipsilateral arm and his leg(s) in case I needed to do a bypass."

That is very interesting because the patient did have an arterial duplex. Can you please interpret these images for me?

- "There is triphasic flow in the subclavian, axillary and proximal brachial artery. There is reduced flow seen in the distal brachial artery suggesting there is some embolus here. At the origin of the radial artery there is monophasic flow, and the distal radial artery also shows very poor monophasic flow. There are very high velocities at the origin of the ulnar artery, and then there does not seem to be any flow in the ulnar artery in the forearm. As such I suspect embolic material has lodged at the brachial bifurcation and it is causing severe flow reduction in the radial and ulnar arteries."

So, what would be your management now?

- "If surgery was appropriate, I would take the patient for a local anaesthetic brachial embolectomy. I would make a lazy S incision, and exposure the brachial bifurcation. I would do a longitudinal arteriotomy at the distal brachial artery. I would expect clot to be present here and would gently lift it out using forceps. I would then do a gentle Fogarty embolectomy of the forearm vessels. At the end, I would do an on-table angiogram and close the arteriotomy with a vein patch."

You seem to have made this brachial embolectomy more complicated than usual. Why not just do a horizontal incision in the antecubital fossa, horizontal arteriotomy in the artery and close primarily?

- "You are correct. This is another option. Indeed on occasion I do follow the approach you have suggested if it is a straightforward case and a big brachial artery. However this case sounds like the brachial bifurcation is involved, the run-off vessels may be occluded and I may be required me to do a bypass. I think the approach I have suggested is still acceptable."

You take the patient to theatre but you are not pleased with the on-table angiogram result. The ulnar artery still is showing filling defects despite multiple balloon trawls. The situation is much the same with the radial artery. What would you do now?

- "I would consider on-table thrombolysis. If that did not work I would consider a bypass onto the best forearm vessel."

Did you review the vein mapping result before taking the patient to theatre?

- "No. But I did say I would do one when you asked me before."

Here is the vein mapping result. Please interpret it for me.

- "The left cephalic vein in the forearm is less than 1.5 mm in diameter and becomes too small to follow in the upper arm. There is 12 cm of suitable calibre basilic vein in the mid to proximal humerus. There is no suitable vein in the right arm. Both lower limbs have sufficient and suitable great saphenous vein from knee to groin level."

So if you needed to do a bypass which vein would you harvest?

- "Preferably I would harvest vein from the lower limb i.e. GSV. For me ipsilateral basilic vein would be a second option."

If you need to do such a vein harvest now, could you do it?

- "It is difficult at the moment because the patient is awake and this is a local anaesthetic case. To harvest the basilic vein would require at least an arm block. Harvesting leg vein would require a general anaesthetic. I would speak to the anaesthetist, update him with the situation and need for a bypass, and then once the patient was asleep I would harvest GSV to do the bypass."

Your FRCS Short Case Ends

JMF Reflections

This is a "mock case" in the sense that you have an antagonistic FRCS examiner who keeps asking you awkward questions that unsettle you. Whatever answer you give will be met with a counter-point, or a question that makes you feel incompetent. The FRCS examiners I had for my exam were on the whole entirely reasonable, but on a few occasions, I did feel like I was being put on the spot and made to sweat a bit. What I hoped to demonstrate in this case is how you can quite easily dig little holes for yourself. For example, I think it is entirely reasonable to suggest an initial conservative management policy for a patient such as this one. However, you must not appear to be committing yourself to this pathway alone, because it is very easy to come across as ageist. You cannot appear to have a blanket policy of depriving elderly patients with multiple comorbidities from an attempt at limb salvage. After all, 90% of vascular patients are elderly and comorbid. If we declined to treat elderly and comorbid patients, vascular surgery as a surgical speciality would no longer exist. Therefore, you need to have an appropriate justification for why you are pursuing a conservative management policy, and you should discuss the other options before committing to a certain strategy. A good way to do this is to always start off by saying you would counsel the patient on the options and get their opinion. If you give the options to the patient and they choose conservative management, then this demonstrates good practice on your part. On the other hand, if you don't discuss the options with the patient and just say you are going to palliate them, you will come across as narrow-minded and harsh.

Similarly, when an examiner asks you what options are available, think carefully before answering. Yes thrombolysis may be an option, as may primary amputation. However, before you mention these theoretical options, ask yourself whether or not they are sensible and appropriate options. In this case, the notion of thrombolysis seems unwise given the recent major surgery and GI bleeding, and similarly, an upper limb amputation also seems entirely premature.

Finally, if you are going to take a patient to theatre, then communicate to the examiner what you would do in real life. For example, in this case, it is very likely (*or at least I hope it is very likely*) that you would have reviewed the vein mapping report, that you would have discussed with the anaesthetist about the possible need for a bypass, and that would have consented the patient for possible vein harvest from leg or arm …. If you say this to the examiner, then you have covered your bases. However, if you don't say it, you lay yourself wide open for criticism and the examiner asking you awkward questions about what does the vein map show, did you speak to the anaesthetist beforehand, etc.

I am sorry to labour the point but this is what the examination can be like. This is also how I was "grilled" by my senior vascular consultant colleagues as I was preparing for the FRCS examination. You are presented with a case, and then you are put on the spot and asked questions. If you have not rehearsed beforehand what you are going to say, you may find yourself saying daft things, or not saying sensible things that would actually be in your routine clinical practice.

PS I am not advocating doing routine bypasses for patients with upper limb embolic ischaemic. I just included the notion of bypass in this case because it was created as a "worse-case scenario" to stretch you out and push your boundaries.

CASE 9.2: Patient with Rutherford 2B Acute Left Leg Ischaemia. No Femoral Pulse. Calf Muscles Tender

- This is a 74-year-old female who presents with a 24-hour history of left leg pain.
- She has pain in her left foot with "pins and needles."
- She is not able to walk because of the pain.
- She says that her GP told her a few years back that she has vascular disease.
- On closer questioning she says she normally gets pain in her left calf muscle on walking about 200 yards.
- She is a smoker, has hypertension, raised cholesterol, and has type 2 diabetes.
- She also suffers from mild angina.
- Her regular medications include aspirin, atorvastatin, metformin, ramipril, and GTN spray.
- She lives at home with her husband and is otherwise independent.
- She has no pulses in the left leg.
- She only has a right femoral pulse, but the right foot is warm and well perfused.
- The left foot is cold with a capillary refill time of 4 seconds.
- There is no fixed mottling.
- She has reduced sensation in the left foot and reduced power in her left toes and ankle.
- Her left calf and anterolateral compartments are slightly tender.
- Her abdomen is soft and non-tender. There is an aortic pulse, and it is not aneurysmal.
- Her upper limb pulses are normal, and she has a regular pulse.

Your FRCS Short Case Begins

What is your management approach?

- "I would first counsel the patient on what I thought the underlying diagnosis was. I suspect she has an acutely ischaemic left leg. I would explain that if we do nothing there is a risk she may lose her leg, and as such I think we should consider revascularisation.

I would make the patient nil by mouth, ensure she had appropriate pain relief, put her on high flow oxygen, and achieve large-bore intravenous access. I would send off urgent bloods: FBC, U&Es, clotting, group and save. I would get an ECG. I would arrange for an urgent CT angiogram from the aortic arch downwards."

Why are you requesting a whole aorta CT angiogram? Why not just scan the abdomen and lower limbs?

- "The patient may have a proximal embolic source such as a thoracic aneurysm. Aortic dissections can also present with lower limb ischaemia."

Would you not check the patient's creatinine kinase or myoglobin levels?

- "No. The up-to-date ESVS guidelines on acute limb ischaemia state that for patients presenting with acute limb ischaemia, it is not recommended to use results of myoglobin and creatine kinase on admission to base the decision to offer revascularisation or primary amputation. As such checking these blood tests would not alter my practice. I think she has an advanced case of limb ischaemia (Rutherford 2B) and her muscle bellies are threatened. In my opinion she needs revascularising quickly, and doing another blood test like this isn't going to change my approach."

Is there something else you would do in the basic management of this patient?

- "I would commence the patient on intravenous heparin."

Please interpret these CT angiogram images.

- "The aortic arch, descending thoracic aorta, abdominal aorta, and mesenteric branches are otherwise clean. There is some calcification affecting the infra-renal aorta and iliac arteries, but they are all patent. The left CFA is occluded which was looks like fresh thrombus. There is also a large amount of calcium and atherosclerotic disease affecting the left CFA. The profunda artery origin appears critically stenosed but is otherwise patent distally. The SFA origin is diseased. The rest of the left SFA is patent but there is evidence of diffuse minor stenotic disease around the adductor canal. There is 2 vessel run-off down to the left ankle via the left AT and PT vessels, although they both appear calcified. The right CFA and profunda origin shows some minor atherosclerotic disease. The right SFA appears chronically occluded in the adductor canal. There is reconstitution in the right below-knee popliteal artery with what looks like 3 vessel run-off down to the ankle. My impression is that this is a patient with pre-existing multi-level peripheral arterial disease. She has all the risk factors for peripheral arterial disease. This CT scan makes me suspect she has had acute in situ thrombosis of her left CFA."

What is your management plan?

"For this I would consider a left CFA thromboendarterectomy and profundaplasty with bovine patch repair and lower limb fasciotomy. I would also do a diagnostic angiogram upon completion of the patch repair, and consider further embolectomy of the SFA if required. I would of course discuss the case with the interventional radiologist on-call and review the CT angiogram with them. The case may require a hybrid approach with subsequent SFA angioplasty/stenting."

OK. You take the patient to theatre and do the fasciotomy and CFA endarterectomy. After the patch is completed, the foot does improve considerably. You do a diagnostic angiogram and it shows there is

a mild/moderate mid-thigh SFA stenosis. The flow past this stenosis seems pretty good however, and the contrast is reaching the foot. What would you do now?

- "There are two options here. One option is to accept that the foot looks better, leave things as they are, put the patient on the VOYAGER regimen post-operatively, and encourage her to exercise. The other option is to cross this lesion with a guidewire, and angioplasty it in the hope we can improve her perfusion further. As for me I do not think there is a right answer here, and I can picture various vascular surgeons/interventional radiologists I know having conflicting opinions. As for me, I remember this phrase: "the enemy of good is perfection. As such, I would leave this non-flow limiting lesion alone."

Well on this day you asked for a second opinion and the advice was to angioplasty this SFA lesion. You did that and you ended up with a flow-limiting dissection. What would you do now?

- "This would need to be stented. Alternatively, one would need to do a bypass."

If you needed to do a bypass, where would you bypass onto?

- "I don't know at this point. I would need to do an angiogram post-dissection to see what the run-off is like. The options would likely be either above-knee popliteal artery, below-knee, or crural vessel."

What would you use as your bypass conduit?

- "Ideally ipsilateral GSV."

Do you know in this case if you have suitable ipsilateral GSV?

- "It is my routine practice to scan the ipsilateral GSV in the anaesthetic room using the ultrasound machine, and I would have counselled and consented the patient beforehand on the possible need for a bypass."

Your FRCS Short Case Ends

JMF Reflections

The first point is that you forgot to commence the patient on intravenous heparin. I will tell you that this is really easy to do in an exam setting because it is something that comes so naturally to you, and no doubt it is something that in an exam setting you probably don't think it is that important to mention …. However, much like doing a driving test, if the examiner does not see you (or hear you) doing the right things, you won't get the marks. Henceforth rehearse the basics! That is why in all of these cases, I keep repeating the same basic points: Large-bore intravenous access, bloods, analgesia, heparin, CT angiogram …. These are easy points that you need to get on your mark sheet.

The second point is that as you progress in the station things get more and more challenging. Things also become more difficult to answer because you realise that whatever you say may be wrong in someone else's opinion. For example, over the course of my career I have worked with "aggressive" interventional radiologists/vascular surgeons who will treat most lesions they see. On the other hand, I have worked with "conservative" interventional radiologists/ vascular surgeons who have a far more cautious approach. As for me, I try to remain pragmatic and sensible. I also try to think out of the box and look backwards from the future onto the current case I am doing. I consider myself doing something and then consider the possible risks and consequences. I also weigh up the benefits of doing this procedure. In this context, I have genuinely seen lots of dissections requiring stents, bypasses, and they have occasionally resulted in the need for a major amputation. As such, if I have improved the patient's lower limb perfusion, I would be reluctant to do something that may completely undo the good work I have just done. My position in cases like this is indeed: "**PERFECTION IS THE ENEMY OF GOOD.**" Of course, if this was a severe SFA stenosis and flow limiting, I would have treated it.

CASE 9.3: Patient with Rutherford 2B Acute Right Leg Ischaemia. No Femoral Pulse

- This is a 68-year-old female patient with an acutely ischaemic right leg.
- Her symptoms started yesterday and have slowly gotten worse.
- She has reduced sensation in the right foot and reduced power.
- Her leg is cool to the lower thigh.
- There is no fixed mottling.
- She has a faint left femoral pulse (i.e. contralateral pulse).
- There is no prior history of claudication, but the patient does not mobilise very far because of severe COPD causing shortness of breath on exertion.

Your FRCS Short Case Begins

Please interpret this CT angiogram.

- "The infra-renal abdominal aorta is slightly calcified but patent. The right CIA is moderately diseased but patent. The right EIA is occluded, this looks fresh. The right IIA is occluded. The right CFA is moderately diseased but patent. The right profunda artery origin is diseased but patent. The right SFA is patent and there is 2-vessel run-off to the right ankle."

What is your management plan?

- "I would take this patient to theatre for a right groin cutdown, CFA endarterectomy and profundaplasty, with over-the-wire thrombectomy of the right iliac system +/− iliac stenting."

OK. You go to theatre and do as you say. You cannot get the guidewire through the right iliac system despite repeated attempts. What would you do now?

- "I would call for help. I would ask an interventional radiologist to come and assist me."

OK. The consultant vascular interventional radiologist comes in 30 minutes later. He cannot cross the right iliac system either. What would you do now?

- "I would consider a femoro-femoral crossover."

Are you sure you are happy with the inflow from the left?

- "You said the patient had a left femoral pulse."

I said the patient had a faint left femoral pulse. Would you like to look at the CT angiogram images again?

- "OK. Fair enough. The left iliac system is quite diseased. It is also heavily calcified. It is also quite small. In this case I would ask the interventional radiologist to stent the left iliac system, and after this I would do a left to right fem-fem crossover."

Did you prep the left groin?

"No. I would re-prep and drape the left groin."

The interventional radiologist crosses the left iliac system and starts off with a balloon angioplasty. All of a sudden the patient's blood pressure drops and she becomes tachycardic. What would you do now?

- "We need to do an urgent angiogram. I suspect the left iliac system has ruptured."

Can you please interpret this angiogram?

- "There is contrast extravasation from outside the left iliac artery. This confirms an iliac artery rupture. The patient needs an emergency covered stent."

OK. The patient's blood pressure is 70/40 mmHg. The anaesthetist is asking if the patient has a valid group and save. Did you request this pre-operatively?

- "I would have done. I am sorry that I did not mention this at the start of the station but this would be part of my routine practice."

OK. The covered stent insertion is successful and a repeat angiogram shows a good result. The patient is transfused blood and her haemodynamic parameters improve. What would you do now?

- "I would make sure that the left iliac system has been effectively treated such that the inflow to the left CFA was optimised for a fem-fem crossover."

OK. The interventional radiologist stents the whole left iliac system. You then do a cutdown onto the left CFA. The artery itself is very diseased. What are you going to do now?

- "Can I look at the CT angiogram again?"

Sure. Here you go.

- "The left CFA is heavily diseased and the left profunda origin is severely stenosed. As such I need to do bilateral femoral endarterectomies and a fem-fem crossover. At this point I would call for help. I would ask the theatre scrub nurse to telephone another vascular surgery consultant."

It is 3 am and none of the other vascular consultants are answering their telephones. What would you do now?

- "I would just have to get on and finish the case myself."

Your FRCS Short Case Ends

JMF Reflections

This is not a real case, but it has been designed to be a "nightmare situation". It basically represents a trap for you not to walk into. Oh, and by the way, in case you did not notice, you did just walk right into it. When everything is straightforward and easy, everything is straightforward and easy. This case, unfortunately for you, is not. The reason to include this case in the book is to teach you important lessons, not just for the examination, but also for real life. Let us start at the beginning:

1. Never, ever, ever, just "take a patient to theatre." That is not how we do things in vascular surgery. Taking a patient to theatre is a big deal, and once you put knife to skin, you better be ready for whatever may ensue. In this case, you completely abandoned all the basics → bloods, group and save, proper interpretation of the CT angiogram, discussing the case with an interventional radiologist beforehand, having a plan B, a plan C, etc. How can you expect to be prepared when you clearly have made no attempts at preparation?

2. Always have a plan for how you are going to call for help. If you are a day one consultant vascular surgeon, then in my opinion you should have some sort of a buddy system. What this means is that there is someone you can call if you need help.

3. It is better to discuss the case with interventional radiology way in advance of you going to theatre for a case like this.

4. When you go to theatre consider "carrying an umbrella". This means setting things up in case it starts raining (i.e. things turn ugly). Prep the patient in a way that allows you to defer to plan B or C. For example, if you think you may need to do a fem-fem crossover, prep the contralateral groin. If you think you may need to go from the aorta, prep the abdomen. If you think you may need brachial access, have the left arm out on an arm board. If you think you may need to do an axillo-femoral bypass, then prep for this possibility. If you think you might need to do a bypass, scan the GSV in the anaesthetic room and prep the leg. Once you find yourself in trouble, it is really awkward to start having to re-position and re-prep the patient ....

5. I am also going to make one final point here that may be self-defeating and controversial. I am going to be perfectly honest here and admit that endovascular surgery is really not my strong point. As such, for myself, if I think I am going to need to be doing endovascular stuff, even if other people think it is really simple, I would still ask an interventional radiologist for their help. I know that there are vascular surgeons who are amazing at endovascular surgery, and for them they may not need any help from interventional radiology at all. If this is you, then this case may not be relevant for you. However, as I see it, I am a vascular surgeon and my strengths reside within open vascular surgery. I am of the opinion that playing to one's strengths is a very sensible idea. On the contrary, I am of the opinion that veering outside of my area of expertise and confidence is risky. For me therefore, in the interest of being safe, I would rather stick to open vascular surgery and call an interventional radiologist for help in these sorts of cases. I don't expect people to agree with me on this point, but this is my position as I write this book.

6. As for vascular surgeons who are good at endovascular surgery, I know quite a few of them myself. I was trained by them, although I don't confess to be anywhere near as good as them. Of the best ones I know, I know that they would never be caught out by a case like this. They would have reviewed the whole CT scan, discussed the case between themselves, and had a plan A and B and C .... I know if they encountered difficulties, they would not hesitate to ask for another vascular surgeon who was good at endovascular surgery (or an interventional radiologist) for help.

7. *Here we go again: Fools rush in where angels fear to tread.*

CASE 9.4: Patient with Rutherford 2B Acute Right Leg Ischaemia. No Femoral Pulse

- This 58-year-old patient presents to A&E @ 1.30 am with acute onset inter-scapular back pain and malignant hypertension.
- The patient's blood pressure is 200/100 mmHg.
- He is otherwise fit and well and works as a car salesman.
- A&E requested a CT scan.
- The patient is referred to you because the patient has a white right leg with no pulses.

Your FRCS Short Case Begins

What is your working diagnosis?

- "It sounds like this patient has an aortic dissection with an acutely ischaemic right leg."

What is your initial management?

- "First of all I would go and see the patient. I would examine the patient from head to toe to assess if there were any perfusion defects related to possible aortic dissection. I would assess for signs of stroke, upper limb ischaemia, mesenteric ischaemia, renal infarction, spinal cord ischaemia, and lower limb ischaemia. If there was indeed evidence of lower limb ischaemia I would want to know the Rutherford status of the limb, if there were calf muscle tenderness, and what the state of the contralateral limb perfusion was. I would review the CT angiogram result and confirm the diagnosis. I would also be trying to ascertain if there were any signs of a type A aortic dissection and its sequelae. If aortic dissection were confirmed the first priority would be to optimise the patient's blood pressure. In my practice this would mean an arterial line, intensive care admission, and intravenous beta-blockade. I would be aiming for a systolic blood pressure < 120 mmHg and a heart rate < 60. I would also ensure the patient had adequate analgesia and was given high flow oxygen."

OK. Can you please interpret the CT angiogram?

- "This appears to be a type B dissection that extends all the way down to the right external iliac artery, almost encroaching into the right common femoral artery. The true lumen has been compressed from just distal to the left subclavian artery. The coeliac axis, SMA and right renal artery come off the true lumen. The left renal artery comes off the false lumen. The left iliac system is being perfused by the false lumen. The right iliac system is occluded. It looks like the false lumen has obliterated the true lumen in the infra-renal aorta and beyond this point the iliac system on the right has occluded. Both kidneys and the bowel seem to be well perfused on the CT."

What is your management plan now?

- "I would confirm if the patient had a decent left femoral pulse. I would also do a point of care ultrasound scan and confirm if there was triphasic flow in the left common femoral artery. I would confirm that the patient had no peritonism or signs of bowel ischaemia, and that the renal function was satisfactory. If the left common femoral artery inflow were satisfactory, I would take the patient to theatre for a left-to-right femoral-femoral crossover +/- right lower limb fasciotomy."

Would you not consider endovascular treatment for the aortic dissection?

- "Not in this setting no. In this case the pressing issue is the ischaemic right leg. The renal and mesenteric perfusion seems satisfactory. My sole purpose in this setting is to restore perfusion to the right leg with the simplest and quickest operation possible. In my opinion that is a femoro-femoral crossover."

You proceed with a left-to-right femoral-femoral cross and right leg fasciotomy. After doing the right CFA longitudinal arteriotomy, the dissection flap is bulging into the distal CFA lumen. It is almost occluding the origins of the SFA and PFA. What would you do in this context?

- "I don't like to poke skunks, but my concern in this setting is that if I leave things as they are my femoro-femoral crossover will either occlude, or the perfusion to the right SFA and PFA will be compromised. As such I would take a knife, make a small stab incision into this dissection flap, and decompress it. I would then tack this flap against the lateral CFA wall using 5-0 or 6-0 prolene."

What would you do if both limbs were ischaemic as a result of the type B dissection?

- "I would confirm if the patient had decent right arm pulses. In this case I would do a right axillo-bifemoral bypass."

Your FRCS Short Case Ends

JMF Reflections

As I was preparing for the FRCS Part B examination, I was being grilled by a bunch of senior vascular surgery consultants and this question came up. It seems to be something of an FRCS classic. It is also a case that does pop up in real life from time to time. Myself and these vascular consultants were sat down in a room around a table discussing this type of case, and I got some very good advice that I pass on to you. As a new vascular surgery consultant, you want to be someone who is safe and makes common sense decisions. You want to be the sort of person who can be trusted to manage patients at 3 o'clock in the morning whilst the rest of the more senior vascular surgery consultant body is fast asleep at home. Your senior colleagues don't want to hand over to you on Friday evening and then come back on Monday morning and find out that you have been doing crazy things during the on-call, and they are now left picking up the pieces. This, for me, is what this case is about. A type B dissection with an ischaemic right leg is an opportunity for you to either be a safe, sensible and pragmatic junior vascular surgical consultant, or a crazy one.

In this case, if you wanted to, you could try some crazy stuff I assure you. Why not do an open surgical repair of the descending thoracic aorta? How about percutaneous fenestration? Why not tell the FRCS examiner about true and false lumen access, intravascular ultrasound, talk about wires passing through the true lumen, into the false lumen, and renal arteries being stented …. This is all genuine vascular surgery practice and I have no problem with it. People out there do this routinely. However, do you really have much experience in this area? Would you be confident doing this? I certainly wouldn't be. And in this case, is it necessary? No, of course not. The patient does not have mesenteric or renal malperfusion. The problem is the ischaemic leg. So focus on treating his ischaemic leg with the simplest most pragmatic option. That is a femoro-femoral crossover in my book.

Indeed, I have chosen not to include loads of complex and "high-end" vascular and endovascular surgery procedures in this book, precisely because I think it is a trap for vascular surgeons at our level. Vascular and endovascular surgery is immensely complicated and it covers an enormous area. However, you (and me) are never going to be experts in all areas of vascular surgery. And we are not meant to be. For me writing this book, and for you reading it, the focus should be on being a safe, sensible junior vascular surgery consultant who can deal with the common "bread and butter" vascular surgery issues. You are also expected to know when to ask for help, when to seek advice, when to refer a case to somebody who is an expert, etc. Of paramount importance is knowing what not to do and when not to do it as well.

This does not mean you are not capable of doing complex "high end" vascular surgery, nor does it mean that you won't go on to become an expert. However, when you are starting off at the bottom of the ladder, just maintain your insight and remember that the big and complex stuff is probably best left for the vascular surgeons in your department with the grey hair, or for vascular surgeons in specialist centres.

Another final piece of advice. If you ever find yourself contemplating doing something that seems crazy, or perhaps you feel that you are being pressured into doing something that seems crazy, maybe you should pick up the telephone and call a fellow vascular surgery consultant colleague. You may find that they will advise you not to do what you are contemplating doing, or that if it does need doing it can wait until morning, or that they will come and assist you.

CASE 9.5: Bilateral Lower Limb Ischaemia

- This is a 49-year-old woman who presents with bilateral white legs.
- Both legs are pulseless.
- Her symptoms started around 8 hours ago.
- Now she can barely feel her feet.
- She cannot move her toes, and her ankle movements are reduced.
- She has painful calf muscles, but they are soft.
- The lower limbs are mottled, but this is not fixed mottling.
- She can bend and straighten her knees.
- She has no arterial handheld Doppler signals in her feet.
- She does have venous signals in her feet.
- She has an regular radial pulse.
- Upper limb pulses are palpable and good volume bilaterally.
- Her ECG is normal.
- She is otherwise fit and well.

Your FRCS Short Case Begins

What is your diagnosis?

- "It sounds like this woman has a saddle aortic embolus. She has acute bilateral lower ischaemia. She has Rutherford 2b ischaemia. Both her legs are immediately threatened."

What is your management plan?

- "Intravenous heparin. Urgent CT angiogram. Analgesia, high flow oxygen. Bloods including FBC, U&Es, clotting and group and save."

You request an urgent CT angiogram but the CT radiographer tells you the patient has to wait until the renal function comes back. What do you say to this?

- "I would personally walk around to CT and speak to the radiologist and the radiographer. I would highlight that this woman has profoundly ischaemic legs and she is at genuine risk of not just bilateral limb loss but also death. I would politely but firmly impress upon the radiology team that this scan needs to happen right now, and we are not waiting for the renal function result."

The CTA shows a saddle embolus at the aortic bifurcation as you described. However, the radiologist also says there is something abnormal in the right colon. He thinks she has a bowel cancer that is invading the right abdominal wall. He also thinks there are some metastatic lesions in the liver and lung. What is your approach now?

- "Arterial thrombosis can be associated with underlying malignancy. Unfortunately, the malignancy is usually advanced, and treatment often has poor results. Limb salvage rates are poor and most patients are not alive six months later. However, the up-to-date ESVS guidelines on acute limb ischaemia recommends that "for patients with acute limb ischaemia and underlying malignant disease, active revascularisation in selected patients should be considered, as the immediate post-operative outcome is comparable to patients without malignancy." It is vitally important to discuss the results of this CT angiogram with the patient and her family and see what they want to do. I would also discuss the case with a colorectal surgeon and/or an oncologist."

The patient's legs are profoundly ischaemic. All those conservations could take hours.

- "You are right, and it is an impossible situation. If I rush into an operation and it all goes wrong I may be criticised for not having these discussions beforehand. If I have all these meaningful conversations and document everything perfectly, I may come up with the perfect plan, but the patient's legs may be non-salvageable by the time I take her to theatre. I think however I could have a few focused discussions in a timely manner and then document things in detail afterwards."

You tell the patient and her partner the results of the CT scan. She and her partner are devastated and start crying. They cannot accept the diagnosis. They don't want her to lose her legs and want you to try and remove the clot. What would you do now?

- "This patient is young. I am not an expert in colorectal surgery or oncology but from my previous general surgery training I know that surgeons can do right hemicolectomies for caecal malignancy, and then refer patients on for chemotherapy etc. There is a genuine possibility that this cancer could be treated, and as such if I had to make a snap decision, it would be to take her to theatre, remove the clot, do bilateral lower limb fasciotomies, and hope for the best. I would make sure that the patient and family were aware of the risks i.e. that her risk of re-thrombosis is still high, that she still may end up with amputations, and that this may indeed all be a palliative approach as her bowel cancer may be very aggressive. I would impress upon the patient and her family the severity of the situation."

What operation would you perform?

- "I would do bilateral groin cutdowns to expose the common femoral arteries. I would do bilateral upstream fogarty embolectomies to achieve torrential inflow. After this I would do bilateral calf fasciotomies. I would ensure that the anaesthetist was forewarned of the risk of a major ischaemic reperfusion injury, and ensure the patient went to intensive care post-operatively."

Your FRCS Short Case Ends

JMF Reflections

This is strictly speaking not a real case. However, I have managed a few patients with acutely ischaemic limbs in the context of metastatic malignancy, and they have been young as well as old. There is never a right answer here. This case is deliberately challenging in the sense that you have very little time to think, the cancer is most certainly not what you expected, and metastatic colorectal malignancy is not your area of expertise. However, in cases like this it comes down to communication, patient counselling, and pragmatic thinking. Perhaps if you were in this FRCS scenario or in real life, you might say revascularisation was inappropriate and the patient should be palliated. However, even though the case is not real, I personally feel that taking her to theatre is acceptable. The patient is young, the risks were made known to her and her partner, there was a viable surgical option, and the ESVS guidelines say that active revascularisation in selected patients should be considered. As such, I feel I could justify my decision to operate in such a context.

CASE 9.6: Thrombosed Popliteal Aneurysm

- A 64-year-old gentleman presents to the acute surgical assessment area with an acutely ischaemic right leg.
- It is 6 pm in the evening now, and the patient developed sudden onset right leg pain earlier on in the morning.
- The patient is a smoker and has a background of hypertension, diabetes, and mild chronic obstructive pulmonary disease.
- He is a farmer and says he walks miles every day and is completely independent.
- On examination the patient has a regular pulse and normal upper limb pulses.
- He has a full complement of left leg pulses, but he clearly has a very large left popliteal aneurysm.
- He only has a right femoral pulse, nil distally.
- There is a large non-pulsatile mass in the right popliteal fossa.
- The right foot is cold with a capillary refill time of 5 seconds.
- There is absent sensation in the forefoot and almost no movement of his toes.
- There is no arterial Doppler signal in the anterior tibial artery, but you can pick up a faint posterior tibial signal.
- There are venous signals in the foot.

Your FRCS Short Case Begins

What is your working diagnosis?

- "Most likely this patient has a thrombosed right popliteal aneurysm. The crural vessels may also be trashed. At the moment he has Rutherford 2B ischaemia. He needs urgent revascularisation."

What is your immediate management?

- "I would counsel the patient on the likely diagnosis. I would explain that his limb is threatened and there was a high risk of limb loss. I would make the patient nil by mouth, give strong analgesia, give high flow oxygen, gain large-bore venous access and send off urgent bloods including clotting and a group and save. I would ask for an ECG. I would get an urgent CT angiogram."

What do you make of these CT images? (examiner hands you a few laminated sheets of paper)

- "There is indeed a very large right popliteal aneurysm that is thrombosed. It is in the popliteal fossa. The below-knee popliteal artery is patent. The posterior tibial artery is patent. The anterior tibial and peroneal arteries are occluded."

What do you make of the occluded crural vessels?

- "They could be acutely occluded. Alternatively, this may represent chronic occlusion of the anterior tibial and peroneal arteries secondary to previous embolic events. I suspect they might be chronically occluded, and the patient's sudden deterioration is as a result of popliteal aneurysm thrombosis."

What would be your management plan then?

- "This is not a straightforward case. I would first review the CT angiogram with the consultant interventional radiologist on-call. I would want their opinion on the run-off. Do they think the run-off vessels are acutely occluded or chronically occluded? I would want to have a good look at the posterior tibial artery as well and confirm it was fully patent. Finally, what does the above-knee popliteal artery/SFA look like? How high does this popliteal aneurysm extend?"

The interventional radiologist thinks the anterior tibial and peroneal arteries are chronically occluded. The posterior tibial appears patent and crosses the ankle. The popliteal aneurysm extends into the adductor canal, but the SFA is normal and patent. What are your thoughts now?

- "It sounds like this patient needs an SFA-PT bypass and exclusion of this popliteal aneurysm via a medial approach. I would confirm the patient had a decent ipsilateral GSV first. But this would be my plan."

What if the radiologist thought the anterior tibial and peroneal arteries were acutely occluded?

- In this case, I would still take the patient to theatre for a plan to do a bypass and exclusion of the popliteal aneurysm. However, I would expose the below-knee popliteal artery and do a Fogarty balloon embolectomy of the AT and peroneal arteries. If this was successful, I could do the bypass onto the below-knee popliteal.

What if all 3 crural vessels were acutely occluded? What would be your options then?

- I would still plan take the patient to theatre for a bypass and exclusion. I would expose the below-knee popliteal artery and trawl all 3 vessels.

What if you could not open all 3 vessels?

- "Pragmatically if I could open 1 or 2 vessels this would be enough. I could try on-table thrombolysis if needed."

You have only mentioned open surgical treatment for this patient. Would you not consider endovascular treatment? Would you not consider catheter-directed thrombolysis? Popliteal aneurysm stenting?

- "No. My concern would be that using thrombolysis to re-open the occluded popliteal aneurysm would not only take too long, but it also carries the risk of causing embolism down the PT. I don't think we have that much time with this patient as he has advanced ischaemia, and I think if is PT was trashed we would lose the only viable bypass target at the target."

When would you consider endovascular strategies with acute limb ischaemia secondary to popliteal aneurysms then?

- "If this was not severe ischaemia (e.g. Rutherford 2a), the popliteal aneurysm was patent and the run-off was acutely occluded, then I might consider catheter-directed thrombolysis to improve the run-off. I would consider a popliteal artery stent after this if the patient was not a good surgical candidate and there was no suitable saphenous vein for a bypass etc. However, even after catheter-directed thrombolysis, ideally I would prefer to do a medial approach popliteal aneurysm exclusion and bypass."

Would you do a fasciotomy for this patient?

- "Definitely."

Your FRCS Short Case Ends

CASE 9.7: Thrombolysis Gone Wrong

- A 59-year-old gentleman presents with sudden onset left foot rest pain and night pain.
- He also has short-distance claudication (can only walk around 50 yards now).
- Prior to 3 days, he had no rest pain or night pain and was about to walk around half a mile.
- There is no tissue loss.
- Last year the patient had a left femoro-above-knee popliteal artery PTFE bypass for intermittent claudication.
- The patient is a smoker and currently works as security guard.
- He has a left femoral pulse but no pulses distally.
- The power and sensation in his left foot is intact.
- He has monophasic arterial Doppler signals in the left foot and venous signals.
- He has no calf muscle tenderness on the left.

Your FRCS Short Case Begins

What is your impression?

- "It sounds like this graft has acutely occluded. The patient has been left with either critical limb ischaemia, or a Rutherford 1 acute ischaemia. Although I question the viability and sensibility of prosthetic doing bypasses for intermittent claudication in the first place, it looks like this patient is going to need something doing in this instance."

What is your immediate management then?

- "Bloods including FBC, U&Es, clotting, group and save. ECG. Analgesia. High flow oxygen. IV heparin. Urgent CT angiogram. Strongly recommend complete smoking cessation. I would also request a vein map of the ipsilateral leg, contralateral leg and possibly the upper limbs. I would also check the patient's ankle pressure, ABPI and toe pressure."

The toe pressure is 29 mmHg. What is the patient's WIfI stage?

- "Based upon what you have told me, the WIfI stage would be 2. He is scoring purely because of the low toe pressure. In this case the patient has a low amputation risk and a moderate potential benefit from revascularisation."

The patient actually has an urgent MR angiogram. Can you interpret these images?

- "This MRA confirms that this prosthetic bypass has occluded. There does not appear to be an inflow issue. The above-knee popliteal artery distal to the distal anastomosis is patent but there is some disease here. The below-knee popliteal artery is patent but similarly diseased. The TPT is diseased. The anterior tibial artery is occluded. The posterior tibial artery is patent down to the ankle but there are some stenoses just above the ankle. The peronealis diffusely diseased but patent. I suspect this bypass has occluded for two main reasons: (1) smoking (2) run-off issues."

What are your options then?

- "Conservative management is potentially an option. However, given the rest pain, night pain, short distance claudication, and the fact that this patient is young and in an active job as a security guard, this does not seem appropriate. The other option is to consider a repeat bypass. However, this does not look very attractive. It is a re-do groin exposure, and the distal bypass targets are not ideal. The other option is thrombolysis to re-open the graft, and then for angioplasty of the run-off vessels."

What would you do?

- "In the real world I would discuss the case in the vascular MDT. However, my gut instinct is to proceed with thrombolysis."

Before committing to thrombolysis what would you check for?

- "Well I would counsel the patient on the CT angiogram result and discuss the meaning of the diagnosis with him. I would highlight the options which include conservative management, repeat bypass, and thrombolysis +/− angioplasty. I discuss the pros and cons of each approach, and see what the patient thought. If I was seriously considering thrombolysis I would also search for any obvious contraindications such as previous bleeding issues, recent major surgery, gastrointestinal bleeding etc."

The patient says his leg symptoms are severe, and he also confirms he has been having to sleep with his leg hanging out of bed for the past 3 nights. He also says he is not going to be able to do his job as a security guard with his leg as it is. Indeed, that was the reason for the original bypass. He had tried to manage things conservatively with best medical therapy and exercise, but his leg did not get better. He says that the surgeon who did his operation looked for vein in his legs and arms and could not find any. He does not report any obvious contraindications to thrombolysis.

- "Fair enough. I would speak to interventional radiology about proceeding with thrombolysis. In my unit we also routinely arrange for a high-dependency bed to be available for the patient whilst they are having thrombolysis so they can be monitored carefully."

The patient goes to interventional radiology for thrombolysis. He has a sheath inserted into the contralateral groin (i.e. retrograde access, up and over approach to left leg) and then is brought back to HDU. You see the patient the following day on the vascular ward round. The nurses are concerned because there is some minor oozing around the right femoral sheath. They are also asking you about the heparin dose and are asking you how often you want the fibrinogen level checked?

- "I would be happy to continue thrombolysis if this was only very minor bleeding, as the benefits seem to outweigh the risks. In terms of checking fibrinogen levels and continuing, the up-to-date ESVS guidelines on acute limb ischaemia do not recommend routine monitoring of plasma fibrinogen, nor continuous systemic therapeutic heparinisation. This is because there is no strong evidence that low fibrinogen levels have a strong predictive value for bleeding during thrombolysis, and that continuous heparin administration is associated with an increased bleeding risk."

The nurses are not happy to stop the intravenous heparin because they insist on following the local guidelines. The patient is also on aspirin 75 mg OD and clopidogrel 75 mg OD which the patient had been started upon last year. Why do you think the patient is on dual antiplatelet therapy?

- "I surmise that the patient was commenced upon dual antiplatelet therapy after his prosthetic bypass last year. The CASPAR trial suggested that dual antiplatelet therapy clopidogrel plus aspirin confers benefit in patients receiving prosthetic grafts in terms of limb outcomes. However, strictly speaking the CASPAR trial was investigating patients with below-knee bypasses, and this patient had an above-knee popliteal bypass."

You decide not to fight with the nursing staff and leave the patient on thrombolysis, dual antiplatelet therapy, and continuous intravenous heparin infusion. The following day you are called urgently to critical care because the patient has dropped his GCS and is not moving his right arm and leg very much. What are your thoughts?

- "It sounds like this patient has had an intra-cerebral haemorrhage. I would assess the patient from head to toe using n ABCDE approach. I would stop the thrombolysis and heparin infusion. I would arrange for an urgent CT brain."

Can you please review these images?

- "Yes. This is a CT head. There is clearly a massive intra-cerebral haemorrhage that is causing midline shift. In this case I would discuss the case urgently with the neurosurgical and stroke teams on-call."

What are the other more common complications of thrombolysis?

- "Groin site bleeding, distal embolization, and possibly compartment syndrome with successful revascularisation."

If this patient became profoundly hypotensive and tachycardic shortly after initiating thrombolysis, but with no exterior signs of haemorrhage, what would be your differential diagnosis?

- "This could be a high or through-and-through puncture of the external iliac artery. The patient could be bleeding into the retroperitoneum. This would present with haemodynamic instability with potentially few exterior signs. The other obvious causes would be gastrointestinal bleeding."

If you suspected a high through-and-through EIA puncture, what would you do?

- "Stop the thrombolysis. Resuscitate the patient. Urgent CT angiogram. Ideally for a covered stent. Alternatively the patient would need to go to theatre for direct haemorrhage control."

Your FRCS Short Case Ends

CHAPTER 10

Aortoiliac Aneurysms

This is a very big topic, and it covers a lot of ground. I have tried to cover the core management principles. I have included the relevant ESVS and NICE guideline recommendations. I have included some interesting case examples. This was the sort of stuff that came up in my FRCS examination, and these cases are drawn from real world experience.

Abdominal Aortic Aneurysm (Non-Ruptured Infra-Renal)

History

- Pulsatile lump in abdomen (noticed in bath by patient classically)
- Back/loin/groin pain?
- Abdominal discomfort?
- *Rapid-fire assessment of risk factors:* "Do you smoke? Do you have high blood pressure? Do you have raised cholesterol? Are you a diabetic?"
- *Rapid-fire assessment of comorbidities:* "Do you have heart disease? Do you have chronic lung disease/COPD? Do you have chronic kidney disease? Have you had a stroke? Do you have pain in your abdomen after eating (i.e. chronic mesenteric disease)?"
- Is there a personal history of previous aneurysms or vascular surgery intervention?
- *Best medical therapy:* "Are you on aspirin or clopidogrel? Are you on a statin to lower your cholesterol?"
- Family history of aneurysms? Any children, how old are they?
- *Social history:* "Where do you live? Who do you live with? Are you independent? Who does the cooking/cleaning/shopping? How active are you normally?"

Examination

- End of bed test
- Auscultate chest and heart sounds (confirm no murmurs)
- Visually inspect abdomen → identify any scars, hernias, and BMI
- Abdominal examination for pulsatile/expansile mass
- Check upper and lower limb pulses
- Check specifically for CFA and popliteal aneurysms

Management Plan (for Asymptomatic Patient)

- Indication for treating AAA → symptomatic AAA of any size, asymptomatic and if size larger than 4.0 cm and has grown by more than 1 cm in 1 year, and asymptomatic and 5.5 cm or larger
- Full set of bloods (FBC, U&Es, LFTs, lipid screen, HBA1c, clotting +/− group, and save if you are contemplating imminent surgery)
- ECG

DOI: 10.1201/b22951-10

- Cardiopulmonary exercise assessment/echocardiogram/pulmonary function tests
- Anaesthetic review
- CT aortogram
- Bilateral lower limb arterial duplex (looking specifically for CFA and popliteal aneurysms)
- Smoking cessation (if relevant)
- Best medical therapy (antiplatelet and statin)
- Optimise diabetes/hypertension (if relevant)
- First-degree relatives aged ≥50 → advise early AAA screening
- Discussion in MDT
- Younger fitter patient → ideally for open AAA repair
- Older less fit patient → ideally for EVAR

Management Plan for Symptomatic Patient

- Same principles as above
- As per ESVS guidelines, symptomatic AAA cases should preferably be done on next available elective vascular surgery theatre list
- Your hand may get forced, but for me, I would try to avoid doing a symptomatic AAA in the night or over the weekend, i.e. you want more people around to support you if there are difficulties/complications

Open AAA VERSUS EVAR Algorithm

Figure 10.1 shows the overview of non-ruptured infra-renal AAA.

Relevant ESVS Guideline Recommendations

- Once the intervention threshold has been reached, the waiting time for vascular surgical care is recommended to be kept to a minimum, with an 8-week pathway as a reasonable upper limit from referral to elective treatment of abdominal aortic aneurysms.
- Ultrasonography is recommended for the first-line diagnosis and surveillance of small abdominal aortic aneurysms.
- The antero-posterior measuring plane with a consistent calliper placement should be considered the preferred method for ultrasound abdominal aortic diameter measurement.
- In patients with abdominal aortic aneurysms computed tomography angiography is recommended for therapeutic decision-making and treatment planning, and for the diagnosis of rupture.
- Aortic diameter measurement with computed tomography angiography should be considered using dedicated post-processing software analysis in three perpendicular planes with a consistent calliper placement.
- It is recommended that patients with incidentally detected abdominal aortic aneurysms are referred to a vascular surgeon for evaluation, except for cases with very limited life expectancy.
- Population screening for abdominal aortic aneurysm with a single ultrasound scan for all men at age 65 years is recommended.

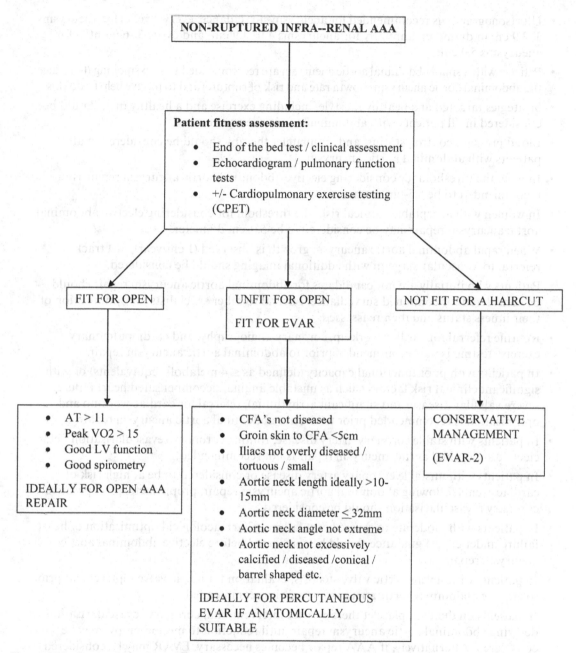

Figure 10.1   Pragmatic overview of management for non-ruptured infra-renal AAA.

- Men with an aorta 2.5–2.9 cm in diameter at initial screening may be considered for rescreening after 5–10 years.
- Population screening for abdominal aortic aneurysm in women is not recommended.
- All men and women aged 50 years and older with a first degree relative with an abdominal aortic aneurysm may be considered for abdominal aortic aneurysm screening at 10-year intervals.
- Screening for abdominal aortic aneurysm at 5–10-year intervals may be considered for all men and women with a true peripheral arterial aneurysm.

- Ultrasonography is recommended for aneurysm surveillance; every 3 years for aneurysms 3–3.9 cm in diameter, annually for aneurysms 4.0–4.9 cm, and every 3–6 months for aneurysms 5.0 cm.
- Patients with a small abdominal aortic aneurysm are recommended to stop smoking (to reduce the abdominal aortic aneurysm growth rate and risk of rupture) and to receive help to do this.
- Strategies targeted at a healthy lifestyle, including exercise and a healthy diet, should be considered in all patients with abdominal aortic aneurysm.
- Blood pressure control, statins, and antiplatelet therapy should be considered in all patients with abdominal aortic aneurysm.
- In men, the threshold for considering elective abdominal aortic aneurysm repair is recommended to be 5.5-cm diameter.
- In women with acceptable surgical risk, the threshold for considering elective abdominal aortic aneurysm repair may be considered to be 5.0-cm diameter.
- When rapid abdominal aortic aneurysm growth is observed (1 cm/year), fast track referral to a vascular surgeon with additional imaging should be considered.
- Patients who initially are not candidates for abdominal aortic aneurysm repair should be considered for continued surveillance, referral to other specialists for optimisation of their fitness status and then reassessed.
- Routine referral for cardiac work-up, coronary angiography, and cardiopulmonary exercise testing is not recommended prior to abdominal aortic aneurysm repair.
- In patients with poor functional capacity (defined as ≤ 4 metabolic equivalents) or with significant clinical risk factors (such as unstable angina, decompensated heart failure, severe valvular disease, and significant arrhythmia), referral for cardiac work-up and optimisation is recommended prior to elective abdominal aortic aneurysm repair.
- In patients with stable coronary artery disease, routine coronary revascularisation before elective abdominal aortic aneurysm repair is not recommended.
- In patients with unstable coronary artery disease or considered to be at high risk of cardiac events following abdominal aortic aneurysm repair, prophylactic pre-operative coronary revascularisation should be considered.
- In patients with moderate to severe heart failure, pharmacological optimisation of heart failure under expert guidance should be considered before elective abdominal aortic aneurysm repair.
- In patients with severe aortic valve stenosis, evaluation for aortic valve replacement prior to elective abdominal aortic aneurysm repair is recommended.
- In patients on dual antiplatelet therapy after interventional coronary revascularisation, delaying abdominal aortic aneurysm repair until reduction to monotherapy, may be considered. Alternatively, if AAA repair becomes necessary, EVAR may be considered under dual antiplatelet therapy.
- In all patients, pulmonary function testing with spirometry prior to elective abdominal aortic aneurysm repair should be considered.
- In patients with risk factors for pulmonary complications or a recent decline in respiratory function, specialist referral for respiratory work-up and optimisation is recommended prior to elective abdominal aortic aneurysm repair.
- In patients undergoing abdominal aortic aneurysm repair, assessment of pre-operative kidney function by measuring serum creatinine and estimating glomerular filtration rate (GFR) is recommended, and those with severe renal impairment (estimated GFR <30 mL/min/1.73 m^2) should be referred to a renal physician.

- Patients with renal impairment should be adequately hydrated before elective abdominal aortic aneurysm repair, and estimated GFR, fluid input, and urine output should be monitored after abdominal aortic aneurysm repair to recognise and manage reduced kidney function.
- Statins are recommended before (if possible, at least 4 weeks) elective abdominal aortic aneurysm surgery to reduce cardiovascular morbidity.
- An established monotherapy with aspirin or thienopyridines (e.g., clopidogrel) is recommended to be continued during the peri-operative period after open and endovascular abdominal aortic aneurysm repair.
- In all patients undergoing open or endovascular abdominal aortic aneurysm repair, peri-operative systemic antibiotic prophylaxis is recommended.
- In patients undergoing open abdominal aortic aneurysm repair, peri-operative epidural analgesia should be considered, to maximise pain relief and minimise early post-operative complications.
- Intra-operative cell salvage and re-transfusion should be considered during open abdominal aortic aneurysm repair.
- Intravenous heparin (50–100 IU/kg) is recommended before aortic cross clamping.
- It is recommended to perform the proximal anastomosis as close as possible to the renal arteries to prevent later aneurysm development in the remaining infra-renal aortic segment.
- An ultrasound-guided percutaneous approach should be considered in endovascular aortic aneurysm repair.
- In most patients with suitable anatomy and reasonable life expectancy, endovascular abdominal aortic aneurysm repair should be considered as the preferred treatment modality.
- In patients with long-life expectancy, open abdominal aortic aneurysm repair should be considered as the preferred treatment modality.
- In patients with limited life expectancy, elective abdominal aortic aneurysm repair is not recommended.
- Emergency referral to a vascular surgeon of patients with symptomatic abdominal aortic aneurysm is recommended.
- Symptomatic non-ruptured abdominal aortic aneurysms should be considered for deferred urgent repair ideally under elective repair conditions.

A Little Note on Aortic Necks and Access for EVAR

- Measurement of the aortic neck should be taken at the level of the lowest renal artery and extended 15 mm caudally in 5-mm segments.
- These measurements should occur using high quality EVAR planning software with the use of a centreline.
- You don't want to be overestimating the size of the aortic neck by using oblique measurements (*i.e. you want to do perpendicular measurements*).
- Endografts should be oversized by 10–20%, which means the actual graft you are using is going to be 3–4 mm larger than the aortic neck.
- Generally speaking, EVAR devices range in diameter from 18 to 36 mm and can accommodate aortic diameters from 16 to 32 mm.
- If your EVAR does not fully appose the aortic neck, you are going to get a type 1A endoleak.

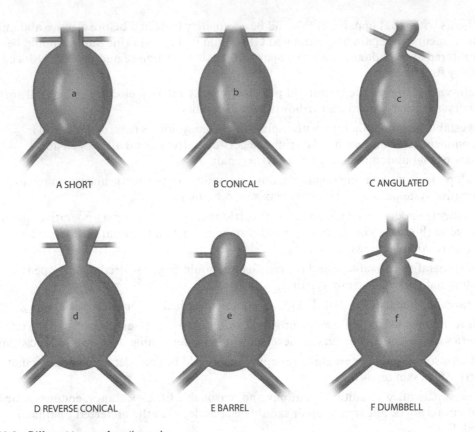

A SHORT   B CONICAL   C ANGULATED

D REVERSE CONICAL   E BARREL   F DUMBBELL

Figure 10.2 Different types of aortic necks.

- If you excessively oversize your EVAR, you will probably get pleating in the fabric which may again lead to a type 1A endoleak.
- Knowing how to describe the infra-renal neck is also important (see Figure 10.2):
  1. Long, straight, less than 32 mm in diameter, and not diseased (ideal—this is what you want)
  2. Short
  3. Conical
  4. Angulated
  5. Reverse conical
  6. Barrell
  7. Dumbbell
  8. Double barrel
  9. Diseased/calcified
  10. The neck may be loaded with thrombus
- Another important point is to have a good grip on whether this is a true infra-renal AAA. If you go sticking an infra-renal EVAR in what is actually a developing para- or supra-renal aneurysm, when the aneurysm continues to expand you are going to have future problems (please see Figure 10.3).
- Generally speaking the instructions for use (IFU) of most current devices suggest a minimum neck length of 10–15 mm and angulation less than 45–60 degrees.

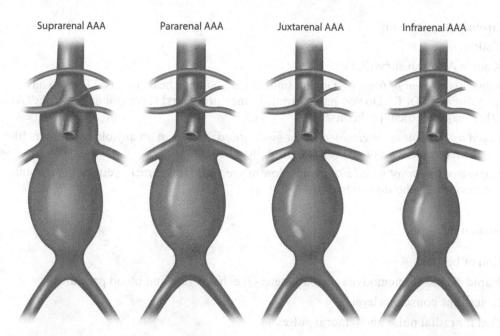

Suprarenal AAA   Pararenal AAA   Juxtarenal AAA   Infrarenal AAA

Figure 10.3 Different types of abdominal aortic aneurysms.

- It is difficult to give strict guidelines on what to make of aortic necks, because the possibilities are endless, and every case is individualised. The endovascular revolution is also rapidly progressing and there are new devices coming out all the time, and there are EVAR devices that can tolerate more extreme aortic neck angulations and even shorter necks ....
- In my real world practice, these aortic cases are all discussed in the aortic MDT by vascular surgeons and interventional radiologists who are cleverer than me and more up-to-date with recent endovascular technological developments.
- Another important point is that all EVAR devices will have compromised outcomes if their anatomical constraints are profoundly exceeded. Henceforth be wary about going "off-IFU."
- Generally speaking, patients with aortic necks less than 10 mm in length should be considered for open surgical repair, fenestrated EVAR, or EVAR with adjunctive endovascular techniques.
- *Concluding remark on aortic necks:* At least as I see it, use some common sense. The dodgier the neck, the more the risk you have of a dodgy outcome. In my book, fit patient plus dodgy neck equals open AAA repair.
- In terms of access for EVAR, I would watch out for severely diseased iliac arteries, small ileofemoral artries, and calcified iliac arteries.
- If you are thinking of percutaneous access, watch out for deep groins (my cut-off is >5 cm from groin skin to anterior CFA wall), anterior calcific femoral artery disease, very diseased femoral arteries (consider cut-down and CFA endarterectomy first), high femoral bifurcations, and previous groin surgery.

Abdominal Aortic Aneurysm (Ruptured Infra-Renal)

History

- Sudden onset pain in abdomen/back/groin
- Loin-to-groin pain (renal colic is classical presentation)

- Groin/testicular pain
- Collapse
- Known AAA on surveillance?
- *Rapid assessment of fitness:* "Do you smoke? Do you have heart disease? Do you have lung disease/COPD? Do you have chronic kidney problems? Have you had a stroke? Any other major medical problems?"
- *Rapid assessment of surgically relevant medications:* "Are you on any blood thinners like warfarin or apixaban or rivaroxaban or dabigatran?"
- *Rapid assessment of social situation:* "How fit are you? How far can you walk? Are you independent? Who do you live with?"

Examination

- End of bed test
- Rapid glance at haemodynamic parameters (i.e. heart rate and blood pressure)
- Determine conscious level
- Feel for radial pulse and femoral pulses
- Visually inspect abdomen → any previous scars?
- Palpate for AAA
- Lower limb pulse assessment
- If there is an ultrasound machine available and the diagnosis is in doubt, do a FAST scan using the curvilinear probe to visualise the aorta.

Immediate Management (for the Exam)

- Arterial blood gas
- Large-bore IV access both antecubital fossa
- *Bloods:* FBC, U&Es, LFTs, coagulation, and group and save sample
- Call blood bank and institute "massive transfusion protocol"
- Urgent CT aorta (thoracic aorta to both groins preferably)
- Permissive hypotension (i.e. avoid loads of intravenous fluids)
- Give blood to maintain consciousness (and/or to keep systolic blood pressure >80 mmHg)

Definitive Management

- Anatomically not suitable for EVAR but "fit" → open repair
- Anatomically suitable for EVAR and "fit" for open repair → NICE guidelines recommend that open repair is likely to provide a better balance of benefits and harms in men under 70. However, EVAR provides more benefit than open repair for most people, especially men over 70 and women of any age.
- Anatomically unsuitable for EVAR and not "fit" for open repair → palliation
- Patient not "fit" for anything → palliation
- Patient does not want anything → palliation

Open Surgical Repair of Ruptured AAA

- General anaesthesia
- Close cooperation between surgeon and anaesthetist
- Surgical team scrubbed up and gowned, surgical field prepped and draped, and ready to start operation as soon as patient intubated
- Midline transperitoneal incision (*quick into the abdomen*)
- Infra-renal clamp (*slow to the neck—avoid injury to left renal vein/IMV/IVC/duodenum*)
- Consider supra-coeliac clamp if infra-renal clamp difficult
- After securing infra-renal clamp allow anaesthetic team time to catch up
- At this stage I would give heparin (note it is difficult to give heparin when patient is shocked and bleeding, but from experience I find clotting complications more challenging to deal with than bleeding in this context. It is a judgement call; however, you make your own decision in the moment)
- Rest of the operation proceeds as with normal elective repair

Endovascular Repair of Ruptured AAA

- Efficiently plan the case using appropriate software.
- Local anaesthesia should be considered anaesthetic of choice.
- In haemodynamically unstable patients consider the placement of aortic balloon occlusion in emergency department.
- Bifurcated device, in preference to aorto-uni-iliac device and femoral-femoral crossover, should be considered whenever anatomically suitable.
- To avoid an intra-operative or late-type 1a endoleak, 30% oversizing is preferable when treating a ruptured AAA assessed by CTA during permissive hypotension.

Relevant ESVS Guideline Recommendations

- In haemodynamically stable patients with suspected ruptured abdominal aortic aneurysm, prompt thoracoabdominal computed tomography angiography is recommended as the imaging modality of choice.
- In haemodynamically unstable patients with suspected ruptured abdominal aortic aneurysm, prompt thoracoabdominal computed tomography angiography, allowing assessment for endovascular repair, should be considered before transferring the patient to the operating room.
- In patients with ruptured abdominal aortic aneurysm, a policy of permissive hypotension, by restricting fluid resuscitation, is recommended in the conscious patient.
- Local anaesthesia should be considered the anaesthetic modality of choice for endovascular repair of ruptured abdominal aortic aneurysm whenever tolerated by the patient.
- Aortic balloon occlusion for proximal control should be considered in haemodynamically unstable ruptured abdominal aortic aneurysm patients undergoing open or endovascular repair.
- In patients undergoing endovascular repair for ruptured abdominal aortic aneurysms, a bifurcated device, in preference to an aorto-uni-iliac device, should be considered whenever anatomically suitable.

- Selection of patients with ruptured abdominal aortic aneurysm for palliation based entirely on scoring systems or solely on advanced age is not recommended.
- In all patients undergoing open or endovascular treatment for ruptured abdominal aortic aneurysm, monitoring of intra-abdominal pressure for early diagnosis and management of intra-abdominal hypertension/abdominal compartment syndrome is recommended.
- In the presence of abdominal compartment syndrome after open or endovascular treatment of ruptured abdominal aortic aneurysm, decompressive laparotomy is recommended.
- In the management of open abdomen following decompression for abdominal compartment syndrome after open or endovascular treatment of ruptured abdominal aortic aneurysm, vacuum-assisted closure system should be considered.
- In patients with ruptured abdominal aortic aneurysm and suitable anatomy, endovascular repair is recommended as a first option.

Juxtarenal AAA

Background

- Juxtarenal AAA is defined as an aneurysm extending up to but not involving the renal arteries, necessitating suprarenal aortic clamping for open surgical repair, i.e. a short neck (<10 mm).
- Minimum threshold for treatment is 5.5 cm.

Basic Management Principles

- Same basic principles as for abdominal aortic aneurysm repair, i.e. fitness tests, best medical therapy, CT angiogram, smoking cessation, look for aneurysms elsewhere (abdominal, thoracic, and popliteal), enquire about family history and advise children to get screened for AAA aged 50 etc.
- Your definitive options are either going to be conservative management with surveillance, open surgical repair, endovascular repair, or consideration of a palliative approach (i.e. no intervention and no surveillance).

Open Surgery

- General anaesthetic
- Transperitoneal or retroperitoneal approach
- Suprarenal clamp (keep clamping time as short as possible)
- Ligation of left renal vein can improve access/exposure of neck
- Alternatively, ligate adrenal/gonadal/lumbar veins to enable further mobilisation of left renal vein

Endovascular Repair

- These are complex aneurysms and as such they take time to plan.
- You may also require a customised stent to be made, and this can take a few weeks.
- The options today include fenestrated repair, branched repair, parallel grafts in a chimney, or snorkel configuration ....

- One might also consider the use of endostaples/endoanchors for infra-renal/juxtarenal aneurysms with short necks. Thus, by using endoanchors, one theoretically can avoid the need for fenestrations etc.
- I think one does need to maintain a degree of caution however ....
- Indeed, the ESVS guidelines recommend centralisation of these cases to specialised high volume centres that can offer both complex open and complex endovascular repair. It also says that in patients with juxtarenal abdominal aortic aneurysm, new techniques/concepts, including endovascular aneurysm seal, endostaples, and in situ laser fenestration, are not recommended as first-line treatment, but should be limited to studies approved by research ethics committees, until adequately evaluated ....
- The NICE guidelines on AAA (2020) also have some interesting things to say about this matter. Essentially, NICE is not so sure if complex EVAR improves peri-operative survival or long term outcomes when compared to open AAA repair, and there needs to be further investigation into the clinical and cost-effectiveness.

Relevant ESVS Guideline Recommendations

- In patients with juxtarenal abdominal aortic aneurysm and acceptable surgical risk, the minimum threshold for elective repair may be considered to be 5.5-cm diameter.
- Centralisation to specialised high volume centres that can offer both complex open and complex endovascular repair for treatment of juxtarenal abdominal aortic aneurysm is recommended.
- In patients with juxtarenal abdominal aortic aneurysm, open repair or complex endovascular repair should be considered based on patient status, anatomy, local routines, team experience, and patient preference.
- In complex endovascular repair of juxtarenal abdominal aortic aneurysm, endovascular repair with fenestrated stent grafts should be considered the preferred treatment option when feasible.
- In complex endovascular repair for juxtarenal abdominal aortic aneurysm, using parallel graft techniques may be considered an alternative in the emergency setting or when fenestrated stent grafts are not indicated or available, or as a bailout, ideally restricted to 2 chimneys.
- In patients with juxtarenal abdominal aortic aneurysm, new techniques/concepts, including endovascular aneurysm seal, endostaples, and in situ laser fenestration, are not recommended as first-line treatment but should be limited to studies approved by research ethics committees, until adequately evaluated.
- In patients undergoing open repair of juxtarenal abdominal aortic aneurysm, a strategy to preserve renal function by means of cold crystalloid renal perfusion may be considered.
- In patients treated for juxtarenal abdominal aortic aneurysm by endovascular repair, a thorough long term follow-up programme including annual computed tomography angiography is recommended.

JMF Reflections

I think for the examination you should have a solid grounding in the core principles of the management of juxtarenal AAA. This is a really big area and there are a lot of endovascular enthusiasts in the world who are doing some pioneering work in this area and pushing various boundaries. As for me, this is not my specialist area. I think the ESVS and NICE guidelines are pretty sensible, and I think they are right about complex endovascular repair for these types of aneurysms. There is definitely a place for complex endovascular repair of juxtarenal/visceral aneurysms, but we need to proceed sensibly and cautiously, we should be doing them in specialist centres, and we need to gather decent data to demonstrate it is genuinely in the patient's best interests and cost-effective in the long term before we wholeheartedly embrace it ....

The reason I mention this is because in the FRCS Part B examination I was asked a question about going "off-IFU" and/or using endoanchors. The case was that of a symptomatic juxtarenal AAA in a borderline high-risk patient. I made the point that going "off-IFU" concerned me as in my practice I have seen various "off-IFU" EVARs that just end up with endoleaks requiring further interventions. I also said I had concerns about endoanchors as I was not certain of the strength of the evidence base behind it. It was an impossible question to answer because if I said I would do an open repair, then this would have exposed me to the criticism that I am doing open surgery on a high-risk patient .... In any case, the patient in this clinical scenario ended up having an emergency EVAR with endoanchors. I was not sure if I said the right thing or wrong thing.

Personally, my approach in these cases is to do the basics properly, i.e. history, examination, CT angiogram, review the images with an interventional radiologist, discuss with my colleagues, put the case through the aortic MDT, and counsel the patient and their family on the options that are available. If I think the patient is fit, my preference would be for open surgical repair. If the patient was not fit, I would refer the case to the interventional radiologists in my department who specialise in this area to see if there was a viable endovascular solution available. If the patient came in with a symptomatic or ruptured juxtarenal AAA I would think on my feet, get some expert help, and do what needed to be done in order to save the patient's life. If this meant going off-IFU and using endoanchors, then so be it.

I would also say in closing that I don't necessarily consider complex endovascular repair of these types of aneurysms as "minimally invasive." These are complex, risky, and lengthy procedures. I have seen patients who have FEVARs and end up with renal failure on dialysis, paraplegic, with ischaemic limbs requiring amputation, with stent graft infections requiring life-long antibiotics, etc. It is all well and good talking about the morbidity and mortality of open surgery, but the door swings both ways.

Iliac Artery Aneurysms

Background

- In general, a common iliac artery (CIA) that is > 18 mm in men and > 15 mm in women, and an internal iliac artery (IIA) > 8 mm is considered aneurysmal.
- IAAs are commonly associated with aneurysmal dilatation of the abdominal aorta, and aorto-iliac aneurysms are present in about 10% of AAA.
- Isolated IAA is an aneurysm of the iliac arteries without an aneurysm of the infrarenal abdominal aorta. This includes aneurysms of the CIA, IIA, EIA, and combinations of those.
- Aneurysms of the EIA, which has a different embryological origin, are rare.
- The threshold for elective repair of isolated iliac artery aneurysm (CIA, IIA, and external iliac artery, or combination thereof) may be considered at a minimum of 3.5-cm diameter.

Clinical Presentation

- Most are asymptomatic.
- Symptoms can be related to local compression of the ureter, sacral plexus, or iliac vein (e.g., urinary symptoms, neurological symptoms, and swollen leg).

- Clinical examination often misses these aneurysms as they are deep in the pelvis, although very large ones might be visible/palpable in the lower abdominal quadrants.
- Clearly, these aneurysms can also rupture and this may be the first presentation.

Basic Management Principles

- Same basic principles as for abdominal aortic aneurysm repair, i.e. fitness tests, best medical therapy, CT angiogram, smoking cessation, look for aneurysms elsewhere (abdominal, thoracic, popliteal), and enquire about family history and advise children to get screened for AAA aged 50.
- Your definitive options are either going to be conservative management with surveillance, open surgical repair, endovascular repair, or consideration of a palliative approach (i.e. no intervention and no surveillance).
- The first-line management approach if you are going to treat is *endovascular.*

Open Surgical Repair

- General anaesthesia
- Transperitoneal or retroperitoneal approach
- Your approach will depend on whether this is an isolated iliac artery aneurysm (and whether CIA/EIA/IIA are involved), whether the contralateral IIA is patent, and if this is also part of an overall aortoiliac artery aneurysm.
- For an isolated CIA aneurysm, one may consider a short iliac tube graft onto the iliac bifurcation.
- For an isolated iliac aneurysm involving the iliac bifurcation itself, one may consider a bifurcated graft onto the EIA and IIA.
- If the contralateral IIA is patent, one could simply ligate the ipsilateral IIA aneurysm and do a tube graft onto the ipsilateral EIA.
- There is also the theoretical option of ligating the iliac aneurysm and doing a crossover graft (i.e. fem-fem or iliac-iliac).
- If the abdominal aorta is also aneurysmal (and/or the contralateral iliac is aneurysmal) this will obviously add to the complexity of the case, but the principles remain much the same.
- What is important to recognise however is that doing these operations is not easy. You are in a deep pelvic location, and open repair of iliac aneurysms can be very technically challenging with an increased risk of iatrogenic injuries of veins, ureter, or nerve, resulting in peri-operative blood loss, morbidity, and mortality.

Endovascular Repair

- The classic endovascular treatment of IAA originally involved embolisation of the IIA and stent graft coverage extending from the CIA to the EIA.
- Involving the infrarenal aorta and the contralateral iliac artery into the repair is sometimes necessary to obtain a proper proximal seal.
- Endovascular techniques have further evolved in recent years from routine embolisation of the IIA in most cases to side branch techniques preserving IIA patency.

Big Deal → The Pelvic Circulation

- Interruption of IIA perfusion is normally well compensated for by collateral artery perfusion via pathways from the contralateral IIA, mesenteric, and femoral arteries.
- However, if this collateral circulation is poorly developed or absent, and you then ligate/cover/embolise the IIA, your patient may get buttock claudication, colonic ischaemia, pelvic necrosis, or erectile dysfunction.
- Therefore, preservation of blood flow to at least one IIA is recommended.
- This is where branched stent grafts are most helpful as they allow preservation of flow in most cases.
- If, on the other hand, you need to embolise the IIA to exclude the aneurysm, the embolising material should preferably be placed in the proximal portion of the IIA in order to maintain communication between its anterior and posterior divisions.
- If you have no choice but to occlude both IIAs, it is wise to try and stage these as two separate procedures to allow collaterals to grow.

Relevant ESVS Guideline Recommendations

- In patients with iliac artery aneurysm endovascular repair may be considered first-line therapy.
- Preserving blood flow to at least one IIA during open surgical and endovascular repair of iliac artery aneurysms is recommended.
- In patients where IIA embolisation or ligation is necessary, occlusion of the proximal main stem of the vessel is recommended if technically feasible, to preserve distal collateral circulation to the pelvis.

CASE 10.1: Symptomatic 7.5-cm Infra-Renal AAA in Fit Patient

History

- A 65-year-old gentleman goes for his AAA screening ultrasound.
- He has been found to have a 6.7-cm AAA.
- At the time of ultrasound, the patient was complaining of left-sided loin pain.
- The patient was referred to A&E immediately.
- The patient is haemodynamically stable.
- *PMH:* Myocardial infarction in 2008, had primary PCI, hypertension. Otherwise, fit and well. Ex-smoker (quit in 2008).
- *Medications:* Aspirin, simvastatin, ramipril, and bisoprolol
- *Social history:* Fit, walks miles, etc. Ex-smoker (quit in 2008). Lives at home with his wife and is independent.
- *On examination:* Haemodynamically stable, looks well, slim build. Abdomen SNT, large palpable AAA, AAA is not tender. No scars (i.e. no previous abdominal surgery).
- Full complement of lower limb pulses

Your FRCS Long Case Begins

What is your impression?

- "This looks like a fit gentleman who arguably has a symptomatic AAA. He sounds like the sort of person I would be considering an open AAA repair on. This would be in-line with the recent NICE guidelines on abdominal aortic aneurysm."

What is your initial management?

- "I would counsel the patient on the diagnosis and discuss the potential options including conservative management, open AAA repair, or EVAR. I would say that at the moment I am worried about his aneurysm, so don't want to send him home. I would get large-bore intravenous access, and send off urgent bloods: FBC, U&Es, LFTs, CRP, amylase, coagulation, group and save. I would get an ECG +/− troponin. If the patient had any urinary symptoms I would consider a urine dip. I would arrange for an urgent CT angiogram aorta."

The ECG is normal. The rest of the bloods are normal. The patient has no urinary symptoms. He has his CT angiogram. Can you please interpret the images?

- "This looks like a large infra-renal AAA. It looks about 8 cm in diameter. It does not look ruptured. I cannot identify any sinister features to suggest imminent rupture. There is an anterior left renal vein. The coeliac and SMA are patent. The IMA looks patent. The para-renal and infra-renal aortic neck is slightly calcified, and there is some posteriorly placed thrombus, and possibly an old dissection flap. There is a fairly large accessory left renal artery. The infra-renal neck is slightly conical and angulated anteriorly by about 40 degrees. The infra-renal neck is about 16 mm in length. The aneurysm extends downwards to the origin of the common iliacs, and the aortic bifurcation does not look suitable for a tube graft, but instead a bifurcated graft. The common iliac arteries are slightly calcified. The internal iliac arteries are both patent. The iliacs are not grossly tortuous, otherwise disease free, and on average the external iliacs are around 1 cm in diameter. Both common femoral arteries are decent size (1 cm), disease free, and around 2–3 cm from the skin surface. This looks like an aneurysm that is potentially suitable for a percuteanous EVAR. However, I am not very happy with the infra-renal neck. Given the patient's youth and fitness, I think he is better suited to an open AAA repair with an infra-renal clamp and bifurcated graft onto his common iliac arteries."

OK. So what would you do now? Would you rush the patient to theatre?

- "No. I would arrange for some urgent fitness tests, an anaesthetic review, and discuss with my vascular surgery and interventional radiology colleagues, ideally in an MDT setting. I would also counsel the patient on the result of the CT, and see what he thinks."

What fitness tests would you do?

- "I would arrange for an urgent echocardiogram and pulmonary function tests."

Would you not consider cardiopulmonary exercise testing?

- "With a symptomatic AAA of this size, I would be worried that CPEX testing may increase the rupture risk, so I would generally avoid. Also, the up-to-date ESVS guidelines on aortoiliac aneurysms do not recommend routine cardiopulmonary exercise testing prior to AAA repair."

In my unit we routinely do CPEX testing for patients being considered for AAA repair. In any case the patient has had a CPEX. Can you please interpret this result?

> *Cycle:* 15 W ramp, reached % predicted
> *Why stopped:* Technician decision due to AAA size, pt obtained sufficient numbers above AT.

Patient started to feel SOB and leg fatigue.
Motivation: Excellent
Exercise Capacity
AT: 14.6 mL/kg/min
Peak VO$_2$: 19.9 mL/kg/min
CVS Function
HR—rest: 70 bpm peak: 131 bpm
BP—rest: 124/76 mmHg peak: 150/80 mmHg
ECG: Sinus Rhythm with isolated VEs
O$_2$ pulse: 96%
Ventilatory Function
FEV1: 2.90 L, 87% predicted
FVC: 4.17 L, 93% predicted
FEV1/FVC: 70%
PEF: 508.9 L/min
VE/VCO$_2$ slope to AT: 30.60
VE/VCO$_2$ slope to peak: 33.99
VE/VCO$_2$ at AT: 33
Breathing Reserve: 38.8 L/min
SpO$_2$: 100%

- "This sounds like a pretty decent result. His AT is 14 and his peak VO$_2$ was around 20. In my eyes this means he is reasonably fit, and suitable for open AAA repair. Oh, and by the way, in my unit CPEX is also routine practice. However, I am aware that the ESVS does not recommend this routinely."

The case is discussed in the vascular MDT. This is the recommendation: "7.4 cm AAA technically suitable for both open and endovascular repair. Patient to be counselled." How would you counsel the patient?

- "I would explain that he has a large AAA and if we leave it alone it is potentially at a high risk of rupture, and this could be life-threatening. The options include an open AAA repair, or EVAR. EVAR is a minimally invasive option that could likely be done as a percutaneous "key hole" approach under local anaesthetic, and he would likely be able to go home day 1 post-op. However, even though in the short term this has its benefits, this is not a definitive repair, and he would require life-long surveillance. He is so at increased risk of needing future interventions. The anatomy of his AAA suggests EVAR is still possible, but the neck of the aneurysm is not ideal, and this could lead to future problems with leak around the stent needing further endovascular procedures. An open repair is a much bigger operation, and in the short term the risks are much bigger. In his case the risks would likely be around his heart and lungs (i.e. heart attack and chest infection/respiratory failure), including all the other surgical risks. However, if he were to get through this operation, he would likely be "sorted" in the long term, and it is arguably a much more durable operation. His fitness tests suggest he is suitable for the open repair, and NICE/ESVS guidelines would also support open AAA repair in this setting. My recommendation would be for open AAA repair."

You mention the NICE and ESVS guidelines on AAA. What evidence are you aware of that backs up your assertions that open AAA repair is better in this setting?

- "There are the long term results from the EVAR-1 trial. Also there is a meta-analysis of the EVAR 1, OVER, ACE and DREAM trials that came to the conclusion that EVAR is arguably better in the short term, but the initial short term benefit is lost after a couple of years mainly because of increased risk of complications and need for further interventions. In the long term, open AAA repair appears to be more durable, henceforth in younger fitter patients like this, open AAA repair should preferably be offered."

The patient wishes to go ahead with open AAA repair. You have just started your night shift and he is on the emergency theatre list. The patient is completely stable. Would you do his case tonight?

- "I would avoid doing an open AAA repair in the late hours and on the emergency list. As per the ESVS guidelines, the recommendation is to try and do these symptomatic cases in the daytime on the next available elective theatre list. Obviously, if his pain suddenly worsened and/he ruptured, I would do him in the middle of the night."

Why wait until daytime?

- "These cases can be very challenging. If something were to go wrong, I would want other senior vascular surgeons to be around to help me. I would also want a dedicated vascular anaesthetist. In the middle of the night this is unlikely to be the case."

If the patient ruptured in the middle of the night would you do an open AAA repair or an EVAR?

- "There is an argument to do an EVAR. I don't think the neck is ideal for this, but it could probably still be done. The recent NICE guidelines on AAA do say that EVAR provides more benefit than open AAA repair for most people with a ruptured AAA. However, the same guidelines say that open AAA repair is likely to provide a better balance of benefits and harms in men under 70. As such for this patient, if he ruptured I would still do an open AAA repair."

Would you do the case on your own?

- "Preferably I would have a second vascular surgery consultant to assist me. As a new vascular consultant I would ideally phone a friend and have them assist me."

Last question. If you did do an EVAR, what is the main complication you would be worried about?

- "Type 1A endoleak because of the diseased infra-renal neck."

Your FRCS Long Case Ends

CASE 10.2: Fit Gentleman with Infra-Renal AAA and Chronic Renal Failure

- A 69-year-old gentleman under surveillance on the National AAA surveillance programme.
- His last AAA surveillance ultrasound a few months previously revealed an AAA of 5.3 cm in diameter.
- Known to also have chronic kidney disease (eGFR now around 29 and slowly deteriorating).
- Patient has not been seen by nephrology team in 5 years.
- Had a recent CT of urinary tract as part of Yorkshire Kidney Screening Trial, which measured his AAA now as 5.7 cm.
- Apart from CKD, patient is generally fit and denied knowledge of any medical issues.

- Ex-smoker, now smoking e-cigarettes. Drinks a moderate amount of alcohol. He drives a car and lives with his wife.
- *Current medication:* Clopidogrel 75 mg, Atorvastatin 20 mg
- *On examination:* Abdomen was soft and non-tender with no palpable aneurysm due to him being slightly overweight. Full complement of normal lower limb pulses with no popliteal aneurysms palpable.

Your FRCS Long Case Begins

What is your impression of the size discrepancy between CT and ultrasound?

- "It is possible that his AAA has grown further over the past few months. However, there is a known discrepancy in measurements between these two imaging modalities, with CT tending to slightly over-call the diameter in comparison to ultrasound. Even if we were basing decisions purely on ultrasound, the patient would likely only be deferred intervention by a few months anyways. As such I would move things forward as if we were considering intervention at this stage."

So what would be your plan at this stage?

- "I would arrange for cardiopulmonary exercise testing, echocardiogram, urgent nephrology team review, anaesthetic review, re-check his bloods including lipid screen. I would aim to optimise his best medical therapy, which would probably include changing him to atorvastatin 80 mg OD. I would also get some dedicated aortic imaging. Usually I would get a CT angiogram, but in this case perhaps an MR angiogram is better given his poor renal function."

Can you please interpret his fitness tests?

- "The echo is reassuring. The patient has normal left ventricular size and an ejection fraction of 55–60%. The CPEX reveals an AT of 14.1 mls/kg/min and a peak VO$_2$ of 21.2 mls/kg/min. These figures suggest to me that this patient is fit for consideration of an open AAA repair."

Can you please review his MR aortogram?

- "There is what looks like a 6 cm infra-renal abdominal aortic aneurysm. There is a mildly conical and diseased infra-renal neck. Small kidneys bilaterally. There are probably two right renal arteries and a single left main renal artery. Reasonable iliacs bilaterally."

Are you happy with this MR angiogram report? Do you wish for any further imaging?

- "If I was contemplating an endovascular AAA repair then I would preferably get a formal CT angiogram. This would require pre-hydration to protect the kidneys. However, this patient sounds pretty fit. If we are considering an open AAA repair, it would likely not be necessary to do any further imaging."

So what would you do at this stage?

- "I would put the case back through the aortic MDT, and also speak to the patient as well. My question would be whether the patient and MDT supported an open AAA repair. If this was the case, I don't think a further CT angiogram would be required. By the sounds of it the infra-renal neck is not ideal, and perhaps therefore an endovascular approach is not in the patient's best interests. To treat this with an endovascular approach would likely require a fenestrated EVAR, which one can argue is not ideal either given his chronic renal failure."

The case is discussed in the aortic MDT again. This is the outcome: "Hostile neck which would be unsuitable for infra-renal EVAR due to thrombus and conical shape. Patient would be fit for open repair but there may be risk of dialysis due to CKD. There would also be an option to continue US surveillance with a higher threshold. To be seen in clinic for risk/benefit discussion for open repair." How would you counsel the patient?

- "Fundamentally, I would explain that his aortic anatomy is not amenable to a conventional endovascular aneurysm repair. Given his chronic kidney disease, a complex fenestrated stent is also likely not an appropriate option for him. He has done well with his fitness tests, and the vascular anaesthetist and MDT would support an open AAA repair. However, this is a big operation, and there are several complications possible. The most pertinent in this case is likely to be his impaired kidney function. There is a chance that the operation may result in him needing either temporary or permanent dialysis. There are also other risks, including: bleeding, infection, injury to other structures in the abdomen such as bowel or blood vessels, hernia, limb ischaemia, limb loss, heart attack, chest infection, DVT/PE, anaesthetic risks, and death. There is a risk of fatal complication overall in the region of 3–5%. I would quote him a 90–95% chance of getting through surgery and recovery thereafter without any serious problem. The average length of hospital stay is around one week, with a couple of nights on the intensive care unit. Most people get back to normal activities within a couple of months, but it can take up to six months to feel back to full strength."

The patient and his wife are very clear that they wish to proceed with open surgery. How would you plan to do this operation?

- "This would be a 2× consultant vascular surgeon operation on an elective list with a dedicated consultant vascular anaesthetist. I would aim to do a supra-umbilical horizontal incision, infra-renal clamp, and bifurcated graft down onto both common iliac arteries."

During the operation you encounter some bleeding from the top end anastomosis. How would you approach such a problem?

- "I would not panic. I would keep the anaesthetist fully informed. If this were serious bleeding I would re-clamp the infra-renal aorta. The possible options include: rescue stitches with pledgets, tightening the aortic anastomotic suture line, applying some haemostatic agents, or simply allowing the body's natural clotting mechanism some time to work by applying swabs around the anastomosis with some finger pressure. In a worse-case scenario I might have to completely take down the anastomosis and re-do it. There is of course always the option to call for further help from another consultant vascular surgeon."

Before the operation the patient had bilateral strong femoral pulses, popliteal pulses, and PT pulses. Upon release of the left iliac anastomosis there is a decent drop in blood pressure, and a good left

femoral pulse. Upon release of the right iliac anastomosis there is no femoral pulse and no significant drop in the patient's blood pressure. What would you do now?

- "I would feel for a pulse in the distal iliac artery beyond my anastomosis. If this were absent I would likely take the anastomosis down, and check there was decent backbleeding from the right iliac artery. I would pump the right femoral artery with my fist and make sure no thrombus came out. If there did not seem to be a load of thrombus occluding the right iliac system, I would copiously flush it with heparinised saline, and re-do the anastomosis."

OK. You do that. However, you find yourself in the same situation. What would you do now?

- "I would consider an upstream femoral embolectomy, and if this did not work, I would do a jump graft down to the right common femoral artery."

OK. You do a jump graft down to the common femoral artery and achieve a good pulse in the graft. However, after looking at the right foot, it looks ischaemic. The anaesthetist says she cannot feel a right posterior tibial pulse. You ask a fellow consultant vascular surgeon to come in and assess the right foot as you are still scrubbed in. She cannot feel a PT pulse, and the foot is cold and looks ischaemic. What would you do now?

- "I would do a diagnostic angiogram from the right groin, with a view to probably having to do a femoral embolectomy."

"OK. You do a diagnostic angiogram. Most of the SFA looks clean. However, there appears to be abrupt embolic occlusion of the TP trunk, and there is occlusion of the AT at its origin. The distal foot perfusion is very poor. What would you do now?"

- "There are 2 options here. One is to re-prep the right leg and do a formal popliteal embolectomy. The second option is to an over-the-wire embolectomy from the groin. I think I would try and the second option, not hesitating to call interventional radiology for help at any stage."

Why not just leave the situation as it is? Could you not just put the patient on intravenous heparin for 24 hours and monitor the right foot?

- "I don't think this is a good idea. I am in theatre now and have the opportunity to do something to improve the right foot perfusion. It already looks ischaemic, we know this is an acute embolic event, and the angiogram shows the perfusion to the foot is poor. No, I don't think conservative management is appropriate here. I think if I tried to manage this conservatively, I would just end up having to take the patient back to theatre in a couple of hours' time anyways."

Your FRCS Long Case Ends

CASE 10.3: Standard Percutaneous EVAR

- 85-year-old reasonably fit gentleman.
- He has been on aneurysm ultrasound surveillance and has hit 5.5 cm threshold.
- Is asymptomatic with non-tender AAA

- *Past medical:* Giant cell arteritis, previous pulmonary embolism, hypertension, and discoid eczema
- *Medications:* Warfarin, prednisolone, methotrexate, atorvastatin, ramipril, amlodipine, and folic acid
- *Social history:* He lives at home with his wife, has good exercise tolerance, walks every morning, does not need a stick, and is independent of activities of daily living.

Your FRCS Long Case Begins

What investigations would you request for this patient if you first saw him in clinic?

- "I would request bloods (FBC, U&Es, LFTs, lipid screen, HBA1c, clotting), ECG, a formal CT angiogram to visualise the aorta from the arch down to both femoral bifurcations, echocardiogram, CPEX. When these results were back I would ask for a formal vascular anaesthetic review, then discuss everything in the aortic MDT."

Can you please interpret this CT angiogram?

- "This looks like a 6 cm infra-renal AAA. The right distal CIA has an aneurysm prior to the iliac bifurcation that measures around 2 cm. Patent IIAs bilaterally. Ectatic CFAs bilaterally. This looks suitable for a standard EVAR with or without CIA aneurysm treatment included. Alternatively one might consider an iliac branched device on the right. In either case I think this could be done under local anaesthetic with a percuteanous approach. The AAA also looks suitable for an open repair, which would either be an infra-renal tube graft and tube repair (with plan to continue to survey CIA aneurysm), or a bifurcated graft to treat this CIA aneurysm all in one sitting."

What is your threshold for treating iliac aneurysms?

- "According to the ESVS guidelines, the threshold is 3.5 cm."

Can you please interpret these fitness tests?

- "His echocardiogram is reassuring with a good left ventricular systolic function (ejection fraction 55-60%) and good right ventricular function. His CPEX is also reassuring. His AT is 16.8 mls/kg/min, and his peak VO_2 is 19.5 mls/kg/min. This means I would consider this patient for open surgery. I consider an AT of less than 11 to be high risk for open AAA repair. His pulmonary function tests are also reassuring with an FEV1 of 2.67 L (115% predicted), an FVC of 3.65 L (115% predicted) with a FEV1: FVC ratio of 73%. As such, given these fitness tests, I conclude he is fit enough to consider an open AAA repair."

The patient is seen by a consultant vascular anaesthetist. The anaesthetist uses the Carlisle Risk Calculator and deems that the patient's risks are as follows:

- 30-Day mortality open repair = 6%
- 30-Day mortality endovascular repair = 2.4%
- Mean Life Expectancy no repair 3.2 years
- Mean Life Expectancy open repair 6.6 years
- Mean Life Expectancy endovascular 6.4 years

What do you make of this?

- "Interesting figures, and these results probably would make one inclined to go for an endovascular repair. However, the 2020 NICE guidelines on AAA state that one should not use the following risk assessment tools to determine whether or not repair is suitable for a person with an asymptomatic unruptured AAA: British Aneurysm Repair score, Carlisle Calculator, Comorbidity Severity Score, Glasgow Aneurysm Scale, Medicare risk prediction tool, Modified Leiden score, Physiological and Operative Severity Score for enumeration of Mortality (POSSUM), Vascular-POSSUM, Vascular Biochemical and Haematological Outcome Model (VBHOM) and Vascular Governance North West (VGNW) risk mode."

OK. So how would you counsel the patient on the risks then?

- "I would have an honest and pragmatic conversation with the patient. I would explain that he has an aneurysm whose natural history is to enlarge and rupture. If rupture were to occur, there is high likelihood this could be a terminal event. However, I would not scare the patient into thinking he has a *ticking time bomb* in his abdomen. I would explain that I have seen a few patients who have never had their aneurysms treated because they were too high risk, and yet they have continued on for over 10 years and remained asymptomatic. Therefore he does not need to feel pressured into making an urgent decision now, and he has time to think. However, he does appear to be a fit candidate, there are definitely viable options to fix this aneurysm, and the evidence and guidelines would support intervention in this case. The two options are either a minimally invasive "keyhole" approach which can probably be done with him awake. If he went for this approach he would likely be in and out of hospital very quickly which is great. However, this type of aneurysm repair requires lifelong surveillance, and there is an increased risk of needing further interventions in the future as it is not as durable beyond a few years. The open repair on the other hand is a much bigger, riskier operation. The risks of death are higher, and in the short term he may struggle. However, if he could get through it, in the long term this is more of a durable option, and he wouldn't need lifelong surveillance. His fitness tests suggest that he is fit for the major operation, therefore this is still on the cards. I would conclude by saying that when it comes to the crunch it is his decision, and it is ultimately about what he thinks is right for him. There is still an option not to have any intervention, although this would not be my advice."

The patient asks what your recommendation is.

- "Given his age, comorbidities requiring immunosuppression, and previous pulmonary embolism, I would be more inclined to pursue an endovascular approach. If the patient wanted an open AAA repair, I would support this also, but I suspect this might be a big hit that he could very well struggle to handle."

The patient and his wife have a talk, and they both say in an ideal world the open repair would be better. However, they acknowledge that he is 85, and although he sounds fit on paper and he feels fit, they are worried the open operation might be too much for him. They would rather pursue the minimally invasive strategy and accept the need for lifelong surveillance. What would you do now?

- "I would confirm the plan in the aortic MDT. I would confirm that endovascular repair is suitable, and if the plan would be for an EVAR with embolization of the right internal iliac and landing the right limb in the external iliac, or for an iliac branch device, or just a standard EVAR."

The aortic MDT acknowledge he was fit for an open AAA repair, but supported the plan for EVAR given his age, prior VTE, rheumatological disease, and use of methotrexate/steroids. The MDT felt that an endovascular approach was in his best interests. The MDT also supported a standard EVAR. Do you agree with this plan?

- "This seems sensible. This is not a massive right common iliac aneurysm, and although it would need to be measured and planned properly, I suspect one could use a flared right iliac limb to achieve a decent seal zone here."

How would you plan this case?

- "I would use EVAR planning software. I also have dedicated EVAR planning sheets which allow me to include all the important elements in EVAR planning that are easy to forget if you don't have a pre-designed structure for planning. These sheets include: patient details, confirm the mesenteric vessels are patent, that the renals are patent, which is the lowest renal artery, what is the length and diameter of the aortic neck, what is the neck actually like (i.e. long/short/straight/conical/calcified/ diseased/heavily angulated ...), length and size measurements of the iliac arteries, are there any access site concerns (iliac stenosis, tortuosity, heavy calcification, very small ....), angles that I would use to best visualise the aortic neck and iliac bifurcations, the main deployment side, the right limb and left limb I have chosen etc. When using the EVAR planning software I make sure I have achieved proper centrelines so that my length measurements are correct. Finally I always draw out the aneurysm and a general description of the salient points relevant to the case so I can see it on the day of the procedure."

You see the patient in clinic to confirm the final plan. The patient and his family are happy to proceed. You notice that the patient's LDL cholesterol level is 2.9 despite being on simvastatin 20 mg daily. What would you do about this?

- "I would commence the patient on atorvastatin 80 mg daily, and ask the GP to re-check the LDL in 3 months. I would ask the GP to add ezetimibe 10 mg daily if the LDL was still not <1.4."

The patient is also on warfarin. What are you going to do about that?

- "The patient would need to stop his warfarin 5 days before the procedure. However, I would discuss the details of this with the haematology team, and confirm what the local guidelines said. I would also want to confirm the post-operative anticoagulation plan i.e. would the haematologists want the patient bridging post-operatively etc."

The patient has a successful percutaneous standard infra-renal EVAR. He is planned to go home the following day. What would your discharge plan be?

- "Resume his warfarin +/− bridging therapy with low molecular weight heparin. I would check his post-EVAR blood tests were OK, mainly being interested in the renal function. He would also require an initial 1 month surveillance CT scan and abdominal X-ray, and then follow the normal post-EVAR follow-up protocol."

Your FRCS Long Case Ends

CASE 10.4: Complex Juxtarenal AAA

- A 69-year-old gentleman with an asymptomatic juxtarenal abdominal aortic aneurysm
- He has been on AAA ultrasound surveillance and reached threshold over 1 year previously.
- Previously offered intervention when AAA size 6 cm, but this was delayed for multiple issues (obesity/family care issues/COVID-19 pandemic patient did not want intervention and requested repeat CT at a later date to monitor aneurysm).
- Most recent CT scan reveals AAA size is 7.3 cm.
- Patient is now willing to proceed with intervention.
- Patient has type 2 diabetes, hypertension, and mild obstructive sleep apnoea.
- *Medications:* Atorvastatin, amlodipine, metformin, losartan, and atenolol
- *Social history:* Lives at home with his wife who he is main carer for. Ex-smoker. Minimal alcohol. Pretty good exercise tolerance according to the patient, thinks he can walk at least a mile on a good day. Independent of activities of daily living.
- *On examination:* Patient still has a fairly raised BMI, but says he has lost a few stone (21 stone down to 17 stone). Abdomen soft and non-tender. No scar from previous abdominal/groin surgery. AAA not tender. Full complement of lower limb pulses, no obvious popliteal aneurysms.

Your FRCS Short Case Begins

Can you please interpret this patient's original CT angiogram.

- "This shows a reasonably large juxtarenal aortic aneurysm. There is a single right renal artery and two left renal arteries. There does not appear to be a genuine infra-renal neck below the inferior accessory left renal artery. The aorta beneath this is atherosclerotic and conical. There are very short common iliac arteries bilaterally, with disease free internal and external iliac arteries bilaterally. However, both iliac systems look quite tortuous. The common femoral arteries look disease free. However, the patient clearly has a very raised BMI. The distance from the groin skin to the femoral arteries is on average 6.5 cm, which is not ideal for a percutaneous approach (my cut-off for percutaneous approach is <5 cm). The distance from the supra-renal aorta to the abdominal skin is around 17 cm. This would make me concerned about the viability of an open AAA repair (pragmatically if this distance was >20 cm I would be very reluctant to proceed with open aortic surgery). Based upon this CT scan, my thoughts would be that the theoretical options would be (1) open AAA repair, supra-renal clamp, and bifurcated graft onto both common iliacs or (2) 4-vessel fenestrated EVAR with bilateral iliac branched devices."

OK. If you were considering bilateral iliac branched devices, what access approach would you use?

- "Given the tortuosity of the iliacs, a brachial approach would probably be required."

What do you think about using endoanchors?

- "Endoanchors are worth considering. However, you need some form of an infra-renal neck, which I do not think this patient has. Also, according to the ESVS guidelines on abdominoiliac aneurysms, recommendation 96 states this: *In complex endovascular repair of juxtarenal abdominal aortic aneurysm, endovascular repair with fenestrated stent grafts should be considered the preferred treatment option when feasible. Recommendation 98 states this: In patients with juxtarenal abdominal aortic aneurysm, new techniques/ concepts, including endovascular aneurysm seal, endostaples, and in situ laser fenestration, are not recommended as first-line treatment, but should be limited to studies approved by research ethics committees, until adequately evaluated.* As such my position would be to avoid endoanchors in this setting, and if endovascular treatment was being considered, it should be for a fenestrated approach."

The patient has had his CPEX and echocardiogram. His AT was 18, his peak VO$_2$ was 21, and his spirometry showed a mild obstructive pattern. His echo reports states he has mild left ventricular systolic dysfunction with an estimated ejection fraction of 50%. What would be your thoughts her?

- "In this instance I think I would be inclined to do an open AAA repair."

Imagine this is a different patient. The AT was 10.2, peak VO$_2$ was 14.1, and spirometry showed a moderate obstructive pattern. Echocardiogram revealed a dilated left ventricular with significantly impaired LV systolic function. There are areas of regional impairment and scarring noted. The left ventricular ejection fraction is at lower end of 35–40%. What would be your thoughts in this context?

- "In this instance I would be inclined to proceed with a complex endovascular repair. In any case, I would not make these decisions in isolation. Interpretation of cardiopulmonary exercise test results is complex and a specialist area. I would value the expert input and opinions of my vascular anaesthetic consultant colleagues. I would also be discussing these cases in the aortic MDT."

Imagine this patient's echocardiogram and CPEX results were "borderline," such that you could make a clear case for either open AAA repair or complex endovascular repair. What would your position be?

- "It is difficult to give an authoritative and confident answer, because I don't think anyone really knows the answers here. The ESVS guidelines on abdominoiliac aneurysms states this in recommendation 95: *In patients with juxtarenal abdominal aortic aneurysm, open repair or complex endovascular repair should be considered based on patient status, anatomy, local routines, team experience, and patient preference.* Henceforth, in light of the ESVS guidelines, one can argue that the final decision is based upon a lot of case-specific variables. On the other hand, recent NICE guidelines on AAA states that: *If both open and complex endovascular repair are suitable, only consider complex EVAR if the risks seem to outweigh the risks of open AAA repair, and that the patient understands there are uncertainties around whether complex EVAR improves peri-operative or long term outcomes when compared to open AAA repair.* A recent meta-analysis by Jones et al (2019) concluded that between open repair and FEVAR for juxtarenal AAA there is no significant difference in 30-day mortality; however, FEVAR was associated with significantly lower morbidity than open surgical repair. On the contrary, long term durability is a concern, with far higher re-intervention rates after FEVAR. As for me personally, I do not like to sit on the fence. If I had a patient in front of me who I thought was arguably "fit for open", and there was a choice between open repair and complex endovascular repair, I would go for open repair. But hey, I am a surgeon, I like operating, so no surprises here."

Your FRCS Short Case Ends

CASE 10.5: EVAR Complications

- A 71-year-old gentleman is in the middle of a percutaneous EVAR.
- It is a local anaesthetic case.
- This is a standard infra-renal aneurysm with a long straight neck.
- The patient was deemed fit for open AAA repair, but the patient chose EVAR.

Your FRCS Short Case Begins

The main body has just been deployed. Can you interpret these images please?

- "I cannot see the renal arteries. As such I suspect the main body has been deployed too high."

How might you manage this?

- "First of all this is a complication that is best prevented as opposed to cured. In any case, I know a few bailout strategies. It might be possible to pull the whole main body down by pulling on a wire that has been placed over the flow-divider, snared, and brought out via the contralateral femoral sheath. Another option is to inflate a large compliant balloon just above the flow divider and apply downwards pressure to try and pull the stent caudally. Depending upon how much of the renal arteries have been covered, it is also possible to come via a brachial approach and place a balloon expandable stent in the renal arteries to restore flow."

What if none of these strategies worked?

- "In terms of open surgery, these are the potential options. One is to do an extra-anatomic bypass via an ileorenal or hepatorenal approach. If this is not possible, one would likely need to explant the main body and do an open AAA repair."

OK. Let's say that you did not cover both renal arteries when deploying the main body. What do you make of this angiographic image?

- "This looks like completion angiogram after the whole EVAR has been completed. At the top end there appears to be a type 1A endoleak."

How do you know it is not a type 2 endoleak?

- "Strictly speaking, I don't know with 100% confidence. However, there is contrast visible outside the EVAR in close vicinity to the proximal seal zone. I would want to know if this endoleak was seen early after contrast injection, as this would then reinforce my impression that this was a type 1A endoleak."

What would you do about this suspected type 1A endoleak then?

- "I would aggressively interrogate it first of all. I would ask for additional magnified views and use different angles if required. However, in general I would treat this. If the distance from the lowest renal artery was less than 3 mm, I would angioplasty the proximal seal zone with a compliant moulding balloon. If the distance was over 5 mm I consider placement of a proximal aortic cuff followed by further compliant balloon angioplasty."

What would you do if the type 1A endoleak persisted even after all of the above?

- "Placement of a giant Palmaz stent should be considered."

Are there any other options?

- "One could consider endoanchors."

Not specifically for this acute case, but in general, are you aware of any other options for managing persistent type 1A endoleaks?

- "There are open surgical options. You can explant the entire EVAR and do an open repair. You can do aortic neck banding. I guess you could also do fenestrated or parallel graft repair."

Can you describe what you see in this angiogram?

- "There is contrast seen outside the proximal left iliac limb within the aneurysm sac. I suspect this is therefore a type 3 endoleak."

What would your management be?

- "I suspect this leak is occurring at the junction of the main body and the left iliac limb. I would consider balloon angioplasty of this area and then repeating the angiogram. However, definitively, this would require endovascular re-lining."

Would you not consider conservative management and observation?

- "No. Type 3 endoleaks expose the aneurysm to direct aortic pressure with subsequent risk of rupture. Therefore, prompt intervention is warranted, primarily by partial or total endovascular relining."

What do you make of this 1-month post-EVAR surveillance CT angiogram?

- "Within the aneurysm sac there is contrast pooling. This is on the left hand side towards the mid/lower segment of the AAA sac. I suspect therefore that this is a type 2 endoleak."

How would you manage this?

- "The long term follow-up of the EVAR trials highlighted that a type II endoleak alone is relatively benign, although type 2 endoleak with sac expansion is concerning given its association with secondary AAA rupture. At this stage, therefore, I would be inclined to sit tight and observe it. If on further surveillance scans the AAA was getting bigger and the type 2 endoleak persisted, I would consider intervention."

What intervention would you consider for a type 2 endoleak?

- "In this case probably transarterial coil embolization of the IMA."

How would you do this?

- "Well, I would not be doing it, the interventional radiologist would. However, one would need to access the middle colic artery via the SMA, which provides retrograde access to the IMA via the arc of Riolan."

What other options are there for treating type 2 endoleaks?

- "Other options for treatment of type 2 endoleaks include coil or glue embolization which can via a transarterial approach, translumbar or transcaval. One can also consider laparoscopic IMA clipping, open surgical ligation of lumbar arteries and IMA ligation, or a complete open surgical conversion with explantation of the EVAR and formal open AAA repair."

Your FRCS Short Case Ends

Relevant ESVS Guideline Recommendations

- In patients with type I endoleak after endovascular abdominal aortic aneurysm repair, re-intervention to achieve a seal, primarily by endovascular means, is recommended.
- Expansion of sac diameter by 1 cm detected during follow up after endovascular abdominal aortic aneurysm repair using the same imaging modality and measurement method may be considered a reasonable threshold for significant growth.
- Re-intervention for type II endoleak after endovascular abdominal aortic aneurysm repair should be considered in the presence of significant aneurysm growth, primarily by endovascular means.
- In patients with type III endoleak after endovascular abdominal aortic aneurysm repair, re-intervention is recommended, primarily by endovascular means.
- Significant aneurysm sac growth after endovascular abdominal aortic aneurysm repair, without visible endoleak on standard imaging, should be considered for further diagnostic evaluation with alternative imaging modalities to exclude the presence of an unidentified endoleak and should be considered for treatment.
- Early (within 30 days) post-operative follow-up after endovascular aortic repair including imaging of the stent graft to assess presence of endoleak, component overlap, and sealing zone length is recommended.

CHAPTER 11

Thoracoabdominal Aortic Aneurysm

I consider this section to be mainly "academic." What I mean by this is that these are complex cases that I do not think a day one vascular consultant would be routinely handling with any degree of confidence or experience. As such, we will discuss the salient points but I am not going to drag you through any case scenarios. Personally, I don't think these cases would commonly show up in the FRCS Part B examination. It may well show up in your Part A examination, however; so it is good to have some working knowledge.

Background

- Use Crawford classification (*see Figure 11.1*).
- A type 1 starts at the level of the left subclavian artery, involves the visceral arteries and ends at the renal arteries.
- A type 2 starts at the same level as a type 1, but involves the entire descending and abdominal aorta. In many patients, especially those suffering from connective tissue diseases and post-dissection aneurysms, the iliac arteries are aneurysmal as well.
- A type 3 starts more distal than type 2 aneurysms, usually at the level of T6, and extends distally as in a type 2.
- A type 4 starts at the level of the diaphragm and involves the entire abdominal aorta, with or without extension to the iliac arteries.
- A type 5 starts below the sixth intercostal space and tapers just above the renal arteries.
- Type 4s can theoretically be treated with just a laparotomy, but all of the rest would require a thoracoabdominal incision and decompression of the left chest for open surgical repair.
- All are associated with potential end organ complications such as paraplegia, renal failure, and visceral ischaemia.
- Open or endovascular repair should be considered for patients at low to moderate surgical risk, with an atherosclerotic or degenerative thoracoabdominal aortic aneurysm of 60 mm or larger diameter, rapid aneurysm enlargement (>10 mm/year), or aneurysm-related symptoms.

Basic Management Principles

- Best medical therapy.
- Smoking cessation (if relevant).
- Consider screening for connective tissue disorders.
- Preoperative cardiac, pulmonary, and renal function should be assessed to estimate surgical risks and initiate therapy to improve the preoperative status.
- These patients requiring extensive preoperative risk assessment and counselling.
- The benefits of intervention should outweigh both the risks of rupture and the risks of intervention.
- It doesn't take a rocket scientist to realise these are complex high-risk cases, and should therefore be managed in a specialist centre if intervention is being considered.

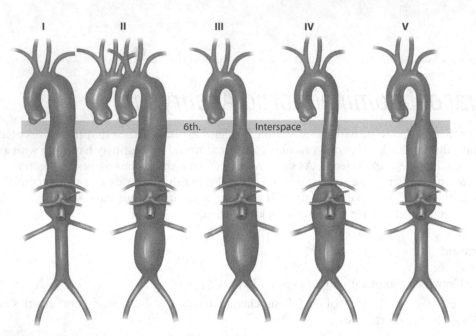

Figure 11.1   Crawford classification of thoracoabdominal aortic aneurysms.

Open Surgical Repair

- Extracorporeal circulation should be considered (including left heart bypass by means of a left atriofemoral bypass circuit or femoral veno-arterial bypass).
- During thoracoabdominal aortic aneurysm repair, the coeliac artery and the superior mesenteric artery should be perfused with blood and both renal arteries should be perfused with either cold crystalloid or blood to reduce end-organ ischaemia.
- One should consider strategies to limit neurological complications including distal aortic perfusion, intercostal artery reimplantation, CSF drainage, spinal cord cooling, and assessment of spinal cord function peri-operatively.

Endovascular Repair

- With the "hybrid approach," visceral perfusion is safeguarded by means of an open surgical extra-anatomic bypass, followed by endovascular exclusion of the entire aneurysm. This approach has the advantage of limiting exposure to a laparotomy while avoiding a thoracotomy, although, this remains a considerable undertaking in unfit patients.
- The second technique is a total endovascular repair using specifically constructed branched modular aortic grafts. Preservation of visceral flow is achieved by means of either fenestrations or branches or a combination of both on the component deployed in the region of the visceral arteries.

Relevant ESVS Guideline Recommendations

- Open or endovascular repair should be considered for patients at low-to-moderate surgical risk, with an atherosclerotic or degenerative thoraco abdominal aortic aneurysm of 60 mm or larger diameter, rapid aneurysm enlargement (>10 mm/year), or aneurysm-related symptoms.

- In patients planned for open or endovascular thoracoabdominal aortic aneurysm repair, preoperative cardiac, pulmonary, and renal function should be assessed to estimate surgical risks and initiate therapy to improve the preoperative status.

- In open type 2, 2, and 3 thoracoabdominal aortic aneurysm surgery, extracorporeal techniques allowing distal aortic and organ perfusion should be considered to reduce ischaemic complications, especially in extensive aneurysms requiring prolonged cross clamping time.

- In patients with extensive thoracoabdominal aortic aneurysm (type 2, 3, 3) undergoing open repair, cerebrospinal fluid drainage should be considered as a measure to decrease the risk of neurological deficit.

- An integrated approach with optimisation of mean and distal aortic arterial pressure, moderate hypothermia, neuromonitoring, and reimplantation of intercostal arteries should be considered to protect the spinal cord during thoracoabdominal aortic aneurysm surgery.

- Centralisation of open repair of thoracoabdominal aortic aneurysm in dedicated high volume centres may be considered.

JMF Reflections

These cases are not straightforward by any means. This is super-specialist vascular surgery. For most day one vascular surgery consultants (or in the FRCS setting), I expect your knowledge and skill level in this area to be mainly academic. You should have an understanding of the Crawford classification, the indications for treatment, the broad options for management, and know when and who to refer to (or just plainly knowing to ask for help). I think you should also have a firm grasp on the realities of intervention, and in particular the risks: Cardiac, pulmonary, renal, end-organ malperfusion, etc. Finally, I would also recommend praying to God that one of these does not come in as a rupture when you are on-call.

CHAPTER 12

Popliteal Aneurysm

This is an absolute FRCS VASC classic. I literally had 4× stations that covered popliteal aneurysm. Make sure you know this like the back of your hand!

History

- Patient has noticed an expansile pulsatile mass in the back of his knee.
- Swelling of leg and/or DVT (due to compression of popliteal vein).
- Cold/painful foot due to embolic occlusion of crural vessel/s.
- Discolouration of toes ("blue toes") due to microembolic phenomena.
- New short distance claudication (secondary to thrombosed popliteal aneurysm).
- Acutely ischaemic foot due to embolic trashing of crural vessels and/or thrombosed popliteal aneurysm (i.e. pain, coldness, reduced sensation, reduced power).
- May present with critically ischaemic foot (rest pain, night pain, sleeping with leg hanging out of bed, short distance claudication, or tissue loss).
- Is patient known to have a popliteal aneurysm?
- Is patient known to have aneurysms elsewhere (e.g. AAA, thoracic aneurysms)?
- Is there a family history of aneurysms?
- *Rapid assessment of cardiovascular risks factors:* "Do you smoke? Do you have raised cholesterol? Do you have high blood pressure? Are you a diabetic?"
- *Rapid assessment of comorbidities:* "Previous heart attack or angina? Chronic lung disease? Chronic kidney disease? Any other major medical comorbidities?"
- *Medications:* Regular medications? Is the patient on best medical therapy?
- *Social history:* How fit/active are you? Who do you live with? Are you independent? What is the patient's job? Do they spend a lot of time with knees bent e.g. gardener? Does the patient mobilise in a wheelchair i.e. legs are always at 90 degrees?

Examination

- End of the bed test.
- Always examine the abdomen in this setting to feel specifically for a AAA.
- Full assessment of lower limb pulses (also look out for CFA and contralateral popliteal aneurysm).
- What does the foot look like? Any signs of embolic events? Chronic or critical ischaemia? Any tissue loss? Any signs of acute ischaemia (not in FRCS exam of course).
- Confirm handheld Doppler waveforms and confirm ABPI.

Investigations (Non-Acute)

- FBC, U&Es, LFTs, HBA1, lipid screen, coagulation
- Lower limb arterial duplex +/− CTA

DOI: 10.1201/b22951-12

Investigations (Acute)

- FBC, U&Es, LFTs, HBA1, lipid screen, coagulation, group & save
- CTA aorta & lower limbs

Management (Non-Acute)

- Popliteal aneurysm > 2.0 cm = consider intervention.
- Popliteal aneurysm with significant thrombus load = consider intervention.
- Popliteal aneurysm with evidence of emboli to crural vessels = consider intervention.
- *Options are:* Conservative management with best medical therapy +/− surveillance, endovascular covered stent, medial approach with exclusion of popliteal aneurysm and bypass, or posterior approach and interposition grafting.
- Patient fitness and anatomical features will influence management approach.

Popliteal Aneurysm Stenting?

- *This question did come up in my FRCS VASC examination, and I was asked about various technical details, so I will include the answers here to the sort of questions I was asked by the two examiners who sat in front of me ....*
  1. Anatomical considerations → Normal proximal and distal landing zones of at least 2 cm in length.
  2. Lack of extensive vessel tortuosity.
  3. Aneurysm should not be extremely large (this makes a stent-graft more prone to kinking and displacement).
  4. Ideally should avoid patients who frequently flex their knees to more than 90 degrees as this increases risk of stent deformation and thrombosis e.g. gardeners, carpenter, people in wheelchairs etc.
- Can be performed either via a percutaneous puncture or a small cut down to expose either the CFA or SFA.
- Covered stent to be used, which is often oversized to about 10–15% more than the internal diameter of the popliteal vessel above and below the aneurysm.
- Probably will be using a 7-French sheath which can be done percutaneously.
- If using larger sheath (i.e. 9–12 French) direct vessel exposure is desirable.
- Make sure patient has been pre-treated with clopidogrel.
- Do a diagnostic angiogram and visualise the run-off vessels.
- Give intravenous heparin.
- Cross the popliteal aneurysm carefully using a 0.035 or 0.018 guidewire.
- If you require more than one stent graft, a maximum of 1 mm size differential between grafts is suggested, and there should be a minimum of 2–3 cm overlap between the stent grafts.
- Try to avoid landing the distal end of the stent graft at the bend of the popliteal artery which is usually a few centimetres above the actual knee joint ....
- Therefore you should make sure you do an angiogram from a lateral position with the knee bent.
- Each stent graft should be moulded with a balloon about the size of the graft, and only inflate the balloon inside the stents.

- Once the procedure is complete you should again do a completion angiogram (including an angiogram with the knee bent).
- If your stent stops at the bend of the popliteal artery, just extend it further down.

Management (Acute)

- If popliteal aneurysm is occluded and there is a patent distal outflow vessel the management is above-knee to below-knee bypass using vein (medial approach with ligation of aneurysm).
- If there is no outflow identified and the limb is not immediately threatened, intra-arterial thrombolysis can be considered to try and restore the crural outflow. Following this the popliteal aneurysm could be treated by either a covered stent or a bypass. *Cases are individualised of course and there is no "correct" answer.*
- If there is no outflow vessel identified and the limb is immediately threatened (i.e. severe sensorimotor compromise), there is no time for thrombolysis. Surgery should be performed immediately. In this setting one would likely be performing a below-knee popliteal artery exposure, thromboembolectomy of the distal popliteal and crural vessels, and this would be followed by ligation of the popliteal aneurysm and bypass (*this is all via a medial approach*). One can also consider direct intra-arterial/on-table thrombolysis of the crural vessels if they are difficult to clear with embolectomy alone.
- One should be strongly considering a fasciotomy in cases of advanced ischaemia.
- If the limb is non-salvageable the options are either major amputation or palliation.
- If the limb is viable and the symptoms are mild (i.e. claudication) there is an argument to manage things conservatively e.g. regular exercise, best medical therapy.

CHAPTER 13

Descending Thoracic Aortic Aneurysm

These cases seem a bit more reasonable for a day one consultant vascular surgeon to handle. I consider these to be "fair game" in both the FRCS examination, and also in your real world practice. As such we will use three examples in the typical FRCS short/long case style to illustrate the salient points. We will also cover the relevant ESVS guideline recommendations.

CASE 13.1: Frail Elderly Gentleman with Incidental Finding of Asymptomatic 9-cm Descending Thoracic Aortic Aneurysm

- This is an 89-year-old gentleman who went for a CT thorax because of issues with shortness of breath, swallowing problems, and weight loss.
- The CT scan has not shown any malignancy but there is a large descending thoracic aortic aneurysm that is causing a 50% compression of the left bronchus.
- *Comorbidities:* Chronic obstructive pulmonary disease, previous myocardial infarction, and chronic kidney disease (eGFR 48).
- *Social history:* Lives alone, but gets a lot of support from his three children. The children do the shopping and cleaning. The patient has a carer come once a day to help with cooking.

Your FRCS Short Case Begins

What would be your immediate management plan?

- "First of all I would counsel the patient. I would explain the diagnosis with the aid of a diagram. I would explain that he has a large aneurysm in his chest that has likely been there a while. However, given its size, there is a high risk for rupture which in his case would likely be a terminal event. I would discuss the potential management options: conservative management, open repair, or endovascular repair with a stent."

The patient is not keen on open repair. He is worried about the risk of rupture, however, and wishes to consider endovascular intervention. How would you approach this?

- "I would start with the basics. First of all I am interested in access. I would confirm if the patient had femoral pulses and upper limb pulses. I would send off blood tests: FBC, U&Es, clotting and group and save. I would request a formal CT angiogram aorta. The scan would ideally go from groins all the way up to the arch of the aorta, carotid vessels, and intra-cranial circulation."

The patient has a CT angiogram. Can you please interpret the scan?

- "This confirms a large 9.5 cm descending thoracic aortic aneurysm. It begins around 3 cm beyond the left subclavian artery. It ends around 1 cm above the diaphragm. The thoracic aorta just beyond the left subclavian artery is about 31 mm in diameter. It looks like this aneurysm is suitable for a thoracic aortic stent. I do not think the patient will require a left carotid-subclavian bypass, nor do I think the coeliac axis will need to be covered."

DOI: 10.1201/b22951-13

If the aneurysm finished less than 15 mm from the coeliac axis, would your plan change?

- "In this case the thoracic aortic stent may need to cover the coeliac artery in order to achieve a satisfactory distal sealing zone."

In what situations would you avoid covering the coeliac artery?

- "Contraindications to CA coverage include the presence of a common coeliaco-mesenteric trunk, the absence of adequate angiographic evidence of collateral circulation, poor portal vein perfusion, and any previous conventional or endovascular procedure that may have compromised the collateral circulation."

If any of the above existed, what would you do to maintain coeliac artery perfusion?

- "One might consider a scallop-designed endograft or the use of a snorkel or chimney technique. Another option is a hybrid type repair with an extra-anatomical bypass onto the coeliac axis prior to thoracic aortic stent insertion. However, in this type of frail comorbid patient, I would generally try to avoid doing a laparotomy."

Would you be worried about spinal cord ischaemia in this case?

- "Yes and I would counsel the patient on the risks of spinal cord ischaemia and paraplegia. However, we are not covering his left subclavian artery. His CT angiogram also shows he has patent lumbar arteries in the infra-renal aorta, his internal iliac arteries are patent, and both his profunda arteries are patent. As such I think the collateral supply to his spinal cord should on the whole be ok."

Would you consider a spinal drain in this case?

- "No. My main focus would be on maintaining a good blood pressure and keeping his haemoglobin > 100. If there were neurological concerns post-TEVAR I would arrange for a spinal drain to be inserted."

In what situations would you consider a spinal drain?

- "Previous abdominal aorta aneurysm (AAA) repair, prolonged hypotension, severe atherosclerosis of the thoracic aorta, occlusion of the left subclavian artery and/or internal iliac arteries, and extensive coverage of the thoracic aorta by the endograft are all associated with an increased risk of spinal cord ischaemia. In these situations I would consider spinal cord protection (including CSF drainage)."

Your FRCS Short Case Ends

Relevant ESVS Guideline Recommendations

- All patients with clinical suspicion of thoracic aortic disease and abnormal chest radiograph should undergo computed tomographic angiography for diagnosis confirmation.
- Multi-detector computed tomographic angiography from thoracic inlet to common femoral arteries should be considered as the first-line diagnostic modality for descending thoracic aortic pathology.

- In fit and unfit patients with favourable anatomy, endovascular repair may be considered for descending thoracic aorta aneurysms between 56 and 59 mm diameter.
- In fit and unfit patients with favourable anatomy, endovascular repair should be considered for descending thoracic aorta aneurysms >60 mm diameter.

CASE 13.2: Ruptured Descending Thoracic Aortic Aneurysm

- A 74-year-old patient presents with sudden onset chest/upper back pain, shortness of breath and collapse.
- He has a background of hypertension, chronic obstructive pulmonary disease, and gout.
- He is a heavy smoker and lives at home with his wife.
- He is otherwise independent and can walk about half a mile usually.
- In A&E resus the patient is awake with a GCS of 15/15.
- His blood pressure is 100/70 mmHg.
- His heart rate is 100.
- The oxygen saturation is 90% on room air and respiratory rate is 22.
- A CT angiogram has been performed which is reported as showing a ruptured 8 cm descending thoracic aortic aneurysm. There is a moderately sized left sided haemothorax.

Your FRCS Short Case Begins

What is your immediate management plan?

- "Large-bore intravenous access. Send off urgent bloods for: FBC, U&Es, coagulation, and institute the major transfusion protocol. I would aim for a permissive hypotension approach currently, avoiding intravenous fluid or blood products so long as the patient was conscious with a systolic blood pressure above 80 mmHg. I would contact the vascular interventional radiologist on-call about an emergency TEVAR."

The A&E consultant advises one of her juniors to insert a left sided chest drain. Would you advise this?

- "No. At the moment the patient is relatively haemodynamically stable with a maintained conscious level. Sticking a chest drain in the left chest may release whatever current tamponade there is, and this may make the patient bleed more and decompensate. I would avoid a chest drain at this stage."

The vascular interventional radiologist comes in and you review the CT angiogram together. Can you please interpret these images for me?

- "There is a large descending thoracic aortic aneurysm that has ruptured. The aneurysm is well below the left subclavian artery, and extends down to around 4cm above the level of the diaphragm. The images also show that there is significant occlusive disease of the common femoral arteries bilaterally. The subclavian arteries however appear patent and disease free."

What would you do now?

- "I would consider a TEVAR via the right axillosubclavian artery."

Would you do this percutaneous or open approach?

- "In this case I would do an open infra-clavicular exposure of the right axillary artery. This would allow safer access for the thoracic stent."

Why not do a supra-clavicular subclavian artery exposure?

- "This is a more complex exposure. There is a risk of phrenic nerve injury, more risk of brachial plexus injury, pneumothorax etc. I think the infra-clavicular exposure is quicker, easier, and safer in this emergency setting."

If you needed to cover the left subclavian artery would you also do a left carotid-subclavian bypass?

- "It depends. If the patient had a dominant (or single) left vertebral artery, or a patent left internal thoracic to coronary artery bypass, then yes I would do a left carotid-subclavian bypass. However, if this was not the case, I would simply plan to plug the left subclavian artery and then cover it with the TEVAR to achieve a decent proximal seal zone."

What if the patient's subclavian arteries were both diseased? Do you have other access options for insertion of the TEVAR?

- "One could consider a Rutherford-Morrison type incision to expose one of the external or common iliac arteries. One might be able to do an iliac conduit."

Your FRCS Short Case Ends

Relevant ESVS Guideline Recommendations

- In patients with ruptured descending thoracic aortic aneurysm, endovascular repair should be the first treatment option when the anatomy is appropriate.
- In emergency ruptured descending thoracic aortic aneurysm in patients with a patent left mammary to coronary bypass or with a dominant or single left vertebral artery, left subclavian artery revascularisation should be performed prior to left subclavian artery coverage.

JMF Reflections

I deliberately set this case example up so it would include all the worst-case scenarios. In fact this is what the FRCS Part B can be like. For example in my FRCS Part B exam I had a case of a patient with a traumatic aortic injury causing transection just beyond the left subclavian artery. However, the CT angiogram showed severe aortoiliac disease. My plan was for a TEVAR, but I didn't understand why the examiners were showing me the CT angiogram with the diseased iliac arteries. I did not give them the answer they wanted, which was to insert the TEVAR via the right subclavian artery. I hope therefore that this case will prepare you for some curveballs that may come up.

CASE 13.3: Fit Middle-Aged Man with Descending Thoracic Aortic Aneurysm

- A 64-year-old patient is found to have a 13 cm descending thoracic aortic aneurysm.
- He was having recurrent chest infections, and over the past few months was complaining of dyspnoea and wheezing.

- The general practitioner requested an outpatient CT thorax which revealed the large aneurysm.
- You are telephoned by the general practitioner with the CT report.
- The patient is currently at home.

Your FRCS Long Case Begins

What is your immediate management plan?

- "The patient requires urgent hospital admission. I would get the patient's phone number from the GP or medical records and ask him to come in today. I would also gain some relevant information from the GP about the past medical history, current medications etc."

The patient has hypertension and is a smoker. He is otherwise fit and well. He is currently on amlodipine and ramipril. The patient comes to the acute surgical assessment area. How would you assess him?

- "I would complete a focused history and examination. I would want to confirm he has no signs/symptoms to suggest this was a symptomatic aneurysm. I would also want to know how his chest is doing i.e. does he have a current chest infection, what is his exercise tolerance like etc. I would want to confirm his medical comorbidities. I would enquire if there was a family history of aneurysms. I would confirm if he was on best medical therapy i.e. antiplatelet and statin. I would examine him from head to toe. I am interested in his upper and lower limb pulse status. I would also check if he had evidence of aneurysms elsewhere e.g. abdominal aortic and popliteal. I would also want to know his baseline observations e.g. heart rate, blood pressure, respiratory rate, oxygen saturations."

The patient does not currently have a chest infection (clinically). He says his chest feels ok. He says he can usually walk miles without getting short of breath. In fact he says that he still plays football every week. He is not a heavy smoker, and says he smokes around 5 cigarettes a day, and not everyday. What would you do now?

- "I would institute some basic investigations. Large-bore intravenous cannula and send off bloods for: FBC, U&Es, clotting, crossmatch 4 units. I would arrange for an ECG. I would request an urgent CT angiogram to cover from the femoral bifurcations all the way up to include the intracranial circulation. I would also finally request an echocardiogram and pulmonary function tests."

The patient has his CT angiogram. Can you please interpret these images?

- "There is what looks like a very large descending thoracic aortic aneurysm. It occupies a large portion of the left chest. It starts a few centimetres beyond the left subclavian artery, and ends around 2 cm above the level of the diaphragm. The aneurysm, because of its size, is quite tortuous. There are no signs of inflammation/fat stranding/rupture. The chest otherwise looks clear."

The patient has his bloods, echocardiogram, and pulmonary function tests. Can you please interpret them?

- "The bloods show a normal full blood count. The renal function shows chronic kidney disease with an eGFR of 62. The creatinine is normal. His echocardiogram shows good left ventricular systolic function. He has no valve stenosis/regurgitation. His pulmonary function tests reveal an obstructive pattern of disease."

What are your thoughts on management?

- "In this setting I do not think conservative management or surveillance is appropriate. This is a very large aneurysm and it carries a high risk of rupture. I also consider him to be a definite candidate for intervention. The options therefore are either endovascular stent repair, or open surgical repair. He sounds pretty fit, and therefore I think both TEVAR and open surgical repair should be considered. I would discuss the case with my consultant colleagues, and ideally put the case through the aortic MDT. I would also counsel the patient on the potential options and see what he thinks."

How would you counsel the patient? What would you say to him?

- "I would explain that he has a large aneurysm in his chest, and the natural history of this aneurysm is to grow, and then eventually rupture. Given its size, it currently has a high risk of rupture. As such, we should seriously consider intervention to treat this. One option is conservative management, but I do not think this is sensible. The other options are a minimally invasive approach with a stent to be inserted via his groin to seal the aneurysm from inside. The other option is a much more invasive and risky operation that would involve opening his chest and repairing the aneurysm with a prosthetic tube graft. I would explain that there are pros and cons to each approach. The benefit of the thoracic stent is that it is minimally invasive and he would likely go home much quicker. However, he would require lifelong surveillance and there are risks of stent graft migration, endoleak, need for further interventions etc. The benefit of the open approach is that it would likely be a "one-off" repair, and if he managed to get through it, he would likely be sorted in the long term. However, it is a very big operation, and the concern would be the stress on his heart, lungs and kidneys. We already know he has some lung and kidney disease, so this may be a much more risky operation for you than the stent."

The patient says he would rather get it over and done with and have the operation. What would you do now?

- "This is not a straightforward situation. The patient may want to get it over and done with, but I would not just proceed blindly. I would discuss the case in the aortic MDT. I would ask for a consultant anaesthetic opinion. I also think that these cases are done fairly infrequently, and an open repair in this setting is probably best done in a specialised centre. I would therefore telephone a vascular surgeon in a specialist centre and discuss the case."

The patient is seen by a consultant anaesthetist. The conclusion is that the patient's lung function is not awful. However, he no doubt has chronic obstructive lung disease according to the spirometry result. Given the recurrent chest infections and active smoking status, he would be at high risk of post-operative chest infection and respiratory failure. He would also be at risk of renal failure given his CKD. The aortic MDT says that the patient is suitable for a TEVAR which could be performed as a local anaesthetic percutaneous approach via either groin. If the patient wants to have an open repair however he will require referral to a regional specialist centre. What would you do now?

- "I would go and speak to the patient again, and try to include the family in the counselling process. I would say that a thoracic stent is possible and this could be performed as a local anaesthetic procedure without the need for any surgical incisions. I would also say that an open repair is another option, but there are concerns about his chest and kidney function post-operatively, and if he wanted this doing he would need to be referred to another specialist centre."

The patient wants to know what your recommendation is.

- "My recommendation would be for a thoracic aortic stent. He may sound relatively fit on paper, but this is a very big operation, and it carries big risks. Our main concern is in regard to his lungs and kidneys. He likely has chronic obstructive pulmonary disease, is still actively smoking, and has evidence of chronic kidney impairment. We know that these are risk factors for post-operative respiratory failure and renal failure. As such, my gut instinct in this case is to go for a thoracic aortic stent."

If the patient had normal renal function and respiratory function, would you consider open repair?

- "I would consider it yes. However, as per the ESVS guidelines on descending thoracic aortic disease, open repair should be limited to those patients who are fit and unsuitable for TEVAR."

Well in what situation would a patient not be suitable for TEVAR then?

1. "If there were no adequate arterial access. For example, absence of adequate femoral or subclavian access, or a contraindication to aortic/iliac conduit graft placement such as the presence of hostile abdomen or severe aortoiliac disease
2. Absence of proximal or distal landing zones
3. Aneurysm associated with a connective tissue disorder such as Marfan's
4. In young and healthy patients without major contraindications to open surgical repair
5. Symptoms related to compression by a large aneurysm on adjacent structures such as the thoracic vertebral bodies (chronic pain syndrome), trachea or left mainstem bronchus (dyspnoea), or oesophagus (dysphagia)."

This patient has compressive symptoms (i.e. dyspnoea), he was initially in favour of open repair, and he has a good exercise tolerance with good cardiac function. Why not refer him to the specialist centre for consideration of open repair?

- "I would have discussed the case with the specialist centre as I previously indicated. If they offered open repair and the patient wished to proceed with this after being appropriately counselled, I would think this approach is acceptable."

Your FRCS Long Case Ends

Relevant ESVS Guideline Recommendations

- CT angiography or MR angiography should be performed for patients planned for descending thoracic aortic repair, to define the extent of the disease and to identify the potential risk of the procedure related to the main intercostal arteries.
- In candidates for open surgical repair of descending thoracic aortic aneurysms with a past medical history of coronary artery disease, additional diagnostic investigations should be considered to define the severity of the underlying heart disease.

- Revascularisation of symptomatic or severe asymptomatic coronary artery disease should be considered before open descending thoracic aorta surgery.

- Stratification of peri-operative risk associated with pulmonary, renal, and cerebrovascular studies should be considered.

- Open repair may be considered for fit patients, with a descending thoracic aorta between 56 and 59 mm in diameter, who are unsuitable for endovascular repair.

- Open repair should be considered for fit patients, with a descending thoracic aorta exceeding 60 mm in diameter, who are unsuitable for endovascular repair.

JMF Reflections

I completely made this case up. It is fictional. However, it illustrates the salient points. From my perspective this is a case that is all about knowing the guidelines, discussing the case with the aortic experts, and patient counselling. I don't think there are any wrong answers here (*well actually, if you said you would rush the patient to theatre for an open repair, then that would be the wrong answer*). If you said you were in favour of open repair, and wished to refer the case to the specialist centre, that would be acceptable. However, if you were worried about the lungs/kidneys, and were in favour of TEVAR, that would also be fine. The important thing here is to come across as sensible and safe. In the real world you know you would speak to your senior colleagues, discuss it in the MDT, and if open repair was seriously being considered you would discuss the case with the specialist centre. From my pragmatic perspective, however, this patient would almost have certainly gotten a TEVAR. Patients may say they can walk miles and think they are fit, but if they are smokers with underlying respiratory/renal compromise, I seriously doubt a thoracotomy is going to be in their best interests. You make your own decision, however.

CHAPTER 14

Type B Aortic Dissection

I am going to go through two FRCS cases here that I think will satisfactorily cover the salient management points. I am not repeating the same points for penetrating aortic ulcers and intra-mural haematoma because they follow the same principles as for type B aortic dissection.

CASE 14.1: Acute Type B Aortic Dissection

- A 58-year-old gentleman presents with sudden onset severe chest and inter-scapular pain.
- He is currently in A&E resus.
- He has a blood pressure of 190/100 mmHg.
- His heart rate is 96.
- He has had an urgent CT aortogram and the A&E consultant is referring him to you with the CT results.

Your FRCS Short Case Begins

Can you please interpret these CT angiogram images?

- "This image is of the aortic arch. There is clearly a large aortic dissection that appears to be originating distal to the left subclavian artery. These 3 images are showing the true and false lumen at the visceral aortic segment. The true lumen is largely compressed by the false lumen. The coelic, SMA and right renal artery are coming off the true lumen, and all appear to be patent. The kidneys appear well perfused. The left renal artery is coming off the false lumen and again appears well perfused. This image shows that both iliac arteries are patent."

How would you assess this patient?

- "Well, firstly I would go and see the patient. I would do a head-to-toe assessment, looking specifically for any signs of malperfusion i.e. stroke, upper limb ischaemia, mesenteric ischaemia, paraplegia, lower limb ischaemia etc."

What would be your immediate management?

- "Blood pressure control with intravenous beta-blockade should be first-line therapy (e.g. labetalol or esmolol). I would aim to reduce the systolic blood pressure to between 100 and 120 mmHg. I would aim for a heart rate < 60 beats/min. I would prescribe good analgesia and also administer high flow oxygen. I would refer the patient to the intensive care team. The patient would need an arterial line to monitor blood pressure and be admitted to high dependency/intensive care for close monitoring and strict blood pressure control."

What if labetolol or esmolol was not effective?

- "Then I would consider second line agents such as calcium channel antagonists, renin-angiotensin inhibitors, sodium nitroprusside and alpha blockers."

DOI: 10.1201/b22951-14

Would you consider a TEVAR in this setting?

- "In my usual practice no. Based upon the CT angiogram that you have shown me, there are no signs of malperfusion. I would only consider TEVAR in complicated acute type B aortic dissection."

What do you mean by complicated type B dissection?

- "I mean those cases with refractory pain, refractory hypertension, malperfusion and aortic rupture ...."

If you had a patient with malperfusion, what would be your management?

- "Ideally TEVAR with endovascular fenestration."

Are there no potential benefits to early stenting in acute uncomplicated type B dissections?

- "Perhaps. There are advocates for TEVAR in the uncomplicated setting .... Some have argued that TEVAR prevents long term aortic dilatation and future rupture. Indeed, ADSORB, the only randomized controlled trial in patients with uncomplicated type B dissection did show higher rates of false lumen thrombosis, and this is associated with fewer late complications and improved aortic remodelling .... Unfortunately, ADSORB was not sufficiently powered for mortality at 1 year of follow-up and it was not a big trial. As such, even though there may indeed be benefits to performing TEVAR in this setting, one must be aware of the potential complications of TEVAR which are not insignificant ...."

OK. What are the potential complications of TEVAR?

- "Stroke, spinal cord ischaemia, aortic rupture during deployment, angulation/ migration/collapse/fracture of the stent graft, false aneurysm formation at the proximal or distal landing zones, graft erosion, graft infection and also retrograde type A aortic dissection."

So would you support TEVAR in this patient? Yes or no?

- "If you force me to give an answer, then my answer is no. The ADSORB trial is the only randomised trial that I am aware of that has looked into this conundrum. The conclusion of this trial was that uncomplicated type B aortic dissection can be safely treated with the Gore TAG device. This seemed to encourage remodelling with thrombosis of the false lumen and reduction of its diameter. However, this was a small trial with only 61 patients, and follow-up was only for 1 year. Even the ADSORB authors concluded that the question remains as to whether endovascular treatment with a stent graft in the acute phase of acute type B aortic dissection is associated with improved survival compared with medical treatment alone, and can only be demonstrated with a larger randomised controlled trial and longer follow-up."

What do the ESVS guidelines say?

- "They say that in order to prevent aortic complications in uncomplicated acute type B aortic dissection, early thoracic endografting may be considered selectively."

If this patient, whilst in ICU, suddenly developed new severe generalised abdominal pain, what would you do?

- "I would get an urgent CT angiogram to assess for progression of the dissection and new visceral malperfusion."

Your FRCS Short Case Ends

Relevant ESVS Guideline Recommendations

- Medical therapy should always be part of the treatment of patients with acute type B dissection.
- In patients with acute type B aortic dissection, β-blockers should be considered the first line of medical therapy.
- In patients with acute type B aortic dissection who do not respond or are intolerant of β-blockers, calcium channel antagonists and/or renin-angiotensin inhibitors may be considered alternatives or complementaries.
- In patients with complicated acute type B aortic dissection, endovascular repair with thoracic endografting should be the first-line intervention.
- In complicated acute type B aortic dissection, endovascular fenestration should be considered to treat malperfusion.
- To prevent aortic complications in uncomplicated acute type B aortic dissection, early thoracic endografting may be considered selectively.
- Patients with acute type B aortic dissection who develop new or recurrent abdominal pain and where there is any suspicion of visceral, renal, and/or limb malperfusion should undergo repeat CT imaging.

CASE 14.2: Chronic Type B Aortic Dissection

- A 58-year-old gentleman had an acute type B aortic dissection 4 years ago.
- He was lost to follow-up.
- He was originally managed medically.
- He presented under the medical team with community-acquired pneumonia at wintertime.
- He has had a routine chest X-ray, and the medical team is ringing you up because the chest X-ray looks abnormal.

Your FRCS Short Case Begins

What do you make of this X-ray?

- "There is a right basal pneumonia. However, there is clearly aortic enlargement in the left chest and I can see calcium deposits here as well."

What would you do at this point?

- "I would gain more details about the patient. Is he well? Does he have chest pain? What is his blood pressure and heart rate? I would recommend a formal CT aortogram."

OK. What do you make of these CT angiogram images?

- "There is aneurysmal degeneration of the descending thoracic aorta. This is quite a large aneurysm, probably about 8 cm. it appears to be beyond the origin of the left subclavian artery. There is evidence of the previous dissection, and it looks like false lumen expansion has resulted in this aneurysm. The false lumen appears to still be patent."

What would you do now?

- "I would go and see the patient and complete a thorough history and examination. I would ensure he was on best medical therapy and his heart rate and blood pressure were optimised."

Would you consider intervention in this patient?

- "Ideally he would recover from his chest infection first of all. However, as this is a large aneurysm and appears to be bigger than 6 cm in diameter, I think there is justification to treat it."

The patient asks you if this could have been prevented.

- "Best medical therapy, appropriate blood pressure control, close surveillance and earlier intervention may have prevented this."

What do you think about TEVAR for chronic type B aortic dissection?

- "The INSTEAD trial randomized patients with sub-acute and chronic dissections to early endovascular repair or best medical management and surveillance. Aortic remodelling was greater in the endovascular group, but there were no statistically significant differences between the groups at 2 years. The original trial therefore concluded that medical management for uncomplicated type B aortic dissection corroborated excellent survival rate with tight blood pressure control and close surveillance. However, the INSTEAD-XL trial suggested that there might be long term beneficial results of TEVAR in sub-acute and chronic dissection. As such, it looks like TEVAR in the sub-acute/chronic setting carries short term risks but potentially long-term benefits."

So in this patient's case, would you have done anything differently?

- "Difficult to say, because I don't know the reasons or him being lost to follow-up. In an ideal world the patient would have received best medical therapy and close surveillance, and if his aorta deteriorated I would have considered a TEVAR."

Didn't the INSTEAD-XL trial suggest that pre-emptive early TEVAR in the sub-acute phase had a better long term outcome as compared to those patients with controlled medical management and optional crossover to TEVAR or open repair when complications emerge?

- "Yes it did. I suppose there is an argument therefore that a proportion of patients with sub-acute dissection may benefit from early endovascular repair, especially in those at risk of further aortic complications."

Which patients then do you think are at higher risk of future aortic complications following an acute type B dissection?

- "Hypertension, an aortic diameter of 40 mm or more in the acute phase, chronic obstructive pulmonary disease, and patency of the false lumen are recognised risk factors for late aneurysmal degeneration. Also, the presence of an entry tear larger than 10 mm in diameter or located in the arch or proximal descending thoracic aorta has also been identified as a predictor of late mortality and need for aortic repair."

If you went back in time, would you consider a TEVAR on this patient in the sub-acute setting?

- "Maybe, maybe not. It is easy to play Captain Hindsight. Perhaps an early TEVAR may have prevented the current situation developing. However, TEVAR still carries risks, including limb and life-threatening risks. Even the INSTEAD-XL authors concluded that there were early hazards associated with TEVAR, and this probably counterbalances the possible prevention of late complications. I think my position is to consider early TEVAR in sub-acute type B dissections on an individualised case-by-case basis."

Your FRCS Short Case Ends

Relevant ESVS Guideline Recommendations

- To prevent aortic complications in uncomplicated acute type B aortic dissection, early thoracic endografting may be considered selectively.

- In patients with chronic aortic dissection, effective antihypertensive therapy should be given to reduce the risk of aortic-related death.

- In patients with chronic dissection, measures to reduce cardiovascular risk (such as treatment of hyperlipidaemia, antiplatelet therapy, management of hypertension, and smoking cessation) should be implemented to reduce the incidence of late cardiovascular death.

- Long term medical treatment with β-blockers should be given to patients with chronic uncomplicated aortic dissection as they reduce the progression of aortic dilatation, the incidence of subsequent hospital admission, and the need for late dissection-related aortic procedures.

- In patients with chronic aortic dissection and acute aortic symptoms, emergency repair should be considered if malperfusion, rupture, or progression of dissection is confirmed on imaging.

- In patients with chronic aortic dissection, a descending thoracic aortic diameter between 56 and 59 mm may be considered an indication for treatment in patients at reasonable surgical risk.

- In patients with chronic aortic dissection, a descending thoracic aortic diameter greater than 60 mm should be considered an indication for treatment in patients at reasonable surgical risk.

- In patients with chronic aortic dissection and thoraco abdominal extension, an aortic diameter greater than 60 mm should be considered an indication for treatment in patients at reasonable surgical risk.

- Open repair of aneurysmal or symptomatic chronic type B aortic dissection in patients with low surgical risk should be considered in dedicated centres with low complication rates.

CHAPTER 15

Symptomatic Carotid Artery Disease

History

- Sudden onset monocular loss of vision.
- Facial weakness / droop.
- Arm weakness / sensory loss.
- Leg weakness / sensory loss.
- Speech disturbance.
- Above symptoms may be permanent or transitory i.e. stroke versus transient ischaemic attack (TIA).
- When did this happen (i.e. get the exact date of last neurological event)?
- Have you experienced chest palpitations before (i.e. looking for atrial fibrillation)?
- *Rapid-fire assessment of risk factors:* "Do you smoke? Do you have high blood pressure? Do you have raised cholesterol? Are you a diabetic?"
- *Rapid-fire assessment of comorbidities:* "Do you have heart disease? Do you have chronic lung disease/COPD? Do you have chronic kidney disease? Have you had a previous stroke? Do you have pain in your abdomen after eating (i.e. chronic mesenteric disease)?"
- Is there a previous history of vascular intervention? Any previous operations on neck?
- *Best medical therapy:* "Are you on aspirin and/or clopidogrel? Are you on a statin to lower your cholesterol?"
- *Social history:* "Where do you live? Who do you live with? Are you independent? Who does the cooking/cleaning/shopping? How active are you normally?"

Examination

- Examine radial pulse (regular or irregular).
- Examine eyes for corneal arcus and xanthelasma.
- Examine neck for signs of previous surgery/thyroid enlargement (thyrotoxicosis can cause atrial fibrillation which can cause stroke/TIA, previous neck surgery may mean you don't offer carotid endarterectomy).
- Auscultate chest to listen for heart murmurs. Confirm whether patient has femoral pulses.
- Determine Rankin score if this was a stroke.

Initial Management

- Full set of bloods (FBC, U&Es, LFTs, lipid screen, HBA1c, coagulation, group & save).
- ECG.
- Carotid duplex (to assess both sides).
- If significant ICA stenosis identified on duplex, for secondary confirmatory imaging.

DOI: 10.1201/b22951-15

- I (JMF) personally prefer CTA, but MRA is the other option.
- Best medical therapy (if a candidate for intervention, I want the patient on dual antiplatelet therapy and high-dose statin).
- Make sure diabetic control and blood pressure control optimised.
- Calculate Carotid Artery Risk Score (CAR Score) or Oxford Risk Score.
- If patient candidate for intervention, ideally discuss in MDT.

Definitive Management Options

1. Conservative management i.e. best medical therapy alone
2. Carotid endarterectomy
3. Carotid stent

Decision-Making around Carotid Intervention (from ESVS Guidelines)

- When revascularisation is considered appropriate in symptomatic patients with 50–99% stenoses, it is recommended that this be performed as soon as possible, preferably within 14 days of symptom onset.
- Patients who are to undergo revascularisation within the first 14 days after onset of symptoms should undergo carotid endarterectomy, rather than carotid stenting.
- In recently symptomatic patients with 50–99% stenoses and anatomical and/or medical comorbidities that are considered by the MDT to make them "higher risk for carotid endarterectomy," carotid stenting should be considered.
- Revascularisation should be deferred in patients with 50–99% stenoses who suffer a disabling stroke (modified Rankin score ≥3), whose area of infarction exceeds one-third of the ipsilateral middle cerebral artery territory, or who have altered consciousness/drowsiness, to minimise the risks of post-operative parenchymal haemorrhage.
- Patients with 50–99% stenoses who present with stroke-in-evolution or crescendo transient ischaemic attacks should be considered for urgent carotid endarterectomy, preferably <24 hours.
- Early carotid endarterectomy (within 14 days) should be considered after intravenous thrombolysis (*for stroke patients*) in symptomatic patients if they make a rapid neurological recovery (i.e. Rankin 0–2), the area of infarction is less than one-third of the ipsilateral middle cerebral artery territory, a previously occluded middle cerebral artery mainstem has been recanalised, there is a 50–99% carotid stenosis, and no evidence of parenchymal haemorrhage or significant brain oedema.
- If patient has had previous neck surgery and you are considering carotid endarterectomy, always ask ENT to check vocal cords are intact or not (i.e. make sure patient gets indirect laryngoscopy). Bilateral recurrent laryngeal *(& hypoglossal)* nerve palsies can be fatal—if a contralateral vocal cord palsy is identified, then the reason for carotid endarterectomy should be urgently reviewed and alternative approach considered (i.e. carotid stent or best medical therapy alone).

Other Considerations

There are apparent sex differences to be aware of. For example, men with significant carotid stenoses seem to derive a clear benefit from carotid endarterectomy, and this seems to persist way beyond 2 weeks. Women with 70–99% also benefit highly from carotid endarterectomy, but beyond 2 weeks the benefit seems to be reduced compared to men. Women with 50–69%

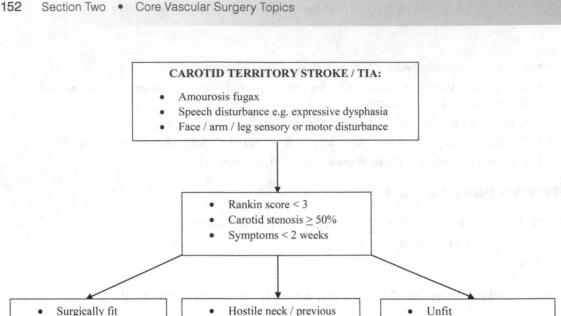

Figure 15.1   Broad management overview for symptomatic carotid disease.

arguably do not derive as much benefit as men and probably not beyond 2 weeks (where carotid endarterectomy is possibly harmful).

This is something of a controversial area however. If you are going to start talking about these sex differences, just make sure you know what you are talking about and can back up your arguments with some decent evidence. As for me, I try to tread carefully around this topic (Figure 15.1).

Technical Aspects of Carotid Endarterectomy

• For carotid endarterectomy, the decision between local anaesthesia and general anaesthesia can be left to the surgical/anaesthetic team's discretion. This is the current position of the ESVS in the 2018 carotid guidelines. However, I expect in the updated

2022 ESVS carotid guidelines this may swing in favour of local anaesthesia. In any case I (JMF) still think GA versus LA should be a decision between surgeon, anaesthetist and patient ....

- Choice of carotid exposure (antegrade/retrojugular) should be left to surgical team's discretion.
- Routine carotid sinus blockade is not recommended.
- Protamine reversal of heparin should be considered to prevent neck haematomas.
- Choice of shunting should be left to discretion of surgeon.
- Routine patching is recommended over routine primary closure.
- The choice between eversion endarterectomy and patched endarterectomy should be left to the discretion of the operating surgeon.

Stroke after Carotid Endarterectomy

This is my (JMF's) plan and it aligns with what you will read in the ESVS guidelines. However, no doubt if you speak to 100 other vascular surgeons, they will all have a different plan ....

- If patient demonstrates new focal neurological deficit or worsening of pre-existing deficit immediately post-operatively (i.e. recovering from anaesthesia in theatre or in shortly afterwards in recovery) → immediate re-exploration to exclude accumulation of thrombus with the endarterectomy zone.
- New neurological symptoms ≥6 hours post-operatively → emergency extracranial and intracranial CTA. This will exclude ICA thrombus which should be removed at re-exploration, or more likely intracerebral oedema, intracerebral haemorrhage, or parenchymal haemorrhage. If CT demonstrates embolic occlusion of middle cerebral artery there should be consideration of mechanical thrombectomy (i.e. ask for neurointerventional radiologist's help if one available). The ESVS guidelines talks about intra-operative thrombolysis for middle or anterior cerebral artery embolism after re-exploration of the endarterectomised zone .... I (JMF) would be scared to do this in regards to bleeding risk frankly ....

Carotid Artery Disease Case Examples

These are a few case examples that should help to illustrate the salient points of management for symptomatic carotid artery disease. They are not real cases, but I hope they reflect the potential complexities of real world practice and are useful for the FRCS examination.

CASE 15.1: Symptomatic Carotid Stenosis

- A 64-year-old gentleman presents with left monocular loss of vision for 5 minutes.
- This event was 2 days ago.
- Past medical history includes type 2 diabetes, hypertension, and peripheral vascular disease.
- He is an ex-smoker.
- He is independent of his activities of daily living.
- He has a reasonable exercise tolerance, walking around 300 yards (which is limited by calf claudication).

Your FRCS Short Case Begins

The patient is referred to you by the stroke physician. He has had a carotid duplex. Can you please interpret this report?

- "This report reveals high velocities in the left ICA, > 230 cm/second. This suggests that there is at least a 70% stenosis according to NASCET criteria. The peak systolic velocity ratio is also > 4, which would also suggest this is at least a 70% stenosis."

How did you calculate the peak systolic velocity ratio?

- "Peak systolic velocity in the ICA divided by the peak systolic velocity in the CCA."

Do you know what St Mary's ratio is for this patient?

- "Yes. The St Mary's ratio is 16. Again, this would support my assertion that this is >70% stenosis."

How did you calculate the St Mary's ratio?

- "Peak systolic velocity in the ICA divided by the end-diastolic velocity in the CCA."

OK. So you think there is a 70% left ICA stenosis. What would you do now?

- "I would request a second confirmatory form of imaging. In my practice that would be a CT angiogram."

Can you please interpret these images?

- "Yes. This confirms a significant left proximal ICA stenosis. The carotid bifurcation appears to be below the angle of the mandible and therefore looks surgically accessible. I would also want to check the patency of the contralateral carotid artery, and confirm the patency of the circle of Willis."

The circle of Willis is patent, but the contralateral ICA is occluded. Does this change your management?

- "I am still at this point considering the patient for a left carotid endarterectomy. The occluded contralateral ICA would not stop me doing the operation. However, as per the GALA trial, there may be added benefit in doing the case under local anaesthetic."

Would you not consider a carotid stent?

- "The evidence suggests that in the acute setting carotid stenting carries a higher procedural risk of stroke than carotid endarterectomy. Therefore, I would still prefer to do a carotid endarterectomy."

How would you plan your left carotid endarterectomy then?

- "Firstly I would need to see the patient, take a history and examine him. I would specifically check his neck for any scars and range of neck movement. I would ensure he was on best medical therapy. I would also need to counsel him on the potential options which include carotid endarterectomy, carotid stenting or just best medical therapy alone. I would run the case through a mini-MDT."

When would you aim to get the operation done?

- "As soon as possible, within 14 days of the index neurological event."

What do you mean by best medical therapy?

- "I mean antiplatelet and statin therapy. In my practice that would mean aspirin 75 mg OD and atorvastatin 80 mg OD. If I was going to do a carotid endarterectomy I would also add in clopidogrel 75 mg."

Would you keep the patient on dual antiplatelet long term following carotid endarterectomy?

- "No. Only for around 1 week post-op, then I would switch back to single antiplatelet therapy."

You examine the patient's neck and he has a scar from a previous thyroidectomy. Would this alter your management?

- "Definitely. I would speak to ENT and ask for an indirect laryngoscopy to ensure his vocal cords were both working. He may have an underlying vocal cord palsy, and if I take him to theatre and cause further cranial nerve injury, this could leave him with a life-threatening airway problem."

If the patient was found to have a contralateral vocal cord palsy, would you still do the operation?

- "No. I would either consider a carotid stent, or best medical therapy alone."

Your FRCS Short Case Ends

Relevant ESVS Guideline Recommendations

- Duplex ultrasound (as first-line), computed tomographic angiography, and/or magnetic resonance angiography are recommended for evaluating the extent and severity of extracranial carotid stenoses.
- When carotid endarterectomy is being considered, it is recommended that duplex ultrasound stenosis estimation be corroborated by computed tomographic angiography or magnetic resonance angiography, or by a repeat Duplex ultrasound performed by a second operator.
- Multidisciplinary assessment is recommended to achieve consensus regarding the indication and optimal treatment of patients by carotid endarterectomy or carotid stenting.
- It is recommended that all patients undergoing carotid endarterectomy should receive antiplatelet therapy throughout the peri-operative period and also in the long term.
- Low-dose aspirin (75–325 mg daily) is recommended rather than higher doses (>625 mg daily) in patients undergoing carotid endarterectomy.
- Early institution of aspirin and clopidogrel after transient ischaemic attack or minor stroke may be considered to reduce early recurrent events in patients with a >50% carotid stenosis awaiting carotid endarterectomy.

- Long term aspirin plus clopidogrel therapy is not recommended in patients undergoing carotid endarterectomy or carotid stenting unless indicated for cardiac reasons.
- Statin therapy is recommended for the prevention of long term stroke, myocardial infarction, and other cardiovascular events in patients with symptomatic carotid disease.
- It is recommended that patients start statin therapy prior to endarterectomy or stenting and that statins should not be stopped during the peri-operative period and should be continued long term.
- Carotid endarterectomy is recommended in patients reporting carotid territory symptoms within the preceding 6 months and who have a 70–99% carotid stenosis, provided the documented procedural death/stroke rate is <6%.
- When revascularisation is considered appropriate in symptomatic patients with 50–99% stenoses, it is recommended that this be performed as soon as possible, preferably within 14 days of symptom onset.
- Patients who are to undergo revascularisation within the first 14 days after onset of symptoms should undergo carotid endarterectomy, rather than carotid stenting.

CASE 15.2: Symptomatic Carotid Stenosis

- A frail 89-year-old woman from a nursing home has had a right cerebral hemisphere TIA 13 days ago.
- Her symptoms were that of left arm weakness and facial droop that lasted 5 minutes then fully resolved.
- Past medical history includes hypertension, ischaemic heart disease, advanced osteoarthritis, and cervical spondylosis.
- She has very poor mobility.
- At the time of this TIA she was not on best medical therapy.
- She has since been started on aspirin and a statin.
- A carotid duplex has reported a right ICA 50% stenosis.
- This plaque is reported to be ulcerated.
- She is referred to you from the TIA clinic by a stroke consultant for consideration of carotid endarterectomy.

Your FRCS Short Case Begins

How would you manage this case?

- "I would go and see the patient, take a history, and examine her. My focus is to determine whether or not I think this patient is a viable candidate for either a carotid endarterectomy or a carotid stent."

What in the history and examination are you particularly interested in?

- "I want to know how fit the patient is. Does she have an accessible neck? Are there scars from previous surgery? Has she had previous radiotherapy around her neck? What is the range of movement of the neck? Does she have capacity? Does she have femoral pulses to allow endovascular access for a possible carotid stent? Would she able to lie flat?"

Let's say the patient has an accessible neck and she has femoral pulses. She is not demented and seems like a potentially viable candidate. She would be willing to consider intervention. What would you do now?

- "Well, if I was seriously considering intervention, I would request a CT angiogram."

The patient has a CT angiogram and it confirms a 50% right ICA stenosis. This is suitable for either an endarterectomy or a carotid stent. What would you do now?

- "I would use a risk tool to calculate her likely future risk of stroke. I routinely use the carotid artery risk score, but there is also the Oxford carotid stenosis risk score."

The patient's Oxford risk score reports a 12.1% 1-year risk of ipsilateral ischaemic stroke, and 30% 5-year risk of stroke. What do you make of this?

- "The patient has a few factors that are definitely increasing her risk of a stroke, notably the fact this is ulcerated plaque, her hypertension and the ischemic heart disease, and her advanced age. There is therefore an argument for intervention based upon these figures. However, my broad understanding is that female patients with 50–69% carotid stenoses do not derive as much benefit from carotid endarterectomy when performed within 2 weeks from the index event, and beyond 2 weeks this is likely even less advantageous (and may be harmful). If we were to intervene on this patient surgically, she would no doubt be outside the 14-day window as it is already day 13."

So what would you do then?

- "As per the ESVS guidelines, I would discuss the case in the vascular MDT. I would also discuss the case with the stroke consultant. The options are still either carotid endarterectomy, carotid stenting, or just best medical therapy alone."

What would be your recommendation?

- "I would be more in favour of best medical therapy. This TIA happened when the patient was not on best medical therapy, and we know that modern best medical therapy is very effective. She is also elderly and frail. This is a 50% carotid stenosis, and if it was only 1% less, I would not be considering intervention at all. Surgical and endovascular interventions are risky, and I am not entirely sure that the benefits of intervention outweigh the risks at the moment."

The patient has a reasonably high 1-year risk of stroke though doesn't she? Don't you think you should be offering surgery if the patient wanted it?

- "I agree that the Oxford score appears to be reasonably high, and therefore there is an argument for intervention. However, this is only one scoring system, and it does not provide all the answers. I am aware of other evidence that I could use to argue against intervention in this context. For example, a recent Cochrane review of the original NASCET, ECST and VASCP trials highlighted that the benefit from carotid endarterectomy is greater in men than women, the benefit from surgery decreased with increased time delay from last neurological symptom, and women had a lower risk of ipsilateral ischaemic stroke with medical treatment and a higher operative risk compared with men. This review also concluded that carotid endarterectomy is very clearly beneficial in women with 70% to 99% symptomatic stenosis, but not in women with 50% to 69% stenosis. The European Carotid Surgery Trialist's Collaboration concluded that, on the whole (now including men and women), surgery was highly beneficial for 70% to 99% stenosis and only moderately beneficial for 50% to 69% stenosis. Therefore the answer to the question of whether we should intervene on this patient is not so straightforward. There are arguments for and against. However, I don't like to sit on the fence for fear of saying the wrong thing. I would rather make a decision and be criticised about it. My decision would be to not do a carotid endarterectomy and instead manage with best medical therapy alone."

What if the vascular MDT and the patient/family supported a carotid endarterectomy i.e. it disagreed with you?

- "I would think this is perfectly acceptable. I never said I had all the answers, nor do I consider myself to be an expert. I would still consider a carotid endarterectomy in this patient, and that is exactly why I referred it to the MDT. If I was going to do a carotid endarterectomy however, I would make sure the patient was properly counselled beforehand and she understood the proposed benefits, risks, and alternatives. I would also involve the family in the discussion ideally as well."

What if the MDT recommended a carotid stent?

- "I respect the opinions of the MDT, but I am aware that the ESVS guidelines recommend that most patients who have suffered carotid territory symptoms within the preceding 6 months and who are aged >70 years and who have 50-99% stenoses should be treated by carotid endarterectomy, rather than carotid stenting."

Do you not think carotid stenting is appropriate here?

- "The pooled results from EVA-3S, SPACE, ICSS and CREST showed that the risk of any stroke or death within 30 days after treatment was higher for the carotid artery stenting compared with carotid endarterectomy (7.3% versus 3.3%). The net conclusion of this paper was that carotid stenting is not as safe as carotid endarterectomy in the treatment of patients with symptomatic stenosis of the ICA irrespective of the timing of treatment. As such, my position is that I would be reluctant offer carotid stenting for this patient. If we were going to offer intervention, I would rather offer carotid endarterectomy."

Your FRCS Short Case Ends

Relevant ESVS Guideline Recommendations

- Carotid endarterectomy is recommended in patients reporting carotid territory symptoms within the preceding 6 months and who have a 70–99% carotid stenosis, provided the documented procedural death/stroke rate is <6%.
- Carotid endarterectomy should be considered in patients reporting carotid territory symptoms within the preceding 6 months and who have a 50–69% carotid stenosis, provided the documented procedural death/stroke rate is <6%.
- It is recommended that most patients who have suffered carotid territory symptoms within the preceding 6 months and who are aged >70 years and who have 50–99% stenoses should be treated by carotid endarterectomy, rather than carotid stenting.

- When revascularisation is indicated in patients who have suffered carotid territory symptoms within the preceding 6 months and who are aged <70 years, carotid stenting may be considered an alternative to endarterectomy, provided the documented procedural death/stroke rate is <6%.
- Patients who are to undergo revascularisation within the first 14 days after onset of symptoms should undergo carotid endarterectomy, rather than carotid stenting.

JMF Reflections

This is not an easy station. I have to admit that I don't find these sorts of scenarios easy. If you have a straightforward fit 70-year-old gentleman with a 90% carotid stenosis within 14 days, then that is a no-brainer, he is going for a carotid endarterectomy. However, frail elderly women with moderate carotid stenoses are genuinely tricky. Once you start getting into the details you can open a whole can of worms. There are so many different factors to consider and again the question of how much women benefit from intervention comes back again. The timing of intervention also becomes tricky. The ESVS guidelines say we should consider intervention for patients with carotid territory symptoms within the past 6 months, and yet at the same time we know we should be aiming to get these cases done within 2 weeks. What happens with patients at 3 weeks then? What if it is a woman beyond 2 weeks? ESVS says on the one hand we should consider carotid stenting in certain circumstances, and yet the evidence shows it is riskier than carotid endarterectomy. What if you start including the carotid artery and oxford risk scoring systems? This brings in another dimension to an already tricky scenario. So what are we supposed to do???!!! Ultimately, I think you just need to present a balanced argument, demonstrate that you are aware of the controversies, and be prepared to discuss the potential options and challenges. For the exam and your real world practice, I would routinely seek second options, use the MDT, discuss with the stroke team, and keep the patient and family firmly in the loop. This is what I hope this case scenario demonstrates.

KEY REFERENCES

Alamowitch S, Eliasziw M, Barnett HJ, North American Symptomatic Carotid Endarterectomy Trial (NASCET); ASA Trial Group; Carotid Endarterectomy (ACE) Trial Group. The Risk and Benefit of Endarterectomy in Women with Symptomatic Internal Carotid Artery Disease. Stroke (2005) 36(1), 27–31.

This paper looked at the original NASCET data and concluded that women and men with >70% symptomatic stenosis had similar long term benefit from CE, although the peri-operative risks were higher for women. Medically treated women with 50–69% stenosis generally had a low risk for stroke and carotid endarterectomy was of no benefit. However, this study identified a small percentage of women with 50–69% stenosis and a high risk factor profile who were at a higher risk for stroke and had a greater chance of benefit. These risk factors included hemispheric (not retinal) event, diabetes, previous stroke, age older than 70 years, stroke (not transient ischemic attack), severe hypertension, and a history of myocardial infarction.

Marulanda-Londoño E, Chaturvedi S. Carotid Stenosis in Women: Time for a Reappraisal. Stroke Vasc Neurol (2016) 1, e000043.

This paper concludes by stating that carotid endarterectomy to prevent stroke is less beneficial for women compared with men. Women with symptomatic carotid disease have a higher peri-procedural risk and a lower risk of recurrent stroke on medical treatment. It also argues that women should be counselled that risk reduction benefit from CEA is less than that for men. In general, women also tend to be undertreated medically, and practitioners should ensure they optimise medical therapy, regardless of whether revascularisation is pursued. It also says that the peri-procedural risk of stroke and death may be higher with carotid stenting than with endarterectomy in women, therefore it is difficult to recommend carotid stenting routinely for women. Finally, which I think is extremely relevant, is the conclusion that ".... the representation of women in stroke clinical trials remains an issue. The fact that women have been under-represented in carotid stenosis trials has led to uncertainty about the optimal treatment for women. A carotid stenosis trial focused on women is one potential solution to this vexing clinical problem."

CASE 15.3: Symptomatic Carotid Stenosis

- A 49-year-old gentleman has been thrombolysed following a right MCA infarct.
- He initially presented 2 days ago under the stroke team with dense left sided hemiplegia.
- Following the thrombolysis he has made a complete neurological recovery.
- He is now 48 hours following thrombolysis.
- He has had an arterial duplex that demonstrates a 60% right ICA stenosis that is reported to show ulcerated plaque.
- He has also had a confirmatory CT angiogram that has confirmed this degree of stenosis.
- The right carotid bifurcation is surgically accessible.

Your FRCS Short Case Begins

What are your thoughts on intervention in this setting?

- "There are many variables to be considered, and I would obviously go and assess the patient for myself first of all. However, based upon what you have told me, I would potentially consider early surgical intervention for this patient. At this stage I would mainly be interested in knowing what the CT brain report was following his thrombolysis. Are there any signs of haemorrhage, significant brain oedema, how much of the MCA territory was affected by the stroke, has the MCA been recanalised? Is the patient's blood pressure control currently satisfactory? I would also want to know if the patient was a suitable surgical candidate i.e. is the neck accessible? Is the patient otherwise well with no significant comorbidities?"

The patient has a background of type 2 diabetes and hypertension. He has a good range of neck movement and no scars in the neck. His CT brain shows no signs of haemorrhage or oedema, the right MCA is patent. What are your thoughts now?

- "The ESVS guidelines on carotid disease states that early carotid endarterectomy (within 14 days) should be considered after intravenous thrombolysis in symptomatic patients if they make a rapid neurological recovery (Rankin 0-2), the area of infarction is less than one-third of the ipsilateral middle cerebral artery territory, a previously occluded middle cerebral artery mainstem has recanalised, there is a 50-99% carotid stenosis and no evidence of parenchymal haemorrhage or significant brain oedema. This patient seems to fit within this context, so yes I would consider early carotid endarterectomy."

What else would you want to check before proceeding to surgery?

- "I would discuss the case in a mini-MDT setting with my vascular surgery, interventional radiology and stroke colleagues. I would ensure the patient was on best medical therapy i.e. antiplatelet and a statin. I would want to make sure the blood pressure was currently well-controlled. I would also counsel the patient on the proposed operation. If the plan was approved, I would speak to the anaesthetist very carefully about how we are going to manage his blood pressure. As a precaution I think an arterial line and post-operative stay in a high dependency setting would be wise."

Why are you worried about the blood pressure?

- "I am mainly worried about the risk of post-reperfusion parenchymal haemorrhage."

What if the patient instead had been thrombolysed, but he was left with a more significant disability?

- I would not rush into early surgery in this setting. The ESVS guidelines recommend that revascularisation should be deferred in patients with 50-99% stenoses who suffer a disabling stroke (modified Rankin score ≥3)"

In this context, when else would you avoid early surgery?

- "If the area of infarction exceeded one-third of the ipsilateral middle cerebral artery territory, and if the patient had altered consciousness/drowsiness. The reason I would not rush in would be to minimise the risks of post-operative parenchymal haemorrhage."

Let's say that such a patient makes a reasonable neurological improvement within about 1 week, however more than one-third of his MCA was affected. When would you intervene surgically?

- "I don't think there is a right answer here. An important concern when performing carotid endarterectomy after intravenous thrombolysis (IVT) is the increased risk of intra-cerebral haemorrhage following reperfusion of ischaemic cerebral tissue. The optimal timing remains unknown. It is essential, however, that patients who undergo treatment within a few days of completing thrombolysis are monitored carefully and treated actively for post-endarterectomy hypertension. In regards to the patient in question who had what sounds like a fairly big neurological event, there is an argument to delay intervention beyond the usual 2-week window. In any case I would discuss the case in the vascular MDT as this is a complex case."

Would you consider carotid stenting in this patient?

- "It is possible. I am sure there are many neuroradiologists who treat acute strokes and do fly-by extra-cranial carotid artery stenting. Therefore it can be considered, and it would potentially be worth a discussion. I am not fully versed in the evidence base for this within this specific context. In general however, I would be more worried about the increased peri-procedural risk of stroke with carotid stenting, therefore I would be more inclined towards carotid endarterectomy."

Final question. If you had a patient referred to you for crescendo TIAs or stroke-in-evolution, what would be your management?

- "I would consider the patient for urgent carotid endarterectomy, preferably within 24 hours."

Your FRCS Short Case Ends

Relevant ESVS Guideline Recommendations

- Revascularisation should be deferred in patients with 50–99% stenoses who suffer a disabling stroke (modified Rankin score ≥3), whose area of infarction exceeds one-third of the ipsilateral middle cerebral artery territory, or who have altered consciousness/drowsiness, to minimise the risks of post-operative parenchymal haemorrhage.

- Patients with 50–99% stenoses who present with stroke-in-evolution or crescendo transient ischaemic attacks should be considered for urgent carotid endarterectomy, preferably <24 hours.

- Early carotid endarterectomy (within 14 days) should be considered after intravenous thrombolysis in symptomatic patients if they make a rapid neurological recovery (Rankin 0–2), the area of infarction is less than one-third of the ipsilateral middle cerebral artery territory, a previously occluded middle cerebral artery mainstem has recanalised, there is a 50–99% carotid stenosis and no evidence of parenchymal haemorrhage or significant brain oedema.

- It is recommended that intravenous heparin and antiplatelet therapy be withheld for 24 hours after completion of intravenous thrombolysis, but antiplatelet therapy should then be commenced before any carotid intervention is undertaken.

- It is recommended that patients undergoing early carotid interventions after thrombolysis should have post-interventional hypertension actively treated to reduce the risks of parenchymal haemorrhage.

JMF Reflections

These are not easy questions to answer. Generally speaking, however, you can still give a decent response by sticking to the guidelines, remembering the core vascular surgery papers, and presenting some reasoned arguments. I would avoid getting sucked into the territory of neurointerventional radiology however. Neurointerventional radiology is an entire speciality of its own and I am not an expert here, and you probably are not either. I am sure when patients come in with acute strokes neurointerventional radiologists must do things like catheter-directed thrombolysis or mechanical thrombectomy, and on occasion must identify an extra-cranial carotid stenosis. Whether they routinely stent or don't stent these lesions I just don't know. What the evidence base for stenting in this exact scenario is (i.e. at the exact time of neurointerventional radiology intervention), again I just don't know. I am not going to try and find out either because this is beyond my speciality frankly. As for me, within the context of vascular surgery, I am aware that carotid stenting carries an increased risk of peri-procedural stroke compared to carotid endarterectomy.

CHAPTER 16

Vascular Access

This is another difficult topic to cover authoritatively in a book like this. Vascular access is an enormous topic, and it really deserves an entire book to be devoted to it! However, in this chapter, I hope to use some reality-based examples that I hope will illustrate the salient points that are relevant for the FRCS examination and your baseline day 1 consultant practice. Hope it helps.

CASE 16.1: Fistula Planning Assessment

- A 40-year-old gentleman with chronic kidney failure stage 4.
- His eGFR is 29.
- He has been referred to your vascular access clinic for consideration of fistula creation.

Your FRCS Long Case Begins

What would you like to know in the history and examination?

- "I would start off by asking if he is left handed or right handed. I would focus on the non-dominant arm and ask if he has had any previous fistulas/grafts/midlines/PICC lines/central lines here. I would also want to know if he has had any DVTs in this arm. In terms of examination, I would examine the entire non-dominant arm from hand up to include the axilla, neck and chest wall. I am interested in the pulse assessment (potentially including an Allen's test, and also the quality of the veins with a tourniquet on. Ideally the room would also be warm to aid with venodilation."

The patient is right handed. He has a full complement of left upper limb pulses. Allen's test suggests his palmar arch is intact. He appears to have a decent cephalic vein from wrist up to the antecubital fossa. Are you happy to plan the fistula?

- "No. I would still examine the contralateral (dominant arm) as a matter of routine, and I would also do a point of care ultrasound assessment of both arms."

OK. Can you please interpret this fistula planning ultrasound report?

- "The left radial artery is 2.5 mm in diameter, and the cephalic vein at the wrist and running up the forearm is consistently around 2.8 mm in diameter. The radial artery is also disease-free and demonstrates triphasic flow. This therefore means that I deem this patient suitable for a left radiocephalic fistula creation. This is the preferred access according to the recent ESVS guidelines on vascular access, and what I would plan to do."

What if the left radial artery was less than 2 mm in diameter, and the cephalic vein at the wrist was 2 mm in diameter. What would you do now?

- "Well, according to this ultrasound report, the brachial artery is 3.1 mm in diameter, disease-free, and demonstrates triphasic flow. The cephalic vein at the antercubital fossa is 3.4 mm in diameter, and remains around this size up towards the shoulder. Therefore I think a left brachiocephalic fistula would be the next fistula I would choose."

What if the cephalic vein at the antecubital fossa was only 2 mm in diameter? Would you be happy with this?

- "No. For myself, I would only really accept a brachiocephalic fistula if the cephalic vein was >2.5 mm. In fact, I would prefer it even bigger."

So what would be your next option?

- "Well, according to this ultrasound report, the left basilic vein appears suitable. It is consistently above 3 mm in diameter from the elbow up towards the axilla. I could therefore consider a basilic vein transposition fistula."

Why not consider a graft instead of this?

- "Well I could do. However, the ESVS guidelines on vascular access states in recommendation 21 that when the upper arm cephalic vein is unavailable, a basilic vein transposition arteriovenous fistula should be considered in preference to an arteriovenous graft because of its improved patency and the reduced risk of infection."

Would you create a basilic vein transposition as a single or two-stage procedure?

- "It depends upon the clinical context. If the basilic vein looked great and the patient needed to go onto dialysis fairly soon, I would do it all in one sitting. On the other hand, if the basilic vein was slightly small, and I had time on my hands, I would do a brachio-basilic fistula to see if the vein matured. If it did mature, then I would complete the second stage probably in around 4–6 weeks time. Generally speaking however, I prefer to do it all in one sitting."

If the left basilic vein did not look great, what would be your next option?

- "Well. The left axillary vein is 4.1 mm in diameter. Therefore, the patient is suitable for a left brachio-axillary graft. However, in his right arm the patient also appears to be suitable for both a radiocephalic and a brachiocephalic fistula. As for me, I would have an honest conservation with the patient and see what he thought. Although focusing on the non-dominant arm is the textbook way to approach vascular access, generally speaking I would try to achieve autologous access in preference to using prosthetic material because of the infection risk. Creating a left brachio-axillary graft also potentially puts the patient at increased risk of steal syndrome. I think therefore that there is a serious argument in favour of a right radiocephalic fistula as opposed to a left arm graft in this situation."

Let's say that the patient does not want you to touch his dominant right arm yet. Let's also say he has a left-sided internal jugular vein tunnelled line in situ at the moment which he is dialysing through. Would you be happy to create a left-sided brachio-axillary graft?

- "No. According to the ESVS guidelines on vascular access, recommendation 20 states that if there is an indwelling central venous catheter or pacemaker the vascular access should be created in the opposite arm because of the risk of central venous stenosis and reduced access patency. As such, this would further persuade me to create a right radiocephalic fistula."

What if the patient told you he had previously had a left-sided central line, but it has since been removed? Does this affect your management?

- "I would want to carefully examine the left neck/chest/axilla to see if there are any signs of central venous obstruction or stenosis."

Can you please interpret this image?

- "This is the left neck/chest/axilla of a patient who clearly has central venous disease. There are many dilated veins across the chest wall. If this was the patient in question I would not do a left sided fistula or graft. I would focus on the right arm instead."

What other options have you got for dialysis access then if not the upper limbs?

- "Peritoneal dialysis can be considered. The lower limbs can be considered. There are complex vascular access procedures such as HERO grafts which can be considered."

Would you not consider a long term tunnelled neck line?

- "No I do not consider this to be a viable option in a young patient like this. The infection risk is high therefore I would not consider this a durable long term option."

OK. If you were planning a lower limb vascular access, what would you be thinking?

- "The options are firstly a femoral vein transposition, and secondly a thigh loop graft."

What are the main complications of each?

- "For femoral vein transposition I would be mainly worried about steal syndrome. For a thigh loop graft I would mainly be worried about infection."

Your FRCS Long Case Ends

Relevant ESVS Guideline Recommendations

- Referral of chronic kidney disease patients to the nephrologist and/or surgeon for preparing vascular access is recommended when they reach stage 4 of chronic kidney disease (glomerular filtration rate <30 ml/min/1.73 m²), especially in cases of rapidly progressing nephropathy.
- A permanent vascular access should be created 3–6 months before the expected start of haemodialysis treatment.
- An autogenous arteriovenous fistula is recommended as the primary option for vascular access.
- The radiocephalic arteriovenous fistula is recommended as the preferred vascular access.
- When vessel suitability is adequate, the non-dominant extremity should be considered as the preferred location for vascular access.
- A lower extremity vascular access should be considered only when upper extremity access is impossible.

- Tunnelled cuffed central venous catheters as a long standing haemodialysis modality should be considered when the creation of arteriovenous fistulas or grafts is impossible or in patients with limited life expectancy.
- Preoperative ultrasonography of bilateral upper extremity arteries and veins is recommended in all patients when planning the creation of a vascular access.
- Patients should be examined prior to surgery with a tourniquet in a warm room and the proposed site of an arteriovenous fistula should be marked preoperatively.
- In adults when the inner radial arterial diameter is less than 2.0 mm and/or the cephalic venous diameter is less than 2.0 mm by ultrasound measurement an alternative site for access should be considered.
- If there is an indwelling central venous catheter or pacemaker, the vascular access should be created in the opposite arm because of the risk of central venous stenosis and reduced access patency.
- When the upper arm cephalic vein is unavailable, a basilic vein transposition arteriovenous fistula should be considered in preference to an arteriovenous graft because of its improved patency and the reduced risk of infection.
- When lower limb vascular access is necessary, a femoral vein transposition should be considered in preference to an arteriovenous graft.

CASE 16.2: Early Access Complication

- A 72-year-old female 1-hour post-op following a left brachiocephalic fistula creation.
- This was done under local anaesthetic.
- You are called to theatre recovery because the patient has severe pain.

Your FRCS Short Case Begins

How would you assess this patient?

- "I would do a focused history and examination. In the history I am interested in the nature of the pain, when did it start, how bad it is. I also want to know if there are related symptoms such as neurological compromise such as reduced power or sensation in the hand or forearm. In the examination I would want to confirm that the fistula had a thrill, that the wound site was OK, the distal pulse status and perfusion status of the hand, and what the power and sensation was like in the hand."

The fistula is working well. There is a good thrill. There is no bleeding and no haematoma. The patient has an intact radial pulse, and the left hand is warm and well perfused. However, she is in a lot of pain around the hand and lower forearm. What are you worried about?

- "I am worried that this patient has ischaemic monomelic neuropathy. I would want to know the neurological findings from the examination."

OK. There is paraesthesia of the left forearm and hand. The patient is unable to move her fingers and wrist. There is clawing of left hand, and the patient is unable to extend the wrist and fingers. There is loss of sensation involving the palm and dorsum of the left hand. Clinical features are suggestive of median, radial, and ulnar nerve palsies.

- "In my opinion this confirms my diagnosis. I would take the patient back to theatre and immediately ligate the fistula."

Would you not consider other diagnoses like stroke? Would you not consider nerve conduction studies first? This is a precious fistula.

- "No. With the information I have been given I believe the diagnosis here is ischaemic monomelic neuropathy. Waiting around for hours (if not days) for a CT brain or nerve conduction studies I suspect will only result in delaying me doing what needs to be done. If this fistula is not ligated quickly the patient will very likely be left with permanent and severe neurological dysfunction in this left arm."

You are struggling to get back into your elective theatre because the day team have already gone home. You speak to the theatre coordinator and ask if you can use the emergency theatre. However, the coordinator says it is not an emergency, and therefore, it should wait until the next day.

- "I would not accept this. This is an emergency, much in the same way as acute limb ischaemia or compartment syndrome is. I would speak to the emergency anaesthetist on-call and explain why I needed to go next into theatre, and if required escalate the case to the theatre matron."

You take the patient back to theatre and ligate the fistula. The neurological symptoms improve rapidly. The patient asks if you can create another fistula on the other arm, so she does not have to come back for another operation.

- "No. I would not do this. This is the emergency theatre list and I was doing an emergency procedure. I would not do anything else at this stage. I would carefully plan the next vascular access procedure at a later date, potentially considering other options such as peritoneal dialysis or maybe even a right radiocephalic fistula if that were possible."

Your FRCS Short Case Ends

Relevant ESVS Guideline Recommendations

- Acute ischaemic neuropathy should be treated by immediate vascular access ligation to prevent further neurological deficit.

JMF Reflections

This is a case where the examiners are seeing what you are made of. The diagnosis of IMN is pretty obvious. However, will you actually ligate the fistula when you are supposed to, or will you faff around for hours or days getting numerous second opinions or requesting different investigations? What if you have to push into the emergency theatre? Will you fight your case, or will you recoil in fear? This case is pretty simple in principle, but complex in its practical application. Essentially, for the exam and for the real world, once you make the diagnosis (which in my opinion is clinical), just ligate the fistula/graft. End of story.

CASE 16.3: Early Access Complication

- It is 2:30 am.
- Your registrar telephones you about a 56-year-old gentleman who is 3 weeks post-op following a left brachio-axillary graft creation.
- The patient has presented to A&E with arterial bleeding from the antecubital fossa wound that has dehisced.
- The patient has a tourniquet on and is currently haemodynamically stable.

Your FRCS Short Case Begins

What is your impression?

- "It sounds like the arterial anastomosis has dehisced. My initial thoughts would be that this is likely to be an infected graft."

What is your management plan?

- "I would first go and assess the patient for myself, starting off with the basics. I would take a history and examine the patient. I would confirm haemodynamic stability. I would want to check the bloods (i.e. FBC, U&Es, clotting, CRP, group and save, crossmatch a few units of blood, blood cultures). I would carefully inspect the wound to see if there was gross evidence of infection. If it were safe, I may also consider releasing the tourniquet temporarily to confirm that this was indeed an arterial bleed."

Can you please describe what you see in this picture?

- "Yes. There is a horizontal scar in the left antecubital fossa. The lateral aspect of the wound has fully healed. However, the medial aspect of the wound has fully dehisced. I can see graft. There is clotted blood evident. The tissues also look generally inflamed and there appears to be purulent fluid coming the wound. The arm also looks erythematous and slightly swollen. In my opinion this is an infected exposed graft and the blood in the wound strongly suggests the arterial anastomosis has been jeopardised."

You temporarily deflate the tourniquet and arterial blood sprays out of the wound. What would you do now?

- "I would quickly reinflate the tourniquet. I would alert the emergency theatre coordinator and emergency anaesthetist on-call. I would counsel/consent the patient for emergency graft ligation and explantation."

The patient asks you to try and save the graft because he does not want to have to go back to using a tunnelled neck line. What would you say to him?

- "I would explain to him that I cannot safely salvage this graft. It is grossly infected and the suture that is holding the graft to the artery has disintegrated. Without the tourniquet he would simply bleed to death and die. Simply re-doing the suture repair would lead to the same problem again, and this would be negligent on my part. Therefore all of this plastic material has to be removed to eradicate the infection. This is not ideal, and you apologise in advance, but this is a life-threatening condition, and this is the recommended safe option."

You take the patient to theatre. The tourniquet is still on, quite high up the arm under the axilla. What would you actually do surgically?

- "I would leave that tourniquet on as it is currently achieving proximal control. I would do the operation in 2 parts (i.e. prep twice). I would first prep the arm below this tourniquet. I would make the antecubital fossa incision larger. If there was any purulent or infected tissue I would take samples for microbiology. I would slope the brachial artery above and below the anastomosis, and apply clamps above and below the anastomosis. Then I would ligate the prosthetic graft above the anastomosis. Now I would take the anastomosis down. I would try to find some vein to harvest for a vein patch i.e. basilic vein/median cubital vein/cephalic vein. I would hand this vein out to the scrub nurse to place in a container filled with heparinised saline. Now I would switch to the second part of the operation. I would ask for the tourniquet to the removed, and then I would completely re-prep the whole arm again so that the axilla is also included in the surgical field. At this point, I would confirm the brachial artery inflow was decent. Then I would do a gentle Fogarty balloon embolectomy of the distal brachial artery and check there was decent backbleeding. I would copiously washout the antecubital fossa wound with 1–2 litres of warmed normal saline. Then I would complete the vein patch repair of the brachial artery arteriotomy using 6-0 prolene. The final part of the operation would involve re-opening the axillary incision, disconnecting the graft from the axillary vein, and then suturing the venous defect using 6-0 prolene. I would remove the entire graft and send samples for microbiology. I would close both wounds to ensure sufficient tissue coverage of the arterial and venous repairs, leaving drains in both wounds."

Why would you insist on removing the whole graft? Why not just disconnect the prosthetic graft at the arterial end and leave it at that? Wouldn't that make the operation much simpler?

- "I guess in one sense you are right. You could sell this as a damage control procedure if the patient were grossly unstable. Ligation alone may also be appropriate if this were a fistula and not a graft. However, the patient is stable. Also, the ESVS guidelines on vascular access states this in recommendation 28: *early peri-operative (<30 days) arteriovenous graft infection with systemic sepsis, purulent discharge, perigraft abscess or haemorrhage should be treated by total graft removal.* This graft is clearly grossly infected, and I think the safest and most sensible option is to just explant it all i.e. do the right thing first time around."

Your FRCS Short Case Ends

Relevant ESVS Guideline Recommendations

- In patients with early peri-operative (<30 days) autogenous arteriovenous fistula infection and absence of haemorrhage or pseudoaneurysm, appropriate antibiotic therapy is recommended.
- Early peri-operative (<30 days) arteriovenous graft infection with systemic sepsis, purulent discharge, perigraft abscess or haemorrhage should be treated by total graft removal.
- For early autogenous arteriovenous fistula infection in the presence of systemic signs, bleeding and involvement of the anastomosis, fistula ligation should be performed.

CASE 16.4: Late Access Complications (Fistula Aneurysm)

- A 59-year-old gentleman presents with a large lobulated pulsatile swelling in his left arm at the site of a left brachiocephalic fistula.
- The patient is not complaining of pain but he says this swelling is unsightly and he wants it fixing.

Your FRCS Short Case Begins

Can you please review this photograph of the patient's arm and describe what you see?

- "This is a photograph of the patient's left upper arm. There is a large lobulated aneurysm of the left brachiocephalic fistula. There are actually 3 parts to the aneurysm, which one can describe as a camel's hump type aneurysm. There is no overlying skin threat, no signs of bleeding, and no signs of infection. I would use describe this as a Valenti Type 2a fistula aneurysm."

What else would you want to know in the history and examination?

- "I would ask about how the patient is dialysing i.e. are there problems with prolonged bleeding after the needles are removed? Is there any re-circulation? Are there high venous pressure? There may be an underlying venous stenosis that is partly responsible for the development of these aneurysmal segments. I would also want to know if these aneurysms have developed at the sites of repeated needling. On examination I would want to confirm if there was decent thrill in the fistula, or is it mainly a pulse. Lack of a thrill would again suggest a venous outflow stenosis. I would want to confirm the pulse status distally i.e. is there a radial pulse. Finally I would examine the chest wall to look for signs of central venous stenosis such as venous collateralisation around the neck/chest/axilla."

Would you like to do any investigations?

- "Yes. I would start off with a fistula ultrasound scan. Depending upon what this showed, I may also need to do further imaging to investigate for a central venous problem. This may require a CT venogram, MR venogram, or possibly going straight for a fistulogram."

The patient has a duplex ultrasound and it confirms these are true aneurysms, and not false aneurysms. There is also no overt evidence of any outflow venous stenosis. Similarly the patient is otherwise dialysing normally without recirculation, high venous pressures or cannulation site bleeding issues. What are your options to manage these fistula aneurysms?

- "There is of course an option to do nothing, and simply manage things conservatively. However, as per the original paper by Valenti et al (2014), I would be more worried about this type of fistula aneurysm. These aneurysms are associated with needling, and they are at significant risk of rupture and need to be monitored carefully or treated prophylactically. The potential surgical procedures include (1) ligation of the aneurysmal section and autologous vein bypass or graft interposition, (2) resection of the aneurysmal section and re-anastomosing the two healthy ends of the vein if it is very redundant, (3) fistula aneurysm aneurysmorrhaphy, and (4) ligate and excise fistula alone with no plan for reconstruction, and for creation of a new vascular access (preferably autologous) on the other arm."

You decide to take the patient to theatre and do a fistula aneurysm aneurysmorrhaphy. How would you do this?

- "I would expose the entire length of the aneurysm/s to so the three aneurysms were fully exposed. I would also expose healthy vein above and below these aneurysms for proximal and distal control. I would open the aneurysms and resect redundant tissue. Then I would ask for a suitable length of chest drain to go inside the fistula, and then do a continuous 5-0 prolene suture repair over this chest drain to ensure the lumen was still big enough. After this if there were redundant skin I would excise this, then close the skin using interrupted 3-0 ethilon vertical mattress sutures."

You create the new fistula but afterwards you cannot feel a thrill. You can only feel a pulse. What would you do now?

- "I would scan the fistula using the ultrasound machine. It sounds like there may be some clot which has embolised upstream into the proximal vein."

The ultrasound shows that the fistula is patent, but there is no colour flow in the cephalic vein at the upper level of the axilla. What would you do now?

- "I would make a short cutdown over the cephalic vein at this site. I would ask for 5000 units of intravenous heparin, control the vein, make a small venotomy, and do a gentle Fogarty balloon embolectomy to trawl this clot. If I achieved decent backbleeding I would simply close the venotomy."

What would you do if no clot was trawled and the backbleeding was not great?

- "I would do an on-table angiogram."

Can you please interpret this angiogram please?

- "This seems to show a tight venous stenosis around the level of the cephalic arch. At this junction I would call for interventional radiology assistance. Usually for venous outflow stenosis the recommendation is for balloon angioplasty. However, as per the ESVS guidelines on vascular access, endovascular treatment with stent grafts should be considered for the treatment of cephalic arch stenosis."

Your FRCS Short Case Ends

Relevant ESVS Guideline Recommendations

- Surgical revision of vascular access aneurysms is recommended if cannulation sites and access diameter can be preserved.
- *Surgical revision of pseudoaneurysms in arteriovenous grafts is recommended when the aneurysm:* Limits the availability of cannulation sites or is associated with pain, poor scar formation, spontaneous bleeding, and rapid expansion.
- Outflow stenosis should be ruled out in symptomatic vascular access aneurysms and treated when present.
- Balloon angioplasty is recommended for the treatment of venous outflow stenosis.
- Endovascular treatment with stent grafts should be considered for the treatment of cephalic arch stenosis.

Case 16.5: Late Access Complications (Thrombosed Graft)

- A 68-year-old woman is referred by the renal team with a thrombosed right brachio-axillary graft.

- This graft is around 1 year old.
- This graft probably occluded 2–3 days ago.
- This occlusion has been confirmed on ultrasound.

Your FRCS Short Case Begins

What would be your management approach for this patient?

- "There are two potential approaches to salvage this graft. One is an open surgical approach with thrombectomy of the graft and on-table imaging of the central venous system +/− central venous endovascular intervention as required. The other option is an entirely endovascular approach with thrombolysis +/− treatment of underlying venous outflow stenosis. The endovascular approach may include catheter-directed thrombolysis, mechanical thrombectomy or thrombo-aspiration."

Which do you think is the best approach?

- "The ESVS guidelines on vascular access suggest that for thrombosed vascular access grafts, surgical thrombectomy and endovascular therapy had comparable results. As such I cannot authoritatively say one approach is better than the other. I think these cases should be individualised depending upon patient, practitioner and individual units. In my practice I would discuss these cases with the interventional radiology team and my consultant colleagues who have a special interest in vascular access before rushing into making a decision. Indeed, with thrombosed grafts, there is less of an urgency in unblocking them. However, if I had to make a decision, I would veer in favour of open surgical intervention."

What if this was a thrombosed brachiocephalic fistula then?

- "This is a different scenario in terms of timing. Treatment needs to be started as soon as possible to prevent organisation of the thrombus and endothelial damage in the vein. Again, the evidence suggests that there is no overwhelming difference between open surgery and endovascular techniques for thrombosed fistulas. For me I think I would be more inclined to treat these with open surgery +/− on-table treatment of any venous outflow lesions. This is because, in general, I think open surgery is faster."

OK. Let's say that you have a thrombosed left brachiocephalic fistula. The patient goes instead for an endovascular attempt at salvage. The interventional radiologists manage to remove the thrombus by way of pharmaco-mechanical thrombectomy. There is a venous outflow stenosis in the mid-upper arm that they angioplasty with a good result. The fistula is now running away. However, the interventional radiologist calls you down to review the angiogram. Can you please describe what you see?

- "There appears to be a juxta-anastomotic stenosis around 2 cm beyond where the cephalic vein joins the brachial artery. It looks like it is around a 50% stenosis."

The interventional radiologist asks what you think they should do. What would you say?

- "I would explain that the ESVS guidelines on vascular access suggests that balloon angioplasty can be used as the primary approach for juxta-anastomotic stenosis. However, the recurrent stenosis rate is higher than after surgery. The options are therefore to not treat this lesion, and instead book the patient for surgery on this admission to revise this short section of vein. However, since we are already here and this lesion looks to be eminently treatable by way of angioplasty, I think this is the pragmatic approach. We can get a surveillance ultrasound in a few weeks' time, and if this lesion recurs we can consider surgical revision at that stage."

What if the interventional radiologist had instead shown you this image instead?

- "This image demonstrates a central venous stenosis i.e. there is a left brachiocephalic vein stenosis."

The interventional radiologist asks you if he should stent this lesion. What would you say?

- "I would explain that the ESVS guidelines on vascular access would primarily support balloon angioplasty as the primary treatment of symptomatic central venous outflow disease is recommended, with repeated interventions if indicated. Therefore this would be my recommendation. However, if recurrence continued to be an issue stenting should be considered."

Stent grafting? Why not consider a bare metal stent?

- "No. Bare metal stents have not demonstrated an advantage in long term patency over balloon angioplasty."

OK. Back-tracking a little .... If this was a thrombosed brachiocephalic fistula or graft that was 2 days old, what would be your management plan?

- "In my opinion early thrombosis will likely be related to technical errors during surgery. As such, my preference would be to take the patient back to theatre. I would explore the wound for any haematoma, probably take down the anastomosis and do a gentle Fogarty embolectomy of the fistula/graft, and then re-do the anastomosis. I would do an on-table angiogram after this to make sure there was no venous outflow problem as well."

Would you not consider endovascular intervention as opposed to open surgery?

- "This is only 2 days following the access creation. As such I think the primary issue here for a fistula is likely to be a technical error, therefore I would rather take the patient back to theatre. If it were instead a graft, also I would suspect there was a technical issue. However, even if I were considering an endovascular approach (i.e. thrombolysis), this is best delayed for at least 7 days after the vascular access creation to allow tissue incorporation to prevent puncture site bleeding."

What if the vascular access (fistula or graft) had occluded 3 weeks post-operatively?

- "In this situation I would consider both open surgical and endovascular options. The ESVS guidelines on vascular access highlights that there are no randomised trials that compare the two approaches, so we cannot draw any definite conclusions on which is the better approach. The guidelines did highlight however that the current evidence did seem to suggest there was a possible advantage in terms of better long term patency with surgical thrombectomy. Again I would judge things on a case by case basis."

Your FRCS Short Case Ends

Relevant ESVS Guideline Recommendations

- Surgery or endovascular methods should be considered for treatment of late thrombosis of vascular accesses depending on the centre's expertise.
- Treatment of vascular access thrombosis should include peri-operative diagnosis and treatment of any associated stenosis.
- Balloon angioplasty as primary treatment of symptomatic central venous outflow disease is recommended, with repeat interventions if indicated.
- The use of stent grafts may be considered for the treatment of central vein stenosis.
- Stenting or repeat balloon angioplasty should be considered if there is significant elastic recoil of the central vein after balloon angioplasty or if the stenosis recurs within 3 months.
- For vascular access salvage after early thrombosis, thrombectomy and revision (if needed) should be performed as soon as possible.
- Thrombolysis should not be used for early vascular access thrombosis within 7 days of creation.

CASE 16.6: Late Access Complication

- A 39-year-old gentleman has a right brachio-axillary graft.
- He has noticed a new lump over the anterior upper arm at one of the needling sites that is painful.
- There is no active bleeding.
- He is systemically well.

Your FRCS Short Case Begins

What is your differential diagnosis?

- "This lump could represent a puncture site haematoma which is otherwise benign. It could be an abscess. It could be a pseudoaneurysm of the graft. These would be my main thoughts."

Can you please describe what you see in this picture?

- "There appears to be a 1.5 cm lump over the anterior upper arm in this gentleman's right arm. There does not appear to be any gross signs of infection. The skin overlying the lump appears intact. There are no signs of bleeding. The skin itself does not look bruised. I can see that this is one of the sites where the graft is routinely needled. My thoughts based upon this image are that this is most likely a graft pseudoaneurysm, likely related to repeated needling. I suspect the button-hole technique is being used for this graft."

How would you confirm the diagnosis?

- "I examine the patient and see if this lump was pulsatile or had a thrill. I would also request an urgent ultrasound duplex of the arm."

The patient has a duplex ultrasound, and it confirms this is a 1.7-cm pseudoaneurysm of the graft. The pseudoaneurysm demonstrates colour flow on the duplex, and it is around 2 mm

below the surface of the skin. The graft is otherwise functioning normally. What would your management be?

- "AV graft pseudoaneurysms are ideally treated by resection and interposition grafting/ bypass. If the graft was infected however it would likely require complete graft excision. There is also the secondary option of inserting a covered stent to exclude this aneurysm, with a plan for needling to occur above and below this covered stent."

Could you not simply manage this pseudoaneurysm conservatively?

- "You can manage anything conservatively. However, this aneurysm is 2 mm away from the skin surface, it is of a reasonable size, and I can really picture this thing rupturing and the patient bleeding to death. I would feel nervous about managing it conservatively."

The patient does not want further surgery, and says he wants to try the covered stent. He is put on the waiting list for this, with a plan for it to be inserted in the next 2 weeks. What would you advise the patient in the meantime?

- "I would strongly advise him, and the dialysis team, to not continue to needle this area. I would also tell the patient that if the skin over this lump breaks down, there are any ulcers or bleeding, that he needs to come back to see a vascular surgeon immediately."

Four days later you are on-call. It is 10:30 pm and you are called from A&E resus. This patient has re-presented because he has had some bleeding from his arm. This was initially mild. The patient got into the shower and then all of a sudden there was torrential bleeding from his arm. A&E are struggling to control the bleeding. How would you manage this?

- "I would first clarify exactly how A&E are trying to manage the bleeding. In this scenario the ideal thing is to get a bottle top cushioned by a piece of gauze, and use a thumb to press it directly down over the bleeding point. This bottle top can then be wrapped securely in place using a crepe bandage. This should stop the bleeding and calm the situation down. What I would not do is put loads of swabs or towels around the area, or apply a poor quality tourniquet around the upper arm as this tends to exacerbate bleeding. I would advise A&E to do this whilst I come to see the patient ...."

OK. This is done. The patient has his bloods taken, IV access, crossmatched a few units of blood, made NBM, etc. What would you do from a vascular surgery perspective?

- "I would primarily consent the patient for urgent ligation of the graft +/− excision. I would do this case tonight and treat it as an emergency."

The patient asks if you can try and save the graft.

- "I would explain to the patient that at the moment he has a life-threatening problem. This is my primary concern. I am mainly focused on stopping him bleeding the death. The safest and most simple option is to ligate the graft. However, I would also explain that if it were possible to save the graft I would consider this. This would only be the case if the patient was haemodynamically stable and there were no obvious signs of infection."

What about endovascular covered stent grafting in the emergency setting?

- "You are correct. This is another potential option that can be considered. It is arguably one way to save the graft. However, in this emergency setting one might err on the side of caution and assume this is an infected bleeding graft pseudoaneurysm. Putting in more prosthetic material may not be a good idea. Also, getting decent access to insert such a covered stent may be challenging. My gut feeling would be to proceed with open surgery, and adhere to core vascular surgery principles (i.e. proximal control, distal control, then to attack the injury. Open surgery would also allow me to confirm if the graft was infected, remove it if necessary, and to get microbiological samples. I feel I could justify my decision to proceed with open surgery."

You take the patient to theatre. How would you tackle this from a surgical perspective?

- "I assume the bottle-top technique is currently achieving haemorrhage control? Therefore I would not disturb this. I would prep the entire arm to include the bottle-top and crepe bandage. I would gain proximal control of the brachial artery in the antecubital fossa. After this I would get distal control of the graft above the crepe bandage. Now I would ask my assistant to hold the arm up whilst I take the crepe bandage down and hand the bottle-top out. I would re-prep the arm again and change my gloves for clean ones. Now I can attack the injury. I would explore the area of bleeding, enlarging my incision so I can identify both the underlying graft and the pseudoaneurysm. The options at this stage would depend upon how stable the patient was, and whether there were obvious signs of infection."

If there were no signs of infection and the patient was completely stable, what are your options?

- "Ligation alone is always an option. There is also the option to simply remove this isolated part of the graft and replace it with a short interposition PTFE graft. Another option is to do a bypass around this area through healthy tissue using PTFE graft."

What if the underlying graft was bathed in pus?

- "I would explant the entire graft and repair the brachial artery arteriotomy site with a vein patch."

Would you not consider a bypass around the infected area through healthy skin using PTFE graft?

- "I don't like playing with fire. This does not sound like a sensible idea. If I did this I would expect this graft to then get infected. I'm sure there are some vascular surgeons who would consider this approach, but I am not one of them. If the graft was bathed in pus my plan would be to explant the graft, not stick in more prosthetic material."

What if the graft looked to be infected but the patient was grossly unstable, i.e., in grade 4 haemorrhagic shock?

- "I would resort to damage control principles in this setting. I would do as short and simple operation as possible to stop bleeding and control contamination, with a plan to bring the patient back for a more definitive procedure once medially optimised.

In this setting that would probably mean ligating the graft above and below the bleeding site, then doing a washout of the bleeding/infected area. I would then consider bringing the patient back to theatre for a definitive explantation when he was physiologically better."

Your FRCS Short Case Ends

Relevant ESV Guideline Recommendations

- *Surgical revision of pseudoaneurysms in arteriovenous grafts is recommended when the aneurysm:* Limits the availability of cannulation sites or is associated with pain, poor scar formation, spontaneous bleeding, and rapid expansion.
- Stent graft exclusion of vascular access aneurysms may be considered in selected patients.
- Access cannulation through a pseudoaneurysm is not recommended.
- In late vascular graft infection, total arteriovenous graft excision is recommended in patients with sepsis, clinical signs of infection, and perigraft fluid around the whole graft.
- Partial excision of an arteriovenous prosthetic graft may be considered in selected cases when sections of the graft are well incorporated and appear to be uninfected.
- The rope ladder technique should be used for cannulation of arteriovenous grafts.

JMF Reflections

These questions were designed to put you on your toes, and see what you are made of. Remember that in the FRCS examination, you are being primarily judged on whether or not you are **safe**. You are also being judged on whether you can come up with common sense plans that adhere to vascular surgery principles. To be perfectly honest, I made all of this case up. It is not real. What you would actually do in reality will be determined by the individual patient that is in front of you. For example, I have used the bottle-top crepe bandage technique with vascular injuries affecting the radial and ulnar arteries, and it did work remarkably well. However, a bottle top was not just dangling in front of me at the time. Somebody in A&E had to go and find it, and it took about 5 minutes for someone to come back. You may find yourself in a situation where nobody can find a bottle top, and so instead you may have to apply a tourniquet to achieve proximal control. Also, how do you prep an arm with this bottle-top/crepe bandage technique? This is how I would do it, but no doubt somebody else has a better approach …. Essentially you just have to think on your feet and make some common sense decisions!

Also, how do you know if a graft is infected or not? I have seen a few patients with anastomotic bleeding following prosthetic bypasses who had no obvious signs of infection, and yet I assumed it was infected and proceeded accordingly (i.e., I ligated the graft and did not reconstruct). Luckily the microbiology came back as confirming infection! In any case, what if you were presented with a case like this one, but there were no obvious signs of infection? Do you reconstruct or do you not reconstruct? I don't know the right answer. However, for the purpose of the FRCS examination, and for the purpose of real life practice, I guess you should always endeavour to be **safe**, and if in doubt err on the side of caution. If you are worried about infection, and that little thing called "instinct" taps you on the shoulder, I would listen up. In these answers, I have tried to demonstrate that above all you want to be demonstrating that you have a firm grasp of the basics: Proximal control, distal control, attack the injury, damage control principles, and being very wary of prosthetic reconstruction in the context of infection.

CASE 16.7: Failure to Mature

- A 58-year-old woman is referred to your vascular access clinic 4 weeks following a left radiocephalic fistula creation.
- The vascular access nurse is concerned because the fistula is not maturing very well.
- She welcomes your expert opinion.

Your FRCS Short Case Begins

What would be your definition of a matured fistula?

- "There is the rule of 6: at least 6 mm vein diameter, 600 ml/min flow, and less than 6 mm vein depth from the skin. In terms of clinical examination findings I would like identify a soft easily compressible vein, a continuous audible bruit, a decent palpable thrill near the anastomosis extending along the vein, with adequate length to allow the fistula to be punctured with two needles."

This fistula has a thrill, but it is very weak. What might be the cause for this?

- "There might be an arterial inflow stenosis, or the anastomosis itself may be narrow. Alternatively there may be venous tributaries that are drawing blood away from the main cephalic vein and thus reducing the flow in the main vein."

What if there was no pulse in the cephalic vein, but instead a pulse?

- "This would suggest an upstream venous stenosis."

How would you investigate this patient?

- "Most of my answers would likely come from the clinical examination and reviewing the fistula planning assessment and operation note. For example, is the radial pulse strong? Are there obvious veins that are coming off the fistula that similarly have a thrill? Is there a pre-operative ultrasound report that comments on the radial artery flow i.e. was it monophasic/biphasic/triphasic? What was the size of the radial artery? Does the operation note state that the radial artery was very small? Does it comment that the cephalic vein was very small? All these factors may be contributing to the failure to mature. However, ultimately I would do a point of care ultrasound assessment in clinic."

Your clinical and ultrasound assessment suggests that there are two large venous tributaries that are drawing a lot of blood away from the main cephalic vein. How would you manage this?

- "I would plan to take the patient to theatre for ligation of these draining venous tributaries under local anaesthetic."

Your ultrasound assessment reveals triphasic flow in the brachial artery, but monophasic flow in the radial artery. How would you manage this?

- "In this case I suspect there is a radial artery inflow stenosis. I would request a fistulogram to confirm this, with a view to balloon angioplasty treatment."

Your clinical findings reveal a pulsatile cephalic vein. As you elevate the arm above the heart the cephalic vein remains pulsatile up the proximal forearm, and it does not collapse. However, above this point, the pulse disappears and the vein appears to collapse. What does this suggest?

- "This suggests that there is a venous stenosis in the cephalic vein in the upper forearm. I would confirm this using ultrasound, and if so I would again request a fistulogram with a view to balloon angioplasty."

What would you do if the cephalic vein was too deep, i.e., it was 1.2 cm beneath the skin?

- "Under local anaesthetic I could do what I describe as an adiposectomy to remove any excessive fat from above the vein."

What if there was no inflow stenosis and outflow stenosis, but the original operation note simply said that the radial artery and cephalic vein were extremely small?

- "In this case there may well be an argument to simply plan a new fistula, such as a brachiocephalic fistula. In such a setting I would probably ligate this radiocephalic fistula in the same setting. I am not saying this is the right course of action, but if a fistula looks genuinely non-viable, it is often worth starting afresh. Ideally however one would not have made this fistula in the first place if the vein and artery were obviously so small."

Final question. You have mentioned duplex ultrasound and catheter angiography for investigating fistulas that are failing to mature. What other radiological options are available?

- "There is CT angiography and MR angiography. These can be considered, but there are potential risks. CT uses iodinated contrast and has a radiation risk. Contrast enhanced MR carries a theoretical risk of causing nephrogenic systemic fibrosis. Henceforth, if these are going to be used, it should only be after carefully weighing the risks and benefits of alternative imaging studies."

Your FRCS Short Case Ends

Relevant ESVS Guideline Recommendations

- Balloon angioplasty is recommended as primary treatment for inflow arterial stenosis of any type of vascular access.
- Balloon angioplasty is recommended for the treatment of venous outflow stenosis.
- If an arteriovenous fistula fails to mature by 6 weeks, additional investigations (like duplex ultrasound) should be considered in order to achieve prompt diagnosis and treatment.
- Duplex ultrasound is recommended as the first-line imaging modality in suspected vascular access dysfunction.
- In vascular access, dysfunction digital subtraction angiography should be performed only when subsequent intervention is anticipated.
- Computed tomographic angiography may be considered in patients with inconclusive ultrasonographic or angiographic results concerning the degree of central venous stenosis.
- Contrast enhanced magnetic resonance angiography is not recommended in patients with end-stage renal disease, because of the potential risk of gadolinium-associated nephrogenic systemic fibrosis.

JMF Reflections

It is worth knowing the ESVS guideline recommendations because on the whole they help streamline your practice. However, I would be ready for some push-back. I remember quoting the ESVS recommendation to avoid MRA in end-stage renal failure patients because of the potential risk of nephrogenic systemic fibrosis. This was in the middle of an MDT. I then found myself in the awkward position of being told by a very experienced and confident interventional radiologist that these risks were very small. I did go away and do some reading about nephrogenic systemic fibrosis after this and found a systematic review and meta-analysis (Woolen et al 2020) that explored this very question. The conclusion from this paper was this: *"This study's findings suggest that the risk of NSF from group II GBCA administration in stage 4 or 5 CKD is likely less than 0.07%. The potential diagnostic harms of withholding group II GBCA for indicated examinations may outweigh the risk of NSF in this population."* The moral of the story here is don't be a smart arse. The other moral of the story is to stick to your speciality. I am not a radiologist, and therefore, I am not going to win a radiology argument with a radiologist. I should just stick to vascular surgery because that is what I am good at (I vaguely think so anyways). This is one of the reasons why I don't have a chapter in this book dedicated to radiology (LOLS).

REFERENCE

Woolen SA, Shankar PR, Gagnier JJ et al. Risk of Nephrogenic Systemic Fibrosis in Patients with Stage 4 or 5 Chronic Kidney Disease Receiving a Group II Gadolinium-Based Contrast Agent: A Systematic Review and Meta-Analysis. JAMA Intern Med (2020) 180(2), 223–230.

STEAL Syndrome

I couldn't do a chapter on vascular access without covering STEAL. However, I am not going to do a case study for this because I think it is too complex. Instead, I thought I would do a brief run through of STEAL (Figure 16.1) to give you a solid grounding in the core principles:

- Severe STEAL occurs in 1% of radial AV fistulas, and in 3–6% of brachial AV fistulas or grafts.
- *Symptoms:* Pain/numbness, persistently cold fingers/hand, decreased sensory or motor function, tissue loss.
- *Main risk factors:* Brachial access, AV grafts, diabetes, female gender, age >60 years, previous steal, peripheral arterial disease, multiple operations in same limb.
- *Differential diagnosis:* Carpal tunnel syndrome, venous hypertension, and IMN should be considered depending upon the clinical context.
- *Classification:*
  Stage 1 = retrograde diastolic flow without complaints
  Stage 2 = pain on exertion, coolness, minimal symptoms
  Stage 3 = rest pain
  Stage 4 = tissue loss (i.e., ulcers and gangrene)
- *Assessment:*
  Clinical → do hand symptoms/signs improve with compression of fistula/graft?
  Doppler ultrasound → with access uncompressed and compressed.
  Wrist or digital arterial pressures: Below 50 mmHg.
  Digital (wrist)/brachial pressure index (DBI): <0.6.
  Pulse oximetry: Oxygen saturations <90%
  Diagnostic angiogram to look for inflow or outflow arterial stenoses (*alternatively can do CTA*).
  Consider nerve conduction studies (*lots of dialysis patients have neuropathy*).

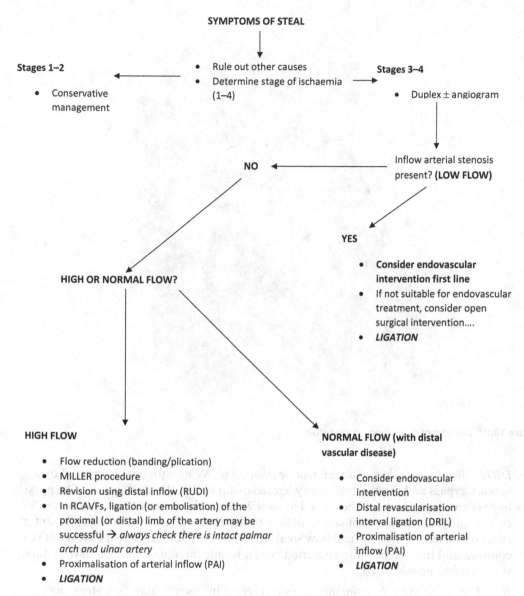

Figure 16.1 General overview of management for vascular access STEAL.

- *Determination of VA flow:*
  - "High flow" (>800 ml/min in native fistula, >1200 ml/min in grafts)
  - "Normal flow"
  - "Low flow" (<400 ml/min in native fistula, <600 ml/min in grafts)

What the heck are all these STEAL procedures about?

- *Banding/plication:* One can excise a portion of vein and plicate with continuous or mattress sutures, and use a cross PTFE band or an interposition of 4 mm PTFE graft. Another option is to trim a piece of Dacron patch into a Christmas tree shape and use it to apply a band around the fistula. This reduces the flow through a high-flow vascular access (Figure 16.2).

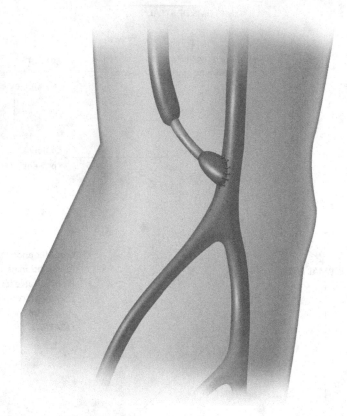

Figure 16.2 Banding of a brachiocephalic fistula.

- *DRIL (distal revascularisation interval ligation):* The AV anastomosis is bridged by a venous bypass and the brachial artery ligated distal to the AV anastomosis. The proximal bypass anastomosis should be placed at least 7–10 cm above the VA anastomosis to ensure adequate deviation of sufficient flow to the distal extremity. DRIL is relevant in cases of normal or near-normal flow steal with distal vascular disease. However, it is a complex and time-consuming operation, and it is only possible when you have suitable vein that can be harvested.

- *RUDI (revision using distal inflow):* This is relevant in cases of high-flow steal secondary to brachial AV access. Closing the anastomosis in the antecubital fossa and interposing a new graft between the forearm radial or ulnar artery has been shown to effectively reduce access flow by up to 50%. Please refer to Figure 16.3 for DRIL and RUDI.

- *PAI (proximalisation of arterial inflow—Figure 16.4):* This again is mainly relevant for brachial AV access steal. It involves disconnecting the current AV anastomosis in the antecubital fossa and using a new graft to extend the anastomosis more proximally, i.e., to the proximal brachial or axillary artery. You are therefore moving the AV anastomosis to a vessel with a larger capacity; hence, the arterial pressure drop distal to the AV anastomosis is significantly lower at the same access flow. By using a longer and tapered graft you will also effectively increase the resistance in the access system. This again should redirect more blood down towards the hand. All this seems a bit counterintuitive and confusing, but for bizarre reason, it does work. Therefore, it is of relevance in both high-flow access steal and in normal flow states but with distal vessel disease (as the overall collateral supply to the hand is improved).

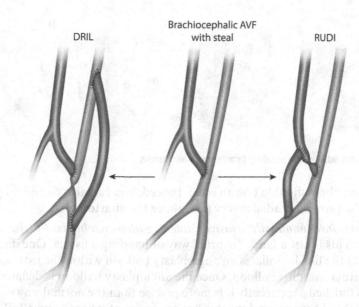

Figure 16.3 DRIL and RUDI procedures for stealing brachiocephalic fistula.

- *Radial artery ligation or embolisation:* If you have a stealing radiocephalic fistula, you can ligate the radial artery distal to the anastomosis (or embolise it). This will prevent the access stealing any blood from the hand. However, this is dangerous. You need to be absolutely certain that the ulnar artery and palmar arch are intact. If you cut off the radial artery supply to the hand and there is no collateral supply, expect there to be some serious ischaemic complications in the hand. However, if the ulnar artery and palmar

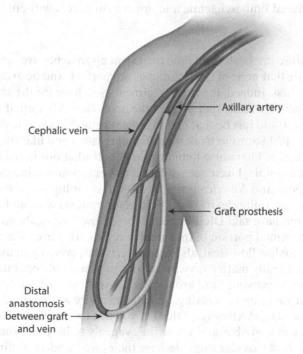

Figure 16.4 Proximalisation procedure for a stealing brachiocephalic fistula using a prosthetic graft to axillary artery.

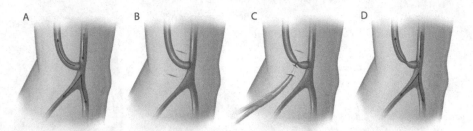

Figure 16.5   Miller procedure for a stealing brachiocephalic fistula.

arch are intact, there shouldn't be an issue. Indeed, you can also consider ligating/ embolising the proximal radial artery (i.e., above the anastomosis).

- *MILLER procedure (minimally invasive limited ligation endoluminal-assisted revision— Figure 16.5):* This is just a fancy "hybrid" way of banding a fistula. One does a little cut down over the fistula, inflates an angioplasty balloon within the fistula, and then ligates the fistula over this balloon. Once the angioplasty balloon is deflated, the banding procedure is finished. Apparently it is more precise than the normal way of banding or placating. I (JMF) have never done this but am aware of it "academically."

Relevant ESVS Guideline Recommendations

- In patients with symptomatic vascular-access-induced extremity ischaemia with arterial inflow, stenosis balloon angioplasty should be considered.
- Symptomatic access-induced extremity ischaemia in patients with high-flow access should be treated by surgical procedures aimed to reduce access flow.
- Distal revascularisation and interval ligation should be considered in patients with vascular-access-induced limb ischaemia and upper arm access without high flow.

JMF Reflections

In my eyes, STEAL is quite complicated, and the treatment approaches are very much "horses for courses." I also surmise that none of the techniques are perfect, and deep down nobody really knows which approach is best. Indeed, the more treatments you have for the same condition usually implies none of them are really that great in the first place. After all, if one treatment was utterly brilliant, there would just be that one treatment right?! There is a lot of overlap in the treatment modalities, e.g., PAI seems to work for different reasons and likewise appears relevant in different access flow situations. I have also found blatant contradictions in the treatment algorithms in varying resources. For example, I have seen different presentations/online videos by respected vascular surgeons (European and American) who say DRIL is for high-flow steal. However, I have seen other guidelines say quite clearly that DRIL is for patients without high flow …. Other respected vascular surgeons have said DRIL is definitely for low flow steal and patients with severe occlusive disease in the proximal portion of the forearm vessels. However, the same person who says DRIL is specifically for low flow steal, also then asserts that even if you use DRIL in a high-flow steal access it does not really matter anyways as long as you do the operation correctly …. Again this is quite difficult to get your head around because different people are saying different things and it all feels a bit vague and confusing, and all you really want is a clear answer! Am I the only person who has noticed this? Anyways, I think if you just have a general understanding of the different treatment strategies available, and where they vaguely fit in, you should be ok in the exam. In the real world, I think most vascular surgeons have their own "understanding" of steal and they have a few chosen treatment strategies that work for them. I hope my algorithm is vaguely sensible, and apologies if you disagree with me. I was caught between a rock and a hard place anyways ….

CHAPTER 17

The IVDU Groin

History

- When last injected?
- What have you injected?
- Any chance there are needles left in your groin?
- Are you using "clean" needles or sharing?
- Have you been injecting elsewhere?
- How long have you been injecting for?
- Have you been screened for HIV/hepatitis?
- Any bleeding from the groin?
- Any fevers/sweats/shakes?
- Noticed any lesions/skin changes affecting your fingers or toes?
- Any shortness of breath?
- Any swelling of your legs?
- Have you had any vascular surgery interventions before?
- Any other medical problems?
- What tablets are you on? Are you on any blood thinners?

Examination

- End of the bed test
- Does the patient look septic?
- Does the patient look anaemic?
- Is the patient shocked?
- *I assume you would notice if blood was hosing from groin....*
- Note heart rate, blood pressure, respiratory rate, temperature, and GCS....
- Any signs of infective endocarditis or DVT?
- Auscultate chest for murmurs etc.
- Assess groin → any sinus/fluctuance/collection/pus discharge/skin threat?
- Assess for venous congestion around groin/abdominal wall
- Assess femoral pulse → feels normal? Obvious pseudoaneurysm? Any thrill (i.e. fistula)?
- Confirm distal pulses and limb viability

Immediate Management for Stable Patient

- IV access (good luck. Probably best using ultrasound. If really struggling will probably need anaesthetist to insert central line).
- Bloods (FBC, U&Es, LFTs, clotting, group & save, and HIV/hepatitis screen).

DOI: 10.1201/b22951-17

- ECG ± CXR if suspect cardiorespiratory pathology.
- Echocardiogram if suspect infective endocarditis ± cardiology review.
- I would always image the femoral vessels unless it was a catastrophic bleed.
- Out of hours → CT angiogram (but need IV access).
- In hours → CT angiogram (but if struggling with IV access ultrasound is next option).

Definitive Management for Stable Patient

- Femoral vessels normal but abscess in groin → try your best to sell to general surgery for incision and drainage.
- Femoral pseudoaneurysm ± infection in groin → generally speaking patient should be considered for femoral vessel ligation.
- Infected femoral vein DVT with gas → this is open to debate. However, my position is this → **do your absolute best to avoid operating**. These cases will get referred to you (usually by the medics) as some vascular emergency. There will be quite a bit of pressure on you to take the patient over and take to theatre urgently etc. I have seen a few of these patients whom my team held their nerve and just treated with antibiotics. The patients got better and avoided an operation. Alternatively, I have heard of cases when other vascular surgeons have chosen to operate, i.e. they have gone in to do a femoral vein thrombectomy etc. All I have heard about these cases is that the vascular surgeon who did it vowed he would never do it again (things tend to bleed horrifically and the veins fall apart …). Don't get me wrong, your hand may get forced and you may have to operate. However, just be wary…
- IVDU patient with incidental finding of foreign body in groin (i.e. a needle). Just say no. Leave the needle where it is. You will only cause more damage by trying to remove it, and only increase your risk of getting a needle stick injury.
- Be wary of the "stable" IVDU patient who has been reported to have had bleeding from the groin (*and has a groin sinus*), a false aneurysm on CT, and is anaemic. There are two possible plans here. One plan is to take to theatre straight away, and the other plan is to resuscitate first and then take to theatre. My position would be to resuscitate and optimise the patient first, and then take to theatre. This would be my preferred plan, especially if it was the middle of the night. However, please be ready for your plan to fail, and be prepared to justify your plan. If you are going to do this, tell the patient to be nil by mouth, crossmatch a few units of blood, transfuse them, tell the patient to stay in bed and not leave the ward (i.e. strict bedrest), alert the nursing staff to look out for any signs of bleeding and to call you immediately if there is, book the patient into theatre pre-emptively, consent and mark the patient, etc. Also document your plan and reason for your plan very clearly. If your plan fails and the patient suddenly starts bleeding, at least you are "ready to go." The reason I would prefer not to rush such a patient to theatre is because in my experience I have seen such patients bleed quite a lot in theatre (venous and arterial bleeding). If they are already anaemic, I am struggling to get control, and there is no one else around to help in the early hours, this could lead to a catastrophic outcome. On the other hand, if the patient is resuscitated and I have surgical back-up around, at least if I run into trouble I am in a better position to overcome such obstacles.

Immediate Management of Unstable Patient (i.e. the Hosing Groin)

- Press on groin (preferably get somebody else to do it).
- Decent IV access.

- Cross-match a load of blood.
- Pray to God patient is not on an anticoagulant. If God is not on your side looks like you are going to have to speak to haematology ....
- Theatre ASAP.
- Rutherford Morrison incision, control external iliac artery.
- Vertical groin incision.
- Start low, find SFA, and sloop / clamp it.
- Work upwards and ideally control profunda.
- Go back to inguinal ligament and identify CFA and control it.
- Don't expect this to be easy → there will likely be a load of haematoma which just makes everything confusing.
- Pragmatically, you may not be able to control the CFA/SFA/PFA in the conventional manner. You may just need to get your assistant to press down using swabs on sticks, open the pseudoaneurysm, and suture the SFA/PFA origins from within the sac. The pseudoaneurysm may be extending above the inguinal ligament and as such you may need to just ligate the distal EIA.
- Be really careful → there might be a needle hanging around in this mess.
- These cases are messy and you just have to do what needs to be done in the moment.
- In my practice, I would avoid reconstructing the femoral arteries in this setting. I am aware of some vascular surgeons joining the SFA and PFA origins to improve collateral flow down the leg. I am not saying this is wrong. From my perspective however, I stick to core principles: I am doing this operation to stop life-threatening bleeding and drain any infection. I assume all tissues in the groin are infected, and I want as few sutures lines as possible. In my eyes, it is a pure damage control operation, and I am not focusing on saving the leg but preserving life. This is open for debate however and I am sure there are people who disagree with me. I am 100% confident however that no one would ever support putting plastic into such a groin in this setting.
- What you do after ligating the femoral arteries is open to debate. Some people leave the groin open, pack it with betadine-soaked gauze and plan for a re-look in 48 hours. Others close the fascial layers, leave the skin open, and apply a VAC. Others do a sartorius flap, leave the skin open, and apply a VAC. Others do a sartorius flap, close the fascial and skin layers, and apply a PICO dressing. I have seen various approaches. I don't think there is a right way or a wrong way, and I doubt if any specific approach is evidence based ....
- I think if you just follow correct general and vascular surgical principles you should be ok: Stop any bleeding, drain/debride any infection, and don't reconstruct arteries in an infected field .... How you deal with the wound is up to you and it depends on what you found in the groin.

Other Technical Considerations for the IVDU Groin

- If the pseudoaneurysm is extending deep into the iliac system you may need to do a laparotomy to get proximal control.
- You can also consider retrograde access from the contralateral CFA for balloon occlusion of ipsilateral iliac system to avoid a laparotomy.
- If the IVDU patient has an infected/disintegrated iliac system with haematoma in the retroperitoneum, **DO NOT** treat the iliac system with a covered stent. The iliac system

will fall to bits and you will only make the bleeding worse. In this case, consider a Rutherford Morrison incision/extended retroperitoneal incision or a full laparotomy to get proximal control and decent access to the proximal iliac vessels.

- Sometimes an IVDU groin pseudoaneurysm will bleed backwards into the retroperitoneal space. I had a patient recently who had a CFA pseudoaneurysm that had bled posteriorly underneath the inguinal ligament and filled the retroperitoneum with a few litres of blood (the kidney was pushed forward by this big haematoma on CT). He had a haemoglobin of 6 and was pale, but he was haemodynamically stable. He was also not actively bleeding. I saw the patient initially at around 11:30 pm. I decided not to take him to theatre in the middle of the night, but instead transfuse him a few units of blood and set him up for a Rutherford Morrison incision and femoral vessel ligation in the morning. I use this as an example of when *not* to rush an IVDU patient to theatre. Don't ever forget that these cases can be tricky and these patients can bleed quite a lot. If you have a chance to optimise them pre-operatively, then do so. You should only be doing these cases as an emergency in the middle of the night if you don't have much of a choice! If your hand gets forced, then so be it.

- If the pseudoaneurysm is not actively bleeding and contained purely within the groin (i.e. below inguinal ligament), then it is definitely worth just making a groin incision. You will probably have no major issues getting CFA control under the inguinal ligament and then just do the operation as normal. However, keep the lower abdomen prepped in case you need to quickly convert to a Rutherford Morrison incision for iliac control.

After the Fact

- After femoral vessel ligation, at least in my experience, most limbs remain viable.
- Expect the patient to have some ischaemic pain/coolness/maybe even reduced sensation.
- I usually give it 48 hours to see how the limb does.
- Whether it is viable or non-viable, it will usually declare itself by this point.
- If non-viable → above-knee amputation most likely will be required.
- If viable, the patient may come back to clinic a few months later complaining of rest pain/ night pain/critical ischaemia. Miraculously, the patient has "cleaned themself up" and has completely stopped taking drugs. The patient sounds genuine. Now you have a dilemma. The question is this: Ileo-profunda/SFA bypass or above-knee amputation? This was a question I had in my FRCS Part B examination. I was shown an MRA with a juicy external iliac artery, a big gap where the CFA had been ligated, and then a lovely PFA and SFA travelling all the way down to supply a perfect 3-vessel run-off to the foot …. You almost feel obliged to say you would do a bypass. I am not going to tell you what I gave as my answer. All I will say is that it depends on whether you are an idealist or a realist, optimist or cynic. If you are feeling like a chicken you could just say: "I will discuss the case in the vascular MDT" at which the examiners may secretly/internally roll their eyes as you demonstrate you are not a decision-maker but a fence-sitter ….

Final Crucial Points

- Always warn the patient about risk of limb loss in this context (unless of course the patient is in extremis and you cannot consent them formally).
- Generally speaking, I would avoid doing lower-limb amputation at the time of emergency femoral vessel ligation. Do the femoral vessel ligation, and then see how the limb does afterwards.

CHAPTER 18

Chronic Venous Disease

We will do some case-based discussions again in an FRCS examination context. These are the sort of cases that routinely pop up in outpatient clinics.

CASE 18.1: Young Gentleman with Bilateral Symptomatic Varicose Veins

- A 26-year-old mechanic presents to your outpatient clinic complaining of bilateral severe varicose veins.
- These veins have been steadily getting worse over the past few years.
- He has been referred by his GP for consideration of intervention.

Your FRCS Long Case Begins

How would you assess this patient?

- "I would begin with a history and examination. I would ask what the exact nature of his symptoms are, how long this has been a problem for, and how much it was affecting his quality of life. Which leg is worse? Has he had a DVT or lower limb fractures before? Has he had any varicose vein interventions before? Is there a family history of varicose veins? Does he have any other medical problems? Is he on any medications? Does he smoke? What is his job? What is his social situation? In terms of examination I am interested in the pattern of the varicose veins. Is this GSV or SSV distribution? Are there signs of skin damage or ulceration? Does the patient have foot pulses? I would also examine the abdominal wall for any signs of deep venous obstruction."

The patient says he is getting a lot of pain, aching, and heaviness in his legs throughout the day that is seriously affecting his ability to work. He has bilateral severe GSV pattern varicosities affecting his calves and thighs. The SSV systems do not appear to be affected. He has no skin damage or ulceration, but both his legs are slightly oedematous to the mid shins. How would you grade this?

- "Using the CEAP system I would grade this as C3 because of the oedema. In terms of the revised Venous Clinical Severity Score (r-VCSS) I would say that for both legs combined he would score around 16."

What would you do now?

- "I would do a point of care ultrasound assessment of both legs, examining mainly the GSV and SSV systems. I also routinely scan the popliteal vein and common femoral vein to look for any obvious deep venous pathology."

How would you specifically do this ultrasound assessment?

- "I would do it with the patient stood upright, with the knee of the patient slightly bent. Using either colour Doppler or pulse wave Doppler, I would stimulate reflux by considerately squeezing the lower calf. The cut off values I use are 1 second for reflux in the common femoral/femoral vein/popliteal vein, and 0.5 seconds in superficial veins. I would map out the refluxing sections, the length of the reflux, and the saphenous vein diameter. I would scan any obvious perforators as well. Finally, I would also draw a venous map in the patient notes and ideally indicate the ideal site for GSV puncturing if I was planning endovenous ablation."

How would you assess for deep venous obstruction?

- "I would place the ultrasound probe over the common femoral vein and look for normal phasic flow with respiration. If this a flat aphasic pattern, this would suggest upstream venous obstruction. However, this is a specialist area. If the clinical assessment and ultrasound findings suggested a deep venous problem I would refer the patient for a formal departmental duplex assessment."

Let's say the patient reported having had a previous car accident and a nasty pelvic fracture, and your ultrasound assessment suggested deep venous obstruction. What would you do now?

- "I would request a formal ultrasound of the abdomen and pelvic veins. After this I might need to request an MR or CT venogram if intervention was being considered."

OK. Going backwards. The deep veins appear normal and the patient has bilateral GSV distribution reflux from the SFJ all the way down to the mid-calf. These varicosities are being supplied by the GSVs. What would be your approach now?

- "Well. This is a young patient who has bilateral C3 GSV distribution reflux. His varicose veins are significantly affecting his quality of life and his work. I would therefore consider him a candidate for intervention. NICE guidelines would primarily support endovenous intervention in this context."

So would you just offer endovenous ablation?

- "No. I would first counsel the patient. I would explain what varicose veins are, the possible causes, the possibility of progression to venous skin changes and ulceration, and the potential treatment options. In my practice this would include conservative management with compression stockings, endothermal ablation, or traditional open surgery. As per NICE I would still encourage the patient to engage in light to moderate physical activity, and to avoid any factors that seem to be provoking his symptoms. If we were going down the intervention route, I would give the patient information leaflets, explain exactly what the interventions involved, with a meaningful discussion of the risks and benefits."

What are NICE's indications for referral to a vascular surgeon?

- "Symptomatic primary or symptomatic recurrent varicose veins, lower-limb skin changes, such as pigmentation or eczema, superficial vein thrombosis, a venous ulcer and a healed venous leg ulcer."

If you were consenting a patient for endovenous ablation, what risks would you mention?

- "Bleeding, infection, neurovascular injury, scarring, recurrence, need for further procedures, DVT/PE, thermal injury, thrombophlebitis, bruising, swelling, itching, and poor cosmesis. I would also ensure these risks were all clearly documented in the patient notes."

What treatments do NICE recommend for varicose veins?

- "For people with confirmed varicose veins and truncal reflux, they should be offered endothermal ablation. If endothermal ablation is unsuitable, the patient should be offered ultrasound-guided foam sclerotherapy. If ultrasound-guided foam sclerotherapy is unsuitable, offer surgery. If incompetent varicose tributaries are to be treated, consider treating them at the same time."

What does NICE say about compression hosiery?

- "It says offer compression hosiery only if interventional treatment is unsuitable."

Are you aware of other recent guidelines?

- "Yes. There are the recent 2022 ESVS guidelines on lower limb chronic venous disease."

What does the ESVS say about our patient then?

- "Exercise should be considered to reduce venous symptoms. It states that in patients with symptomatic chronic venous disease, elastic compression stockings, exerting a pressure of at least 15 mmHg at the ankle, are recommended to reduce venous symptoms. It then makes a further recommendation that for C3 patients with oedema, compression treatment which exerts a pressure of 20–40 mmHg at the ankle, is recommended to reduce oedema."

So what would you do here?

- "I would offer the patient either class 2 or class 3 compression stockings whether I was considering intervention or not. In this patient's case, above-knee stockings would be ideal."

How do you grade compression stockings?

- "Stockings prescribed in primary care follow the British standard for class of compression:

  Class 1 stockings (light compression) exert an ankle pressure of 14–17 mmHg.
  Class 2 stockings (medium compression) exert an ankle pressure of 18–24 mmHg.
  Class 3 stockings (high compression) exert an ankle pressure of 25–35 mmHg."

Are you aware of any contraindications to compression stockings?

- "As per the recent ESVS guidelines: severe lower extremity PAD with an ABPI < 0.6 and/or ankle pressure < 60 mmHg, extra-anatomic or superficially tunnelled arterial bypass at the site of intended compression, severe heart failure, NYHA Class IV, confirmed allergy to compression material, severe diabetic neuropathy with the risk of skin necrosis."

If the patient's venous duplex suggested both superficial and deep venous reflux, would you still consider endovascular or open surgical intervention?

- "Yes I would. The original ESCHAR trial suggested that even in patients with superficial and deep reflux, treating the superficial venous system still resulted in reduced ulcer recurrence and improved ulcer free time when compared with compression alone. This is not the exact clinical context we are talking about, but it does demonstrate the treating the superficial system even with deep reflux can still be beneficial. Similarly, the 2022 ESVS guidelines states that in patients with chronic venous disease, caused by combined superficial and deep venous incompetence, treatment of incompetent superficial veins should be considered."

Final question. If this was an 80-year-old patient with bilateral GSV reflux on duplex with bilateral lower limb oedema, but no significant varicosities or venous type symptoms, would you still proceed directly to intervention?

- "No. If the patient's main presenting complaint was just bilateral lower limb oedema, I would consider other pathologies. In an elderly patient I would be considering other causes like heart failure and renal failure etc. The GSV reflux may be a red-herring."

Your FRCS Long Case Ends

Relevant ESVS Guideline Recommendations

- For patients with chronic venous disease, the use of the Clinical, Etiological, Anatomical, Pathophysiological (CEAP) classification is recommended for clinical audit and research.
- For patients with chronic venous disease, grading of clinical severity, and evaluation of treatment success using the revised Venous Clinical Severity Score (r-VCSS) and the Villalta scale for post-thrombotic syndrome should be considered for clinical audit and research.
- For diagnosis and treatment planning in patients with suspected or clinically evident chronic venous disease, full lower limb venous duplex ultrasound is recommended as the primary imaging modality.
- For patients with suspected supra-inguinal venous obstruction, in addition to full leg duplex assessment, ultrasound of the abdominal and pelvic veins should be considered, as part of the initial assessment.
- When an intervention is contemplated in patients with suspected supra-inguinal venous obstruction, cross-sectional imaging by magnetic resonance venography or computed tomography is recommended in addition to duplex ultrasound assessment.
- For patients with symptomatic chronic venous disease, exercise should be considered to reduce venous symptoms.
- For patients with symptomatic chronic venous disease, elastic compression stockings, exerting a pressure of at least 15 mmHg at the ankle, are recommended to reduce venous symptoms.
- For patients with chronic venous disease and oedema (CEAP clinical class C3), compression treatment using below-knee elastic compression stockings, inelastic bandages, or adjustable compression garments, exerting a pressure of 20–40 mmHg at the ankle, is recommended to reduce oedema.

- For patients with chronic venous disease and lipodermatosclerosis and/or atrophie blanche (CEAP clinical class C4b), using below-knee elastic compression stockings, exerting a pressure of 20–40 mmHg at the ankle, is recommended to reduce skin induration.
- For patients with superficial venous incompetence presenting with symptomatic varicose veins (CEAP clinical class C2S), interventional treatment is recommended.
- For patients with superficial venous incompetence presenting with oedema (CEAP clinical class C3), other non-venous causes of oedema should be considered before planning interventional treatment.
- For patients with great saphenous vein incompetence requiring treatment, endovenous thermal ablation is recommended as first choice treatment in preference to high ligation/stripping and ultrasound guided foam sclerotherapy.
- For patients with great saphenous vein incompetence requiring treatment, high ligation/stripping should be considered if endovenous thermal ablation options are not available.
- In patients with chronic venous disease, caused by combined superficial and deep venous incompetence, treatment of incompetent superficial veins should be considered.

CASE 18.2: Patient with Venous Leg Ulceration

- A 68-year-old woman presents to your outpatient clinic with an ulcer around her right medial malleolus.
- It has been present for around 3 weeks.

Your FRCS Short Case Begins

Can you please describe what you see in this picture?

- "There is a 2 × 3 cm ulcer around the medial gaiter region, just above the medial malleolus. This is superficial and there is no tendon or bone involved. The border is slightly irregular, and there is a small amount of slough present. There are no gross signs of infection. I can see surrounding venous skin changes with haemosiderin desposition. There are also reticular veins present in the surrounding skin."

What pattern of reflux would likely be responsible for this ulcer?

- "GSV distribution reflux."

What are other potential causes for such an ulcer?

- "You can get mixed arteriovenous ulceration i.e. if there is additional peripheral arterial disease. Other less common causes include malignancy and rheumatological conditions like pyoderma gangrenosum."

The patient has had a venous duplex. Can you please interpret this for me?

- "Yes. It shows that the deep system of veins appears intact with no obvious reflux or obstruction. The short saphenous system is competent. The SFJ is incompetent, and the main trunk of the GSV in the thigh and calf is also incompetent. The report says that the GSV is on average 6 mm in diameter, and straight. It sounds like it is suitable for GSV endovenous ablation therefore, which I would consider in light of the EVRA trial."

What did the EVRA trial show?

- "It showed that early endovenous ablation of superficial venous reflux as an adjunct to compression therapy was associated with a significantly shorter time to healing of venous leg ulcers than compression therapy alone. Patients assigned to the early-intervention group also had longer ulcer-free time. The long term results of the EVRA trial also showed that early endovenous ablation of superficial venous reflux was highly likely to be cost-effective over a 3-year horizon compared with deferred intervention."

How would you classify this venous leg ulcer?

- "By way of the CEAP classification, this would be C6."

Would you give this patient antibiotics for this venous leg ulcer?

- "No. As per the 202 ESVS guidelines, for patients with active venous leg ulceration without infection, the use of local or systemic antibiotics to improve ulcer healing is not recommended."

After a discussion with the patient she seems keen for endovenous treatment. You mentioned compression in regards to the EVRA trial. Would you still employ compression here even though you are considering intervention?

- "I would still use compression. The 2022 ESVS guidelines recommend compression for patients with active venous leg ulceration to improve ulcer healing."

What sort of compression would you be aiming for? What types of compression are available?

- "I would first want to confirm the patient had foot pulses before I committed to full compression. However, if I was happy with the leg perfusion, I would be aiming for a target pressure of 40 mmHg at the ankle. The options for compression are numerous, but generally speaking there are multilayer, inelastic bandages or adjustable compression garments. For small and recent onset venous ulcers elastic compression stockings exerting a target pressure up to 40 mmHg at the ankle can also be considered."

What if you could not feel the patient's foot pulses, and she had an ABPI of 0.75 and an ankle pressure of 70 mmHg?

- "In this case I would try modified/reduced compression therapy under close clinical supervision."

If this venous leg ulcer healed on its own with compression, even before you proceeded to do endovenous ablation, what would you do then? Would you continue compression? Would you still proceed to endovenous ablation?

- "I would obviously counsel the patient and not decide on anything without involving the patient. However, the 2022 ESVS guidelines highlights that for patients with healed venous leg ulceration, long term compression therapy should be considered to reduce the risk of ulcer recurrence. The same guidelines also recommend intervention to treat the incompetent vein to reduce the risk of future recurrence. Henceforth my general position would be to say yes, I would consider long term compression and endovenous intervention even if the venous ulcer was healed."

You offer the patient intervention, but she does not like the sound of endovenous intervention. The notion of multiple injections is off-putting. She thinks having the case performed under local anaesthetic is scary. She is asking you if you would recommend open surgery instead, which would be better because it can be done under general anaesthesia?

- "As part of my patient counselling process I would routinely discuss all of the valid options that are available. This would include endovenous treatments, foam sclerotherapy, conservative management and open surgery. I would provide the patient with information leaflets, and discuss the individual risks and benefits. However, it would also be my routine practice to try and adhere to guideline recommendations. As such, I would explain to the patient that NICE guidelines would primarily support endovenous treatment first, then foam sclerotherapy, and then open surgery. The 2022 ESVS guidelines also recommends endovenous ablation as first-line treatment, over foam sclerotherapy and open surgery."

The patient still would prefer traditional open surgery under general anaesthesia.

- "This is acceptable in my opinion. However, I would want to first ensure open surgery was safe i.e. from a comorbidity/anaesthetic perspective. I would also clearly document in the patient notes that my recommendation was for endovenous intervention in line with the NICE and ESVS guidelines."

Do you have to do high tie and stripping under general anaesthesia?

- "Apparently not. The 2022 ESVS guidelines states that for patients with superficial venous incompetence undergoing high ligation/stripping, ultrasound guided tumescent anaesthesia may be considered, as an alternative to general or regional anaesthesia."

If you did a high tie and strip, or endovenous ablation or foam sclerotherapy, what are your thoughts on compression afterwards?

- "Irrespective of the procedure I would routinely dress the leg with an adhesive elastic bandage which stays on for 2–3 days, which is followed by 2 weeks of class 2 above-knee compression stockings."

Your FRCS Short Case Ends

Relevant ESVS Guideline Recommendations

- For patients with superficial venous incompetence presenting with skin changes as a result of chronic venous disease (CEAP clinical class C4–C6), interventional treatment of venous incompetence is recommended.
- For patients with superficial venous incompetence undergoing high ligation / stripping, ultrasound guided tumescent anaesthesia may be considered as an alternative to general or regional anaesthesia.
- For patients with superficial venous incompetence undergoing ultrasound guided foam sclerotherapy or endovenous thermal ablation of a saphenous trunk, post-procedural compression treatment should be considered.

- For patients with superficial venous incompetence undergoing stripping and/or extensive phlebectomies, immediate post-procedural compression treatment is recommended.
- For patients with superficial venous incompetence undergoing intervention, the duration of post-intervention compression used to minimise post-operative local complications, should be decided on an individual basis.
- For patients with great saphenous vein incompetence requiring treatment, endovenous thermal ablation is recommended as first choice treatment in preference to high ligation / stripping and ultrasound guided foam sclerotherapy.
- For patients with great saphenous vein incompetence requiring treatment, high ligation / stripping should be considered if endovenous thermal ablation options are not available.
- For patients with active venous leg ulceration, compression therapy is recommended to improve ulcer healing.
- For patients with active venous leg ulceration, multilayer or inelastic bandages or adjustable compression garments, exerting a target pressure of at least 40 mmHg at the ankle, are recommended to improve ulcer healing.
- For patients with active venous leg ulceration, super-imposed elastic compression stockings exerting a target pressure up to 40 mmHg at the ankle should be considered for small and recent onset ulcers.
- For patients with active venous leg ulceration with ankle pressure less than 60 mmHg, toe pressure less than 30 mmHg, or ankle brachial index lower than 0.6, sustained compression therapy is not recommended.
- For patients with a mixed ulcer caused by coexisting arterial and venous disease, modified compression therapy under close clinical supervision with a compression pressure less than 40 mmHg may be considered, provided the ankle pressure is higher than 60 mmHg.
- For patients with healed venous leg ulceration, long term compression therapy should be considered to reduce the risk of ulcer recurrence.
- For patients with active venous leg ulceration and superficial venous incompetence, early endovenous ablation is recommended to accelerate ulcer healing.
- For patients with superficial venous incompetence and healed venous leg ulceration, treatment of the incompetent veins is recommended to reduce the risk of ulcer recurrence.
- For patients with active leg ulceration, objective arterial assessment is recommended.

CASE 18.3: Deep Venous Obstruction

- A 30 year old presents to your outpatient clinic complaining of left leg chronic swelling and discomfort when walking.
- She has also developed a new ulcer around her medial malleolar region in the past few weeks.
- She says she had a left leg DVT around 1 year ago a week after giving birth to her second child.
- This DVT was managed with warfarin for 6 months.
- She is otherwise fit and well.

Your FRCS Short Case Begins

What are your thoughts as to the diagnosis?

- "Given the previous ipsilateral DVT, it sounds like this patient has post-thrombotic syndrome."

What are the classic symptoms and signs of PTS?

- "Typical symptoms are pain, heaviness, fatigue, itching, cramping, and venous claudication. Typical signs are pain with calf compression, varicose veins, oedema, and skin changes including venous ulceration."

Is it common after DVT?

- "It occurs in 20–50% of DVT patients, of whom 5–10% will develop severe PTS, including venous ulceration."

How would you investigate this patient?

- "First of all I would carry out a detailed clinical assessment. I am not only interested in the leg, but also the abdominal wall to look for any collaterals that suggest a supra-inguinal deep venous problem. After this I would request a formal departmental ultrasound to look at both the infra-inguinal veins and the supra-inguinal veins."

Your ultrasound request is rejected because there are no ultra-sonographers trained to do supra-inguinal venous scanning.

- "I would request cross-sectional imaging then, such as a CT or MR venogram."

The patient has a left leg venous duplex and an MR venogram. The duplex does not report any significant reflux in the superficial venous systems. The femoro-popliteal deep veins appear patent and relatively disease-free. However, in the proximal femoral vein and the common femoral vein there is loss of normal phasic flow with respiration, and there appears to be scarring and fibrosis here. The MRV is reported as showing stenotic disease of the left external iliac vein, which is around 70% narrowed. What would be your management approach?

- "I think this patient should be considered for intervention. She is young and fit, and by the sounds of it she has genuine severe PTS. However, deep venous disease is a specialist area. I would discuss the case in the vascular MDT and ideally refer the patient on to a clinician with a specialist interest in this area. What I can do however is counsel the patient on the broad options for management, and at the very least prescribe her some compression stockings."

Well, what are the treatment options?

- "In this case either conservative management with compression stockings, and/or endovascular recannalisation and angioplasty / stenting."

Are there not open surgical options?

- "Yes I am sure that there are. But again, this is complex and highly-specialised surgery. I am not familiar with this type of surgery, and would not be offering it myself. Again, I would refer the case to the vascular MDT and experts in this area if required."

What if the patient's symptoms were minor and she did not have a venous ulcer?

- "I would be extremely reluctant to be offering intervention. In fact, the 2022 ESVS guidelines states that for patients with iliac vein outflow obstruction, without severe symptoms, neither endovascular nor surgical interventions are recommended."

If the patient's investigations had revealed GSV reflux and deep venous obstruction, would you not consider just treating the superficial venous reflux and leaving the deep venous problem alone?

- "It depends. In patients with superficial reflux and deep vein obstruction, the GSV rarely functions as a collateral. It also does not contribute to leg drainage if there is gross reflux in the GSV. Therefore, in this context, the main question is whether the GSV is playing any role in limb drainage. An expert venous duplex assessment or venography would help to assess the drainage pattern. If there was no significant drainage via the GSV, arguably it could be ablated without risk of compromising venous drainage of the limb. However, ablation of a competent and large GSV with antegrade flow would likely worsen the situation by compromising venous outflow of the leg in case of femoro-popliteal occlusion. For iliac or ilio-femoral occlusion, the cranial extent of ipsi- or contralateral GSV ablation may have to be limited to preserve inflow and outflow of cross pubic collateral circulation."

You are a bit of a nerd aren't you?

- "No. I am actually very cool and extremely popular (*as if*). All joking aside though, I do know the ESVS guidelines like the back of my hand. Indeed, to reinforce my original position, these are complex cases, and I would not be managing them in isolation. I would be discussing them in the vascular MDT and referring them to experts in the field of deep venous disease."

Can you please describe to me how you perform deep venous stenting?

- "No. I do not know how to do it. This is a highly specialised area and I think it is way beyond the requirements of a day one consultant vascular surgeon. I have an academic understanding of the principles of management, but would not want to step outside of my area of expertise."

Your FRCS Short Case Ends

Relevant ESVS Guideline Recommendations

- For patients with iliac vein outflow obstruction and severe symptoms/signs, endovascular treatment should be considered as the first choice of treatment.
- For patients with iliac vein outflow obstruction suffering from a recalcitrant venous ulcer, severe post-thrombotic syndrome, or disabling venous claudication, surgical or hybrid deep venous reconstruction may be considered when endovascular options alone are not appropriate.
- For patients with iliac vein outflow obstruction without severe symptoms, neither endovascular nor surgical interventions are recommended.
- For patients with iliac vein outflow obstruction, management by a multidisciplinary team is recommended.
- For patients with extensive axial deep venous incompetence and severe persistent symptoms and signs where previous management has failed, surgical repair of valvular incompetence may be considered in specialised centres.
- For patients with post-thrombotic syndrome, below-knee elastic compression stockings, exerting a pressure of 20–40 mmHg at the ankle, should be considered to reduce severity.

CHAPTER 19

Lower Limb Venous Thromboembolism

This is again a very big area, and I could devote an entire textbook to this topic. However, people have already done this, and if you wish to know the minutiae, please refer to other specialist texts. As per usual, I will keep things focused and as high yield as possible. I think it is again a good idea to use some real life case examples, and run through some mock FRCS Part B short and long cases. In this section, we will cover what I consider to be the sort of the lower DVT stuff that is particularly pertinent to a vascular surgeon for both the exam and in the real world.

CASE 19.1: Ileo-Femoral DVT

This patient is referred to you by a general practitioner. You see her in the surgical assessment unit.

History

- This is a 23-year-old Afro-Caribbean female patient.
- She presents with an acutely swollen right leg.
- The entire leg is swollen up to the groin.
- This started 48 hours ago, and the swelling has progressed upwards.
- She is not in any pain, but the right leg is slightly uncomfortable and feels congested.
- She feels well in herself.
- She is not reporting fevers/sweats/shakes/weight loss/poor appetite.
- She has no other red flag features to suggest underlying malignancy (breathing OK, bowels OK, no swallowing problems, no lumps in her breasts or under her armpits or in his groins, no urinary symptoms).
- She is not reporting back pain, and the swelling does not seem to have progressed proximally to cause abdominal swelling.
- She is a smoker.
- She reports having chronic issues with heavy periods and is chronically anaemic.
- She is currently on her period and her bleeding is quite heavy—she is having to use multiple pads.
- She has no other medical problems.
- There is no personal history of venous thromboembolism, lower limb fracture, recent long-haul travel, no family history of venous thromboembolism.
- Her regular medications include iron tablets. She says she has only recently started taking the combined oral contraceptive pill mainly to help with her heavy periods (started it last week).
- Social history—is studying architecture at university.

Examination

- Patient is systemically well, does not appear to be in any pain, not in respiratory distress.
- Right leg is more swollen than the left, but certainly not massively swollen.

DOI: 10.1201/b22951-19

- Upper limb examination NAD.
- No palpable lymph nodes in axilla or neck.
- *Breast examination not done in this setting but should be considered in certain contexts if you are considering malignancy and always use a female chaperone.*
- Chest sounds clear.
- Abdomen soft and non-tender, no masses.
- Groins again do not obviously demonstrate any lymphadenopathy.
- Can feel foot pulses in both legs, warm, and well perfused feet, triphasic handheld Doppler signals.
- Right leg on the whole is 2 cm larger than the left.
- Right leg is moderately oedematous all the way up to the right upper thigh.
- Power 5/5.
- Sensation completely intact.
- No signs of compartment syndrome.
- No obvious bruising/blistering/skin necrosis.

Your FRCS Long Case Begins

What is your working diagnosis?

- "I suspect that this patient has a right-sided ileofemoral DVT. This is likely secondary to starting the combined oral contraceptive pill one week ago, which is a known risk factor. At the moment I am not overtly concerned that the patient has any limb threat. Given the pigment of her skin it is difficult to authoritatively say that she does not have phlegmasia alba dolens or phlegmasia cerula dolens, but pragmatically I do not think she does."

What is your immediate management plan?

- "I would first counsel the patient on my suspected diagnosis, and discuss some of the potential therapeutic strategies, including their risks and benefits. I would admit the patient to a normal vascular surgery ward and advise strict bedrest and leg elevation in order to get the swelling down. I would gain large-bore intravenous access and send of urgent bloods for: FBC, U&Es, clotting, and group and save. I would also request a right leg venous duplex scan to confirm my diagnosis. In the meantime I would probably commence the patient on low-dose intravenous heparin as well."

What about her menorrhagia? Would you still commence on anticoagulation at this stage?

- "This is a challenging clinical case. I would of course discuss the pros and cons of anticoagulation with the patient, and I would also discuss the case with the haematology and gynaecology teams. From my perspective however, intravenous heparin can be given at a low dose, the therapeutic effect can be monitored carefully with APTT levels, and it wears off after only a few hours. This patient looks like she has a fairly large thrombus burden, and there is a risk of further progression and potentially the risk of a fatal pulmonary embolism. As such my decision would be to commence the patient on IV heparin and keep a close eye on her from a bleeding perspective."

The ultrasound scan reveals what you expected. It shows DVT affecting the right femoropopliteal vein that is extending up to the common femoral vein/external iliac vein. The patient's haemoglobin is 84, and this is a chronic trend observed over the past few months. What would your approach be now?

- "I have two conflicting thought processes currently. On the one hand this is a young, fit, independent patient with a provoked ileofemoral DVT. Generally speaking this is the exact sort of patient I would consider thrombolysis on in order to improve her symptoms and hopefully reduce the future risk of severe post-thrombotic syndrome. However, she has a current bleeding problem that has already made her chronically anaemic. My major worry would be that if we were to consider thrombolysis we might potentially cause even worse menstrual bleeding, which in the worst-case scenario may be difficult to control. In this situation I would discuss with my fellow consultant vascular surgery colleagues and interventional radiology colleagues. I would also discuss with the patient and gain her thoughts. As for me, my decision at this stage would be to hold-off thrombolysis as the bleeding risk concerns me and I don't think her symptoms are bad enough currently to force my hand. Her DVT only developed 2 days ago, and I think it would be reasonable to allow her heavy period to settle, and then reconsider catheter-directed thrombolysis later on. As long as we could get this procedure done within 2 weeks from the onset of the ileofemoral DVT I think that would be a safe compromise. In the meantime I would recommend limb elevation, anticoagulation and a compression stocking."

Are you aware of any relevant randomised controlled trials in this area?

- "Yes. I am aware of the CaVenT, ATTRACT, CAVA, and TORPEDO trials. These trials looked at mainly catheter-directed thrombolysis in comparison to anticoagulation alone for lower limb DVT and what the outcomes were like in terms of bleeding risk, symptomatic improvement, and the development of PTS. A meta-analysis of these trials concluded that early thrombus removal was more effective than anticoagulation alone in preventing any PTS and in particular moderate to severe PTS. However, there is a significantly increased risk of major bleeding."

The vascular MDT agrees with your plan, and so does the patient. Five days later she goes for right leg catheter-directed thrombolysis when her menorrhagia has settled. The infusion is running for 12 hours when the patient suddenly develops speech disturbance, a left-sided facial droop, and left-sided weakness in her upper and lower limbs. How would you approach this case?

- "My primary concern is that this patient has an intra-cerebral bleed. I would immediately go to assess the patient and examine her with an ABCDE approach. I would stop the thrombolysis infusion immediately and also stop any other anticoagulation that might be running e.g. intravenous heparin. I would ensure large-bore intravenous access and send off urgent bloods for: FBC, U&Es, clotting, fibrinogen, and sent a group and save sample. I would immediately contact the stroke team on call and arrange for an urgent CT brain."

The CT brain confirms a large right-sided intra-cerebral haematoma with significant mass effect and midline shift. What would you do now?

- "I would contact the neurosurgical on-call team and ask for an urgent review. They may consider urgent craniotomy for decompression."

Was there another option you might have considered in this patient in regards to her bleeding risks?

- "We could have simply pursued a conservative management approach with compression stockings and oral anticoagulation. Alternatively, we could have considered a formal surgical thrombectomy via a CFV venotomy and fogarty thrombectomy. However, this operation is rarely done in my experience, and I would only really consider it in an emergency setting where I felt thrombolysis were not possible."

Your FRCS Long Case Ends

Relevant ESVS Guideline Recommendations

- For patients with suspected deep vein thrombosis requiring imaging, ultrasound is recommended as the first modality.
- For patients with proximal deep vein thrombosis, early compression at 30–40 mmHg with either multilayer bandaging or compression hosiery, applied within 24 hours, is recommended to reduce pain, oedema, and residual venous obstruction.
- For patients with proximal deep vein thrombosis, use of below-knee compression stockings should be considered in order to reduce the risk of post-thrombotic syndrome.
- In selected patients with symptomatic iliofemoral deep vein thrombosis, early thrombus removal strategies should be considered.
- For patients with deep vein thrombosis limited to femoral, popliteal, or calf veins, early thrombus removal is not recommended.

CASE 19.2: Phlegmasia Cerula Dolens

You get a phone call from a consultant colorectal surgeon. He is worried that a patient he has just operated on has an ileo-femoral DVT.

History/Examination Findings as per Telephone Discussion

- You are told that this is a 46-year-old female who has a pelvic exenteration operation yesterday. It was a 12 hour operation and ran into the later evening (case started at 10:30 am and finished at 11 pm).
- The patient has been in theatre recovery overnight waiting for an intensive care bed.
- This surgeon has just been to see the patient this morning (it is now 9 am the following day).
- The case was that of an aggressive colorectal cancer that had locally invaded various structures in the pelvis. The operation involved an AP resection with removal of various pelvic structures, including the uterus, part of the bladder, ureter, and part of the lumbar spine. The internal iliac vein on the right was ligated, and there was also an injury to the right common iliac vein. There was significant bleeding secondary to this injury and the common iliac vein was repaired using some interrupted prolene stitches.
- The surgeon explains that when the common iliac vein repair was done, the vein was clearly left stenosed.
- Overnight the patient's right leg has swollen considerably. The entire leg is oedematous and purple. The patient is reporting a lot of pain. She has pins and needles in her right foot and her sensation is reduced. She can barely move her right ankle or toes. Her calf muscles/shin muscles are diffusely tender.

- She is not doing well from an anaesthetic perspective. She is hypotensive requiring vasoconstrictors. She is tachycardia. She looks unwell. She has spiked a temperature. Because she lost so much blood she is being transfused a few units now, and her last haemoglobin was 94.

Your FRCS Long Case Begins

What is your working diagnosis?

- "I suspect the pelvic exenteration surgery itself largely obliterated most of the pelvic venous collaterals. The common iliac vein sounds like it has been battered and bruised, and the suture repair probably left it critically stenosed. I suspect the ileo-femoral system thrombosed post-operatively, and the patient now has what sounds like phlegmasia cerula dolens. She is systemically unwell and is at risk of not just limb loss but also death."

What is your immediate management plan?

- "I would immediately go and assess the patient myself. What am I mainly interested in confirming is whether this is phlegmasia cerula dolens, and does the patient have compartment syndrome."

The right leg is significantly swollen compared to the right. It has a deep purple appearance that extends up to the upper thigh. She has sensory disturbance in her right foot. She does have weakened right foot/ankle movement. Her calf and shin muscles are tense and tender. Her whole leg is engorged. Does this confirm your diagnosis?

- "That is enough for me to diagnose phlegmasia cerula dolens (clinically). However, I would also want to confirm the lower limb pulse status to be sure there is not an arterial component as well. The iliac artery could have been simultaneously injured during the pelvic exenteration as well. Does the patient have a femoral pulse and distal pulses? Are there decent handheld Doppler signals in the right foot?"

Yes the arterial perfusion is intact. Would you request any further investigations?

- "Yes. I would discuss the case with the vascular interventional radiology consultant on-call first, but provisionally I would request an urgent CT venogram."

You are handed some relevant CT venogram images. You are asked to interpret them.

- "The right ileofemoral system has thrombosed. The clot is extending all the down the right femoropopliteal system. There is also a narrowing of the right common iliac vein at the site where the suture repair took place. The thrombus extends up to this level but as of yet does not appear to have extended into the inferior vena cava."

What would your management plan be at this stage?

- "From my perspective, conservative management does not feel appropriate. This is a young woman. I recognise that she has had surgery for a horrific colorectal malignancy, but I still believe we should try our best for her and an aggressive approach is indicated. Catheter-directed thrombolysis is inappropriate. Her bleeding risk is too high. In this sitting I would defer to traditional open vascular surgery. In my hands this would potentially include a right lower limb fasciotomy, common femoral vein venotomy, fogarty thrombectomy up and down to clear the deep venous system, and then ask my expert interventional radiology consultant colleague to stent the right common iliac vein. I would also likely consider an IVC filter in this setting as she is unlikely to be on formal anticoagulation given the recent major surgery. Of course, I would not commit to any of this without first discussing with the patient and/or a close family member, and I would aim to get informed consent to proceed."

Please take us through your approach in doing such a venous thrombectomy

1. "General anaesthesia.
2. Longitudinal groin incision to enable exposure of the common femoral vein, superficial femoral vein, sapheno-femoral junction, and profunda femoral vein.
3. Longitudinal venotomy is made in the common femoral vein that will enable access into the great saphenous and profunda femoral veins.
4. As there is infra-inguinal thrombus present in this case, I would now elevate the right leg and use an Esmark bandage to tightly wrap the entire leg from foot all the way up to the proximal thigh.
5. This would ideally squeeze much of the infra-inguinal clot burden out from the venotomy site.
6. If this were not sufficient, I would consider a cutdown at the ankle to expose the posterior tibial vein. I would advance a fogarty embolectomy catheter from the ankle all the way to the common femoral vein and out of the pre-existing venotomy.
7. At this point I would use the silastic stem of an intravenous catheter (12–14 ga) that had been amputated from its hub. I would insert the fogarty balloon in one end of this silastic stem. After this I would get another fogarty balloon and insert this into the other end of the silastic stem. Both balloons would be inflated to ensure that both fogarty balloon catheters remain within this silastic sheath. The fogarty balloon catheter can then be carefully drawn down the leg from the groin to the posterior tibial vein site.
8. Now I would be able to perform a balloon thrombectomy from the posterior tibial vein all the way up to the common femoral vein and would be going in the direction of the venous valves.
9. After withdrawing a large amount of clot I would copiously flush the posterior tibial vein upwards using vigorous heparinised saline injection. The hydraulic force should force any residual thrombus out from the deep venous system.
10. One the infra-inguinal venous system has been cleared, I would apply a vascular clamp just below the common femoral vein venotomy site.
11. I would then fill the infra-inguinal venous system with dilute plasminogen activator solution from the posterior tibial vein, and could be left to work as I complete the rest of the procedure.
12. Alternatively, if one wanted to avoid a direct posterior tibial vein exposure, one could consider an over-the-wire balloon thrombectomy of the infra-inguinal veins via the CFV. This would require the passage of a floppy guidewire from the CFV down to the ankle.
13. I would do a profunda vein thrombectomy if this were now required.
14. Now we turn our attention to the proximal venous system. A larger venous thrombectomy balloon can be passed partially into the iliac vein for several passes to remove the bulk of the thrombus.
15. At this stage I would hand over the case to the interventional radiologist. Any clot around the right common iliac vein should be removed under fluoroscopic guidance. There is also

a critical right common iliac vein stenosis which would likely need to be crossed carefully under fluoroscopic guidance. Close cooperation with the anaesthetist would also be required. If there was still clot around this area, positive end-expiratory pressure should be applied to reduce the risk of clot shooting upwards and causing a pulmonary embolism.

16. After completion of the ileo-femoral venous thrombectomy, an angiogram would be performed to ascertain the exact nature and position of this critical right common iliac vein stenosis. In the context of recent trauma and suture repair, I would not entertain the notion of just doing a balloon angioplasty in this setting. This would no doubt just lead to iliac vein tearing / rupture and pelvic bleeding. I would of course get the expert opinion of the interventional radiology consultant, but my thoughts would be to insert a covered stent at this level.

17. At the end of the operation I would simply ligate the posterior tibial vein.

18. I would also consider doing a small arteriovenous fistula creation from the proximal great saphenous vein to the superficial/common femoral artery. This would be to increase venous velocity and reduce the risk of recurrent deep venous thrombosis.

19. In this context I would also consider an inferior vena cava filter.

20. I would also strongly consider proceeding to do fasciotomies in this context"

What would your post-operative plan be?

- If an inferior vena cava filter was not inserted and the patient's bleeding risk improved, I would commence the patient on intravenous heparin post-operatively.
- Oral anticoagulation would be begun in a few days depending upon her surgical progress.
- I would use intermittent pneumatic compression garments for both legs whilst she were non-ambulating.
- If I had done calf fasciotomies, these would be managed as with cases of acute arterial limb ischaemia (i.e. ideally closed when any swelling settles down).
- Upon discharge I would change to 40 mmHg ankle-gradient below-knee compression stockings.
- If an IVC filter had been used I would arrange for early removal (i.e., as soon as the major surgery episode were over and she was able to go back onto anticoagulation).
- I would also arrange for a face-to-face outpatient review in 4–6 weeks' time to check on her progress.

Your FRCS Long Case Ends

Relevant ESVS Guideline Recommendation

- For patients who are anticoagulated for deep vein thrombosis, the routine use of inferior vena cava filters is not recommended.

CASE 19.3: May-Thurner Syndrome

This is a young female patient you see in your outpatient clinic.

History

- This is a 23-year-old female patient complaining of a chronic left leg discomfort and swelling.

- These symptoms have been present for a few years and she generally has "just put up with it."
- The symptoms are a moderate inconvenience to her quality of life, but they are getting worse.
- She is not reporting any varicose veins, leg ulcers, pain in her legs when walking.
- She neither reports any previous episodes of venous thromboembolism, lower limb trauma or fractures, nor a family history of venous problems.
- She is otherwise fit and well.
- She is not on any regular medications.
- She is currently a student at university studying chemistry.

Examination

- The patient looks very well.
- She is fit and healthy.
- The left leg is reported to be symptomatic but it actually looks normal.
- There is no gross venous congestion in the leg.
- There are no varicose veins.
- There are no areas of venous ulceration.
- She has easily palpable foot pulses and warm well perfused feet.
- The left leg is not swollen compared to the right.
- There are no varicosities around the upper thigh or abdominal wall.

Your FRCS Short Case Begins

What is your impression?

- "I am not overly worried at the moment. I have not identified any grossly concerning clinical findings. However, this patient says she has symptoms, and according to her they are moderately affecting her quality of life, and they are progressing. As such I think it is reasonable to consider further investigation."

What further investigations would you request?

- "I would start off with a formal lower limb venous duplex to assess the deep and superficial venous systems."

The patient has this and it comes back as normal. The patient says her symptoms are getting worse. What would you do now?

- "This could potentially be a more proximal venous problem, so I would request an MRV."

The MRV is performed, and it is reported as showing compression of the left common iliac vein by the overlying right common iliac artery. What would you do now?

- "Based upon this report the patient potentially has a diagnosis of May Thurner's syndrome. However, it must be recognised that there have been post-mortem studies done in the early 20th century that have revealed a 22%-32% incidence of left iliac vein compression. Modern CT imaging studies have also revealed that in asymptomatic patients, there is an average amount of compression of the left iliac vein in 35%, and that

24% of this population demonstrated compression of more than 50%. Therefore, one should not be overtly alarmed by radiological reports, nor should one assume that this is the cause of the symptoms. On the other hand, it is well known that left leg ileofemoral DVT is more common than the right, and that compression of the left iliac vein does increase the risks of ileofemoral DVT. In this case the patient does have radiological evidence of left iliac vein compression, she does have venous congestion-type symptoms that seem to be genuinely affecting her quality of life, and she is theoretically at increased risk of an ileofemoral DVT."

So would you treat her?

- "Her youth concerns me. Theoretically yes there is the option to do a left iliac vein stent to improve the venous return in her left leg. This may improve her symptoms. However, stents do not last forever. She may initially have a good result, but this may be short-lived. The stent may occlude. There are also risks related to the proposed procedure including: groin complications, contrast allergy and nephropathy, DVT, PE, bleeding, infection. I know that in a young fit person these sound like relatively minor risks, but they are still real risks. Also, if the stent were to occlude or stenose, she could end up in a worse situation than she is currently in. Inserting the stent may result in her getting an ileofemoral DVT. My gut feeling would be to try and avoid intervention at such a young age if at all possible. However, I would discuss the case in the vascular MDT, and get a further expert opinion from someone in my unit with a special interest in deep venous disease. I could also seek an expert opinion from someone outside my unit if this was necessary. Naturally, the most important person to speak to is also the patient. Her decision would be of paramount importance also."

The vascular MDT and the patient decide on conservative management. However, she returns as an emergency admission 8 months later with a significant left-sided ileo-femoral DVT. What would you do now?

- "In this situation I think it would be fair to arrange for catheter-directed thrombolysis followed by left iliac vein stenting."

Your FRCS Short Case Ends

JMF Reflections

This was a real case of mine from a few months ago. She did have left iliac vein compression on an MRA and had vague congestion-type symptoms in the left leg. Intervention was discussed, but the longevity of iliac stenting was a concern given her youth. It was put through the vascular MDT and the general consensus was to avoid stenting at this stage. The patient was referred to one of our interventional radiology consultants who has a deep venous specialist interest, but the patient did not show up for her outpatient review… A difficult one to know how to answer. I suspect there will be a body of vascular surgeons and interventional radiologists who would not stent this patient. Likewise, there may be a body of clinicians who would stent. As for me, I would prefer not to stent given her youth and relatively minor symptoms. The patient has not come in with an ileo-femoral DVT as of yet, I made this part up for the sake of case discussion ….

CASE 19.4: Superficial Venous Thrombosis

This is a patient who is referred in acutely by his general practitioner for a swollen, tender vein in his right leg.

History

- This is a 57-year-old gentleman who is known to have bilateral lower limb varicose veins.
- These are being managed conservatively with compression stockings which he routinely wears in the daytime.
- Over the past 48 hours his right inner calf has become acutely painful and erythematous.
- There is also a palpable tender cord in his inner leg and this is spreading upwards.
- The patient feels well in himself.
- He does not say that the whole leg itself is swollen.
- He has no fevers/sweats/shakes.
- He reports no trauma.
- He reports no recent long-haul travel or lower limb surgery.
- He is not reporting any weight loss, poor appetite, change in bowel habit. He has no shortness of breath, blood in his urine etc.
- His other medical comorbidities include hypertension and diet-controlled type 2 diabetes.
- His only medication is ramipril.
- In the social history he works as an accountant and is otherwise fit, well, and independent.

Examination

- The patient is systemically well.
- There is no respiratory distress.
- His lower limb pulses are intact.
- The right leg is no grossly swollen or oedematous.
- There are no areas of ulceration around the ankle.
- He has varicosities on the medial side of the calf and thigh in the great saphenous vein distribution.
- There is erythema along the course of the great saphenous vein, and it is a leash of these varicosities that are inflamed, tender, and swollen.
- The erythema runs from the mid-calf to the mid-thigh.

Your FRCS Short Case Begins

What is your suspected diagnosis?

- "I suspect this patient has superficial venous thrombosis (or thrombophlebitis) of his great saphenous vein."

Would you do any further investigations at this point?

- "I would check routine blood tests, including: FBC, U&Es, clotting, and D-dimer. I would refer the patient for an urgent whole leg ultrasound to determine thrombus extent and exclude asymptomatic DVT."

The duplex confirms SVT but no DVT. What would your management plan be?

- "My main worry in these patients is related to a high risk of further venous thromboembolic events (i.e. DVT and PE). The mainstay of treatment at this stage is anticoagulation. My approach would be determined by the distance of the SVT from the saphenofemoral junction. If the SVT were ≥ 3 cm away from the junction with the deep veins and extending ≥ 5 cm in length I would commence the patient on 45 days of fondaparinux 2.5 mg OD. If the SVT were < 3 cm away from the junction with the deep veins, I would commence the patient on therapeutic anticoagulation for 3 months. In either case I would consider ablation of incompetent superficial veins once the acute inflammatory and prothrombotic phase has settled, at least three months after the most recent thrombotic event."

If the SVT was very close to the junction, for example, 1 cm away, would you consider surgical intervention?

- "I would never say never, but generally speaking my position would be to say no. High ligation of the saphenofemoral junction was frequently used in the past to treat SVT approaching the deep venous system. However, anticoagulation is a less expensive and possibly safer method, and has largely replaced this strategy."

Are there any other medications relevant for treatment of SVT?

- "Yes nonsteroidal anti-inflammatory medications can be considered. NSAIDs may potentially provide symptomatic relief, but also reduce the risk of SVT extension and recurrence."

How would you approach a patient who presented with SVT unrelated to varicose veins?

- "It would depend on the context. SVT can be related to trauma e.g. intravenous drug abuse, cannulation in a healthcare setting etc. The treatment may be much the same as above in terms of anticoagulation, NSAIDs etc. Sometimes patients present with septic thrombophlebitis, and this is associated with the use of intravenous cannulas. In this case I would remove the cannula and commence intravenous antibiotics via a different line. In another context the SVT may be related to an underlying condition such as a hypercoagulable state or underlying malignancy. If this was a possibility I would carry out a focused clinical assessment. I would consider a CT chest/abdomen/pelvis if considering underlying malignancy. I may also liaise with haematology about doing special blood tests to look for clotting abnormalities."

Your FRCS Short Case Ends

Relevant ESVS Guideline Recommendations on SVT

- For patients with suspected lower limb superficial vein thrombosis, a whole leg ultrasound scan is recommended to determine thrombus extent and exclude asymptomatic deep vein thrombosis.
- For patients with isolated lower limb superficial vein thrombosis <5 cm in length on ultrasound and lacking high risk features, such as malignancy, thrombophilia, or proximity to the deep venous system, anticoagulation is not recommended.

- For patients with lower limb superficial vein thrombosis ≥3 cm away from the junction with the deep veins and extending ≥5 cm in length, fondaparinux 2.5 mg once daily is recommended.
- For patients with lower limb superficial vein thrombosis ≥3 cm away from the junction with the deep veins and extending ≥5 cm in length, an intermediate dose of a low molecular weight heparin should be considered as an alternative to fondaparinux.
- For patients with lower limb superficial vein thrombosis extending ≥5 cm in length on ultrasound and extending ≥3 cm from the junction with the deep veins, 45 days of anticoagulation treatment is recommended.
- For patients with superficial vein thrombosis of the leg, which exhibits high risk clinical and/or anatomical features, a 3-month course of anticoagulation may be considered.
- For patients with lower limb superficial vein thrombosis, acute superficial venous intervention is not recommended.
- For patients with lower limb superficial vein thrombosis, ablation of incompetent superficial veins should be considered once the acute inflammatory and prothrombotic phase has settled, at least 3 months after the most recent thrombotic event.

CHAPTER 20

Mesenteric Arterial Disease

One of these cases turned up in my FRCS Part B Examination as a short case. There were a few questions around this topic in the Part A Examination as well. Also, in the past few years, I have dealt with a few cases of mesenteric ischaemia that had to go to theatre for laparotomies and mesenteric embolectomy/bypass/retrograde stenting, etc. For the most part, however, mesenteric ischaemia cases are in the chronic setting, and they often are managed by endovascular means. I don't think this is a "common" topic, but I still consider it a core topic. I will use my own experiences to create some FRCS case examples and we will go through them and draw out the important principles of management.

CASE 20.1: Elderly Woman with Chronic Mesenteric Ischaemia

- A 78-year-old woman is referred to your outpatient clinic with weight loss and abdominal pain after eating.
- She has already had an ultrasound scan, upper GI endoscopy, and abdominal CT scan after being investigated and discharged by the general surgery team.
- The referral later states that this patient has suspected chronic mesenteric ischaemia.

Your FRCS Long Case Begins

Please take a history and examine this patient, and present your findings to me afterwards.

- "This is a 78 year old patient who presents with postprandial abdominal pain. The pain begins 20–30 minutes after eating and lasts 1-2 hours. She also has a fear of eating and reports significant weight loss. She is smoker, diabetic, has hypertension and is on treatment for raised cholesterol. In terms of comorbidities she has ischaemic disease, previous TIA, chronic obstructive pulmonary disease, chronic kidney disease and peripheral vascular disease. It sounds like she has had previous angioplasty/stenting to her right leg, and a left carotid endarterectomy following a TIA 7 years ago. She is currently on best medical therapy with aspirin and high-dose atorvastatin. In the social history she lives at home with her husband, she is independent of activities of daily living, although she has a poor exercise tolerance because of mainly intermittent claudication. She is a heavy smoker. On examination she is systemically well, but looks like she as lost a lot of weight. Her trousers are loose. Her abdomen is soft and non-tender, it is scaphoid in appearance, and she has a midline laparotomy scar. Pulse assessment reveals a full complement of upper limb pulses, but only femoral pulses. There are no signs of chronic limb-threatening ischaemia. My impression is that this patient is a true vasculopath with evidence of atherosclerosis in multiple territories. She has all the risk factors for atherosclerotic disease. The symptoms and signs I would consider to represent a classic presentation of chronic mesenteric ischaemia."

What would be your initial management plan?

- "Bloods (FBC, U&Es, LFTs, lipid screen, clotting, HBA1c), ECG, duplex ultrasound of the mesenteric arteries and/or CT angiography. I would strongly recommend smoking cessation. It sounds like she is already on best medical therapy. After this I would discuss the case in the vascular MDT depending upon the radiology results."

Can you please review these CT angiogram images?

- "Based upon these images, there appears to be severe stenotic disease of both the coeliac artery origin and the proximal SMA. This is obviously not a full CT for me to interpret, but the supra-renal aorta looks like calcified and diseased, and the infra-renal aorta and iliac arteries also look diseased as well."

What are the management options if you were considering intervention?

- "There are three broad options: conservative management, endovascular intervention, or open surgery. This looks like genuine chronic mesenteric ischaemia, and therefore I do not think conservative management alone is a viable option. I also don't think open surgery looks ideal. Therefore I would primarily support an endovascular approach."

How would you approach endovascular intervention?

- "I would review the CT images in the vascular MDT and with interventional radiology. The most important points are access, and the anatomical pattern of disease. The patient has upper limb and femoral pulses, so we could approach the mesenteric vessels from above and below. I would also be interested in reviewing the angles of the SMA and coeliac axis as they come off the aorta. If the angles were awkward, a brachial approach might be better."

Which vessels are you mainly interested in targeting?

- "The SMA."

Would you support balloon angioplasty or stenting?

- "In these cases I would support routine mesenteric stenting as opposed to balloon angioplasty alone."

Would you not consider open surgery in this patient?

- "Yes I would consider it. However, in this case I think endovascular is more appropriate. The patient has had a previous laparotomy which would make surgery more challenging, and the aorta and iliacs are diseased which would make mesenteric bypass more challenging. She also looks like a good candidate for endovascular treatment."

When would you be more inclined to offer open surgery then?

- "Failed endovascular therapy, patients who are not candidates for endovascular therapy because of long occlusions, extensive calcification or access difficulties. Also in younger fitter patients as one can argue that open surgery is potentially a more durable option."

If this patient had an isolated coeliac artery stenosis, and the SMA and IMA were disease free, would you consider intervention?

- "I think you are possibly suggesting median arcuate ligament syndrome. Generally speaking, for coeliac artery lesions angioplasty and stenting carries a higher rate of re-stenosis and should not be performed if there is active compression by the median arcuate ligament. Coeliac stenting might be an option if the vessel was not being compressed or if the median arcuate ligament had been surgically released already either by a laparoscopic or open surgical technique. In any case I would not rush into this. I would discuss it in the MDT, and probably consider further duplex assessment of the coeliac artery to ascertain the significance of the disease with flow/velocity measurements."

Your FRCS Long Case Ends

Relevant ESVS Guideline Recommendations

- In patients with suspected CMI, DUS of the mesenteric arteries is recommended as the first-line examination.

- In patients with a moderate-to-high suspicion of CMI, CTA is recommended to map the occlusive disease, and to detect or exclude other intra-abdominal pathology.

- MRA may be considered an alternative to CTA for the diagnosis of suspected CMI, although there is some evidence that images obtained with MRA are not as accurate or complete as those obtained with CTA.

- The diagnosis of CMI should be considered less likely in the absence of multi-vessel stenosis or occlusion and warrants careful investigation for alternative causes.

- In patients with otherwise unexplained abdominal symptoms, and occlusive disease of two or three mesenteric arteries, CMI should be considered to be the cause of the symptoms.

- In patients with symptomatic chronic mesenteric ischaemia caused by multi-vessel occlusive disease, revascularisation is recommended.

- In patients with symptomatic single vessel disease, revascularisation may be considered.

- In patients with advanced disease (severe weight loss, diarrhoea, continuous pain), it is not recommended to delay revascularisation in order to improve nutritional status first.

- In patients requiring intervention, the superior long term results of open surgery must be offset against a possible early benefit of endovascular intervention with regard to peri-procedural mortality and morbidity.

- The SMA should be the main target vessel to revascularise.

- If endovascular treatment is required, routine mesenteric stenting should be used as opposed to plain balloon angioplasty.

- In patients requiring mesenteric artery stenting, covered stents, as opposed to bare metal stents, may be considered.

- In patients with chronic mesenteric ischaemia, open revascularisation should be considered in the following situations:
  1. Failed endovascular therapy.
  2. Patients who are not candidates for endovascular therapy because of long occlusions and extensive calcification that precludes safe angioplasty and stenting.
  3. In young patients with complex non-atherosclerotic lesions caused by vasculitis or mid-aortic syndrome.

- Patients with CMI should preferably be investigated and treated at specialised centres that can offer a multidisciplinary assessment, as well as both open and endovascular treatment.

CASE 20.2: Middle-Aged Gentleman with Chronic Mesenteric Ischaemia

- A 61-year-old gentleman presents with abdominal pain, weight loss, and diarrhoea.
- These symptoms have been progressing for a few months.
- He has had a previous left to right femoro-femoral crossover for intermittent claudication 10 years ago.
- He also has hypertension, diabetes, raised cholesterol, and is a heavy smoker.
- H denies any previous abdominal surgery.
- He works as an oil rig manager in South Africa and is currently visiting family in the United Kingdom.
- He lives with his wife and says he is otherwise independent.

Your FRCS Short Case Begins

Can you please review these CT images?

- "This image shows severe stenotic disease of the SMA. The sagittal and coronal images suggest there is a 2–3 cm length of heavy atherosclerotic disease of the proximal SMA. The coeliac artery also has what looks like a 50% stenosis at the origin. The IMA appears occluded. There is also a femoro-femoral crossover that is occluded. The right iliac artery is occluded and the left iliac artery is severely diseased and calcified."

The case is discussed in the vascular MDT and the recommendation is for endovascular treatment. What would be your plan in this context?

- "Firstly I would start off with the basics i.e. recommend smoking cessation, and ensure he was on best medical therapy. I would counsel the patient carefully and highlight that an endovascular approach is minimally invasive and has been recommended by the MDT, however it still carries risks and there are alternatives which include open surgery. I would specifically mention that there is a risk of making the blood supply to his gut worse with an endovascular approach, and that this could be life-threatening. Indeed, if that happened, we would likely need to proceed to open surgery."

OK fair enough. But how would you access the mesenteric vessels?

- "Well, femoral access does not look viable. Does the patient have upper limb pulses? (the examiner nods their head). Therefore, I would adopt a brachial access approach."

The patient goes for an endovascular approach the morning after the MDT. Unfortunately, the interventional radiologist cannot cross the SMA lesion. However, the coeliac artery stenosis is crossed and stented. You are called to see the patient on the vascular ward 4 hours later as he is complaining of severe abdominal pain. How would you approach this?

- "Focused history and examination. What are the abdominal examination findings? …. Strong analgesia, high flow oxygen, large-bore IV access. Urgent blood tests including D-dimer and arterial blood gas. Urgent repeat CT angiogram."

The patient is not peritonitic but he is complaining of severe generalised abdominal pain. Can you please review these investigation results?

- "The WBC and CRP and slightly raised. The lactate and pH are normal. The CT shows occlusion of the proximal SMA now, but the coeliac stent is still patent."

Why did you ask for a D-dimer?

- "The ESVS guidelines recommend D-dimer assessment in patients with acute abdominal pain to exclude acute mesenteric ischaemia."

Are you reassured by the normal lactate?

- "Not in the slightest. Raised lactate is a sign of global tissue malperfusion, and I would expect it to be raised at the later stage when probably bowel ischaemia was already fully established. Again, as per the ESVS guidelines, use of L-lactate measurement is not recommended to diagnose or rule out acute occlusive mesenteric ischaemia."

What is your management plan then?

- "In my opinion this patient has acute mesenteric ischaemia. The proximal SMA has thrombosed and occluded. This is a failed endovascular attempt. Therefore I think the patient needs open surgery."

Would you not consider another endovascular attempt?

- "Well it did not work the first time, why would it work a second time?"

Don't the ESVS guidelines on mesenteric disease recommend endovascular therapy as first-line treatment for acute SMA thrombotic occlusion?

- "Yes it does. However, these are guidelines. The authors of these guidelines still expect their readers to have common sense. Repeating techniques that did not work the first time equals flailing in my book. I am not wasting time with this patient. He needs a laparotomy end of story."

What are your options for open surgery then?

- "In terms of restoring mesenteric perfusion I think the options are either a bypass or retrograde SMA stenting."

How would you do a bypass?

- "The options are either prosthetic or using autologous vein (i.e. GSV or femoral vein). However, I need a bypass source. His iliacs looked terrible on the CT angiogram, so I don't think a retrograde bypass is possible. The other options include an antegrade bypass from the infra-renal or supra-coeliac aorta."

Please review these images.

- "His infra-renal and supra-coeliac aorta look pretty calcified. I would not want to go clamping them."

So what would you do?

- "I would take the patient to theatre, do a laparotomy, expose the SMA at the route of the mesentery, and ask interventional radiology to stent the proximal SMA from here. After this I would put some warm wet packs over the bowel, wait for 15 minutes, and check its viability. If the bowel was non-viable I would resect it and leave the ends in situ, leave a laparostomy, and come back in 24–48 hours for a re-look. Even if the bowel did look viable, I probably would still leave a laparostomy and plan for further re-look."

Would you do this case on your own?

- "No. I would ask for a general surgery consultant to be present, a second senior vascular surgery consultant to be present, and also for a consultant interventional radiologist to be present."

When you were doing the laparotomy what would you be particularly wary of?

- "It does not matter as much in this case, but I would be careful not to cut the femoro-femoral crossover in half. If this crossover was patent and that happened there would be massive life-threatening bleeding."

This is a pretty complex case. Do you not think you should wait for a formal MDT discussion before you took the patient to theatre?

- "A rapid 'mini-MDT' could take place and would be what I would do in real life. However, this is a life-threatening time-sensitive vascular surgery emergency. This is the time to be restoring mesenteric perfusion, not spending 3 hours talking about restoring mesenteric perfusion. Time is tissue."

Your FRCS Short Case Ends

Shout out to Duncan, great job here. You know who you are.

Relevant ESVS Guideline Recommendations

- In patients with acute abdominal pain, D-dimer measurement is recommended to exclude acute mesenteric ischaemia.
- Use of L-lactate measurement is not recommended to diagnose or rule out acute occlusive mesenteric ischaemia.
- In patients with suspected AMI, triphasic CTA with 1-mm slices (or thinner) should be used to detect mesenteric arterial occlusion.
- In patients with suspected AMI and elevated creatinine values, CTA might be considered, accepting the risk of contrast-induced renal failure, to save life.
- In patients with acute mesenteric arterial ischaemia, open or endovascular revascularisation should be considered before bowel surgery.
- In patients undergoing mesenteric revascularisation, completion imaging with angiography or transit time flow measurements should be considered.

- In patients undergoing laparotomy for AMI, clinical judgement should be considered the preferred method for assessing bowel viability.
- In patients undergoing acute intestinal revascularisation, second-look laparotomy and damage control surgery should be considered.
- In patients with acute thrombotic SMA occlusion, endovascular therapy should be considered first-line therapy because of lower mortality and bowel resection rates compared with open revascularisation.
- In patients surviving AMI, secondary medical prevention, including smoking cessation, statin therapy, and antiplatelet or anticoagulation treatment, is recommended.

CASE 20.3: Young Gentleman with Acute Mesenteric Ischaemia

- A 40-year-old gentleman is admitted under the general surgical team with sudden onset generalised abdominal pain.
- He does not have peritonitis.
- His routine blood tests are normal, including amylase and CRP.
- He has had a CT abdomen.
- He is referred urgently to you by the general surgical registrar on-call.

Your FRCS Short Case Begins

The general surgical registrar informs you over the telephone that this patient has had a CT angiogram which has been reported as showing embolic occlusion of the mid-SMA. The scan also says that there are signs of small bowel malperfusion. What would be your approach to this case?

- "I would immediately go and assess the patient. I would carry out a focused history and examination. Is there an obvious source for embolism for atrial fibrillation such as an irregular pulse? Does the patient have any other comorbidities? Is he on any regular medications? How well is the patient? What are the abdominal examination findings? Has he had previous abdominal surgery? Does he have any hernias?"

The patient is completely fit and well. He is not on any medications. His abdomen is completely soft but generally tender. There are no signs of previous surgery or hernias. He has a regular pulse.

- "I would review the CT angiogram myself in the real world."

Here you go (examiner hands you some CT images on laminated white paper).

- "The coeliac artery appears disease free and patent. The proximal SMA appears similarly disease free and patent. The coronal and sagittal images demonstrate occlusion of the SMA around 4 cm from the SMA origin. Again, there is no obvious atherosclerotic or calcific disease of the SMA to suggest chronic disease. Otherwise the arteries appear pristine. In my opinion this would be consistent with acute mesenteric ischaemia secondary to SMA embolism."

What would be your management approach?

- "Make the patient nil by mouth. Ensure large-bore intravenous access and ensure the patient has his clotting checked and a valid group and save. ECG. Intravenous heparin. My plan this juncture would be to take the patient to theatre for a laparotomy and SMA embolectomy."

What CT signs are you most worried about in this context?

- "The presence of intestinal wall or porto-mesenteric gas on CTA is a sign of severe transmural ischaemia."

If the CT showed this, would you palliate the patient?

- "No. This is not necessarily associated with a fatal outcome if treated in a timely fashion."

Would you not consider an endovascular attempt to restore perfusion followed by a diagnostic laparoscopy to examine the bowel?

- "These are options which can be considered, but I think a laparotomy is quicker and safer."

How would you do an SMA embolectomy then?

- "I would ask for the assistance of another senior vascular surgery consultant. I would also ask for a general surgery consultant to be involved in the case to help evaluate the bowel. I would do a full midline laparotomy, lift up the transverse mesocolon and omentum, and expose the route of the mesentery. Hopefully I would still be able to feel an SMA pulse at the base of the mesentery. I would make a 4–5 cm transverse incision in the visceral peritoneum/transverse mesocolon in the root of the mesentery, and then carefully dissect downwards and sloop the SMA twice (proximally and distally). I would be careful not to injure any branches coming off the SMA or the SMV. I would make a small horizontal arteriotomy and proceed with a gentle Fogarty balloon embolectomy. I would focus on the inflow first, and then clear the outflow. After this I would do a 6-0 prolene suture repair of the arteriotomy. I would also do an on-table diagnostic angiogram. Of note, if there SMA was small or diseased, I would do a longitudinal arteriotomy and repair with a vein patch."

What if the on-table angiogram showed that the very distal parts of SMA were still affected by some embolus?

- "Then I would consider on-table thrombolysis. However, if the main proximal part of the SMA and the large proximal branches were patent, I would be inclined to sit tight."

What would you do after this?

- "I would put some warm packs around the bowel and return the viscera into the abdomen, waiting for 15–20 minutes. After this I would ask the general surgeon to have a look at the bowel, and we would make a decision on the need for bowel resection."

The small bowel and right colon look reasonably well-perfused after 20 minutes. Part of the mid-small bowel looks suspicious, but the general surgeon feels positive about it. The general surgeon is keen to close the abdomen. What are your thoughts?

- "I would be inclined to leave the abdomen open as a laparostomy, and plan to bring the patient back for a re-look laparotomy in 24–48 hours time. This segment of small bowel may well become frankly ischaemic and declare itself by then when it would likely need to be resected."

What else would be in your post-operative plan?

- "Continue IV heparin. 2 post-op doses of intravenous antibiotics. The patient would go back to intensive care, and I would highlight to the critical care team that there may a systemic response as a consequence of reperfusion injury. If the ECG was normal then as it stands we do not have a cause for the embolic event. I would therefore request a CT angiogram of the thoracic aorta, 24-hour ECG, and echocardiogram. The patient will likely require long term anticoagulation."

Your FRCS Short Case Ends

CASE 20.4: Elderly Woman with Acute Mesenteric Ischaemia

- A 78-year-old woman presents under the general surgeons with acute generalised abdominal pain for the past 24 hours.
- *She is comorbid:* Ischaemic heart disease, hypertension, type 2 diabetes, chronic kidney disease stage 3, raised BMI, and osteoarthritis.
- She lives at home with her husband.
- She has poor mobility due to advanced osteoarthritis of her knees.
- On presentation, she had an initial CT angiogram which demonstrated severe disease of the coeliac and SMA origins. The IMA was occluded. There was CT evidence of ischaemia in the coeliac territory with gallbladder ischaemia and splenic ischaemia. The small bowel also looked globally malperfused, but not frankly ischaemic.
- The patient was referred directly to interventional radiology by the general surgeons.
- She went for an endovascular attempt at revascularisation.
- The coeliac artery has been stented, but the SMA lesion could not be crossed.
- *This is now 24 hours later, and the general surgical team are referring the case to you the vascular consultant on-call.*

Your FRCS Long Case Begins

The general surgery consultant telephones you and explains the above story. He says that the patient has worsening abdominal pain and a repeat CT scan shows that the proximal SMA is now occluded. The coeliac stent is still patent but the gallbladder is showing worsening signs of ischaemia. The small bowel also looks generally malperfused. The patient is now on intensive care with increasing inotropic requirements. The patient is not peritonitic, but generally very tender. The lactate is slightly raised at 2.4. What are your thoughts?

- "It sounds like this patient needs a laparotomy."

Fair enough. If you were to take the patient to theatre, what would be your plan?

- "From the beginning I would go and see the patient myself. I would look at the CT scan myself, and review it with a consultant interventional radiologist. I would ask for a senior vascular surgery consultant to be involved. I am thinking of doing either a retrograde open SMA stent or a mesenteric bypass to revascularise the SMA. I also think the patient needs a cholecystectomy and there is a high chance she will need bowel resecting. I would therefore keep the general surgeons involved as well."

Are there other surgical options?

- "Theoretically one could divide the SMA distal to the occlusive lesion and re-implant it onto the infra-renal aorta, or one could consider thromboendarterectomy of the SMA with patch angioplasty."

Would you consider this in such a case?

- "Probably not. You told me that the proximal SMA was occluded. Getting access here to do an endarterectomy and patch repair does not look like a viable option. Similarly, clamping the aorta in this patient is probably not a good idea. She is already pretty comorbid and sick, and I doubt clamping her aorta is going to help."

So where would you take a bypass from?

- "The options include the supra-coeliac aorta, infra-renal aorta or the iliacs. In my experience the aorta is rarely an option in these patients because they are not the fittest candidates, and the aortas are usually heavily calcified/diseased. I also would not to clamp the supra-coeliac aorta as I would be worried about the coeliac stent thrombosing."

Can you please review these images? (*You are handed some more CT images on laminated bits of paper*)

- "As I said the supra-coeliac is very calcified. I would not clamp that. The infra-renal aorta is also diseased and calcified. The right common iliac artery looks relatively disease free. Therefore this is where I would my bypass from."

How would you do such a bypass?

- "First of all I would counsel the patient very carefully and involve the family in the discussions. I would explain that this is complex risky surgery, and there is a very high risk of death even despite a successful revascularisation attempt. I would also not do this on my own. I would get a second consultant vascular surgeon to assist me along with a general surgery consultant. The patient would get a full midline laparotomy and I would use an Omnitract to improve exposure."

As soon as you enter the abdomen, the majority of the small bowel looks generally malperfused, but not frankly ischaemic. The right colon also looks malperfused, but still viable. There is no bowel perforation. There is segment of mid-small bowel that looks worse than the rest of the areas with some more frank ischaemic patches. The gallbladder is frankly ischemic and necrotic and grossly

oedematous, but not perforated. The spleen on the whole looks viable, and not overtly ischaemic. Would you revascularise the gut first?

- "In principle revascularisation should take place first. However, this gallbladder sounds like it is about to perforate, and I would rather remove it first to avoid causing any intra-abdominal contamination. After this I would do the bypass."

How would you do the bypass?

- "I would expose the SMA at the route of the mesentery and the right common iliac artery. I would use a long C-shaped PTFE ring-enforced graft with end-to-side anastomoses to both the SMA and CIA. I would also cover the SMA anastomosis with an omental flap."

Would you not rather use an autologous vein bypass such as GSV harvested from the leg?

- "This is an emergency setting, the patient is unwell, and the whole small bowel and right colon look ischaemic. Autologous vein bypass sounds like the correct plan in theory, but this is the real world and I am interested in restoring mesenteric perfusion as soon as possible. Also, vein grafts originating from the iliac artery are prone to kinking, which is why I think prosthetic is better."

You do the bypass. What's next?

- "I would ask for a handheld Doppler and confirm decent flow in the SMA distal to my anastomosis. I would also put warm wet packs around the bowel and return everything into the abdomen and wait for 15–20 minutes."

After 20 minutes, most of the small bowel and right colon improve and develop a nice healthy pink appearance. The segment of mid-small bowel you were worrying about also pinks up. However, there are a few small ischaemic patches that are slightly concerning. The general surgeon does not wish to resect. What would you do now?

- "I would leave the abdomen open as a laparostomy, with a plan to bring back in 24 hours time."

The patient deteriorates on ICU. She is brought back to theatre within 24 hours. This segment of small bowel is resected. The rest of the small bowel and right colon look viable. There is still a pulse in the graft and the SMA. The transverse colon and left colon also look viable. The liver and spleen look otherwise reassuring. As she is still unwell, the small bowel is not re-anastomosed. The laparostomy is maintained and she goes back to ICU again. The patient dies 24 hours later of multi-organ failure. What are your thoughts?

- "This was an elderly comorbid patient with significant ischaemia involving the coeliac and SMA distributions. As per my original discussion with the patient and family there was a high risk of mortality despite a successful revascularisation. Upon reperfusion of the SMA there may well have been a profound reperfusion injury which accelerated her demise."

Another vascular surgeon asks how you did the bypass? Why did you not do a bypass using GSV or femoral vein? Since you used plastic, why did you not use a vein patch for the SMA anastomosis? ...

Your FRCS Long Case Ends

JMF Reflections

Cases like these are not easy, especially not in real life. Whatever you do, don't be surprised if the outcome is not great. I would recommend having in your mind what your approach to tackling these sorts of problems is going to be ahead of time. Also be prepared to justify your approach as well, whatever you choose to do in such a setting. Finally, don't forget that it is easy to play Captain Hindsight with cases like these. My advice would be to do the best job you can.

CHAPTER 21

Vascular Trauma

Vascular trauma is an enormous topic, and one cannot authoritatively cover it in a single chapter. However, I do remember the questions I got asked in regards to vascular trauma in the FRCS examination, and I also work in a major trauma unit. Henceforth, I hope to use this chapter to give you some common sense, pragmatic, and real world guidance on how to handle vascular trauma. I have chosen to design this chapter with a few case-based discussions which will hopefully map out the principles of management that will be transferrable to other scenarios. I am just going to describe these cases as if you and I were actually there, in the moment, as first persons.

Laparoscopic Port Injury to Major Retroperitoneal Vessel with Unstable Patient

- In this context, you are being telephoned by a frantic anaesthetic registrar at 10 pm.
- The case is that of a young woman who was having a diagnostic laparoscopy for a case of suspected ovarian torsion.
- The case is being performed by a junior gynaecology registrar.
- A veress needle was used to enter the abdomen when suddenly the patient became haemodynamically unstable and developed abdominal swelling.
- The gynaecology registrar thinks he has damaged a major vessel and the patient is unstable. The gynaecology consultant is coming in urgently but advised urgent vascular surgery input.
- The first thing to do is stay calm and not panic!
- Get some decent information from the person who is telephoning you. Chances are it will be an anaesthetist or a theatre nurse who is calling you in panic at the request of the operating surgeon who is in the middle of a panic attack themselves!
- What is the problem? Get as much information as you can. What was the intended operation? What has happened? Is the patient stable or unstable? What has been done so far?
- Where is the problem? Which theatre? Is it in another hospital? If it is in another hospital, try and get some information in regards to how you are actually going to find the operating theatre, and contact details for someone who can direct you to the theatre in question.
- *Give some instructions:* If it is a suspected major vascular injury related to a laparoscopic port injury, this would be my advice: "Do a laparotomy, put your finger on the bleeding point, call for assistance from a senior general surgeon who is available, institute the massive blood transfusion protocol, try and open a major vascular tray and have some aortic clamps available, ideally get an omnitract if you have one available, that it is going to be 15–30 minutes until you get there, and the priority is to stop the bleeding in the meantime …"
- Next thing is for you to put your clothes on and get in the car.
- **DON'T SPEED**. If you are in a car accident and harm yourself or another person, you will look back with regret. Even if all you get is a speeding ticket, I doubt the authorities who issued you the speeding ticket will empathise with you in any shape or form.
- When you arrive in the hospital, now you are in that really awkward position. Where are the operating theatres? Where are the changing rooms? Hopefully there is someone at main reception who can help direct you. Or perhaps you took the mobile phone number

of the person in theatre who originally rang you who can come down and help direct you to where you need to be ....

- Eventually you arrive in the theatre. Expect there to be commotion and panic.
- I would go and introduce myself to the anaesthetist first and ask how the patient is doing. What is the haemodynamic status? What is the lactate? What is the temperature of the patient? Do we know what the clotting is like? Are we in a damage control situation?
- After this I would introduce myself to the surgeon and get an update.
- After this I would introduce myself to the rest of the team.
- Then I would scrub in.
- Assuming we are dealing with a zone 1 injury (i.e., aortic injury), and a laparotomy has taken place already, with the abdomen being packed, this would be my plan ....
- I would consider extending the laparotomy upwards (i.e., cutting along the xiphisternum to open up the gap between it and the costal margin).
- I would expect to see a belly full of blood → this would require some suctioning and evacuation.
- If an omnitract were available, I would insert it now to improve exposure.
- Gain supra-coeliac control. I would ask the anaesthetist to insert a naso/orogastric tube to help me to identify the oesophagus. I would dissect the left triangular ligament of the liver and try to move the left lobe of the liver to the patient's right. I would dissect through the lesser omentum and feel for an aortic pulse just below the diaphragmatic crura. This may require some sharp and blunt dissection. I would apply the aortic clamp and push it backwards so it settles on the vertebra (*easier said than done, and we all know it probably won't look anything like this when you do it as everything is unstable and uncontrolled*).
- Once the supra-coeliac aorta is controlled, I would **STOP THE OPERATION**.
- The anaesthetist is updated by myself and I ask for them to "catch-up." This means instituting the major transfusion protocol and transfusing the patient with blood, platelets, and fresh frozen plasma in a ratio of 1:1:1.
- I would give some time for the anaesthetist to get settled. I would also make sure to ask the anaesthetic registrar to call their consultant in to come and assist.
- *Call for further help* → Are there any other senior surgeons around who can come and assist?
- After a little bit of time, we need to start doing some actual vascular surgery ....
- The abdominal packs are going to have to be removed (if they haven't been already), and we are going to need to do some exploring around zone 1.
- If this is an infra-renal aortic injury, I would probably just eviscerate the small bowel over to the right, liberate the fourth part of the duodenum by taking down the ligament of Trietz, and clamp the infra-renal aorta below the left renal vein. This would allow me to release the supra-coeliac clamp and restore mesenteric perfusion ....
- Then I would probably use a combination of finger dissection and/or suction dissection to feel for the iliac arteries and clamp them (the haematoma would hopefully have done most of the dissection for me).
- *Remember the overall plan for vascular injury is this:* Proximal control, distal control, and then attack the injury.
- Once proximal and distal control has been achieved, I would enter the haematoma and identify the injury.
- Given the nature of the original surgery, I would expect there to be a hole in the infra-renal aorta that I would hopefully be able to repair using a few 3-0 prolene sutures. If this were possible, I would do so, and then leave it at that!

- Assuming I were able to repair the aortic injury, I would then continue with damage control principles → keep the operation focused on stopping haemorrhage and controlling contamination.

- I would do a rapid laparotomy to ensure there was no visceral injury (i.e., run the large bowel, small bowel, stomach, and gallbladder). If there were bowel injury, I would just suture any small holes, or staple bowel ends off and leave the ends in the abdomen.

- Next job is to do a laparostomy and get the patient to intensive care as soon as possible. All this I would try and get done within 1.5 hours.

- This is all on the basis that the patient is unstable, and we are in damage control mode.

- The definitive plan would be to optimise the patient in intensive care over the next 24–48 hours, and then take the patient back for a re-look and hopefully definitive closure.

JMF's Personal Notes

- From experience, and in particular experience learned from other people's mistakes, I would just remember to stick to basic vascular surgery and damage control surgery principles.

- If the patient is in extremis, keep things simple and remember your priority is to stop bleeding, control contamination, and do as little operating as possible.

- Vascular injury = proximal control, distal control, then attack the injury. Don't attack the injury first!

- Packing does not work for an aortic (or iliac injury) → put a damn finger on the hole and press, as opposed to five packs that will just absorb the patient's blood volume!

- Recognise when you should be in damage control mode. Yes be aware of hypothermia, lactic acidosis, and deranged clotting. But also read the scene → has the patient lost a load of blood, do the anaesthetic team look really worried and are they pumping in loads of nasty vasoconstrictors, does the bowel look unhealthy and poorly perfused, do you feel like the patient is really in trouble? If you think you should be in damage control mode, you probably should be. So don't spend 4 hours in the operating room trying to do a "definitive job." You should be focusing on doing the bare minimum to save the patient's life and then getting them to intensive care ASAP!

- Be aware of your other options. In this case, I talked about doing a standard infra-renal aortic exposure. However, you can always consider the left medial visceral rotation ... we will revisit this approach later on in a different context.

Self-Harm Knife Injury to Antecubital Fossa with Reported Brachial Artery Laceration, Stable Patient with Tourniquet In Situ

- *First point* → Just because you have been told this is a brachial artery injury, it does not mean it is ....

- On more than one occasion I have been called down to A&E resus for a "major vascular injury" and the patient has a tourniquet in situ. I am usually cynical at the best of times, and henceforth usually ask for the tourniquet to be taken down to allow me to assess the injury for myself. It is not uncommon for the "brachial artery injury" to actually be nothing more than a superficial venous injury. Anyways, I have made this point now, so let us continue as if this is a genuine brachial artery injury ....

- *Eyeball the patient* → Do they look like there has been a major haemorrhage? Is the patient pale, sweaty, clammy, anxious? Is there blood over and around the patient? What is the patient's GCS?

- Make sure the ABCDE's are OK.
- Ensure good intravenous access (contralateral arm preferably).
- *Ensure bloods have been sent urgently:* FBC, U&Es, clotting, group & save (+/− crossmatch).
- I guess you should listen to the paramedic handover. They will usually tell you there was a load of blood on the scene and there was arterial bleeding .... I would take this with a big pinch of salt however .... You could have a paper cut and the paramedics would put a tourniquet on and call the case a major haemorrhage ....
- I would always release the tourniquet and get confirmation this is a vascular injury. You will know pretty quickly! However, before you release the tourniquet, I would take advantage of the situation and assess the forearm for suitable veins that you might use as a conduit for a possible bypass—the tourniquet should have made the veins nice and juicy.
- I would say trust your instincts and clinical acumen. If there is a deep gash in the antecubital fossa or medial arm with blood hosing out then no surprises as to the diagnosis. If the tourniquet comes off and there is no bleeding, no expanding haematoma, and an intact radial pulse distally, I would breathe a big sigh of relief ....
- On the other hand, I have seen genuine brachial artery injuries where the artery has been completely transected, and yet there has been absolutely no bleeding. The patient however had no distal pulses and a cold hand, i.e., it was ischaemic .... Henceforth, don't always think there has to be massive bleeding in a case of significant vascular trauma.
- Let's assume there is an obvious vascular injury however, and there is active bleeding .... put the tourniquet back on!
- Counsel and consent the patient for a left arm exploration and brachial artery repair (include need to harvest vein from arm or leg).
- Transfer the patient to emergency theatre.
- I would not do such a case under a local anaesthetic or an arm block, as far as I am concerned this is a general anaesthetic case.
- *Same principles as with last case* → Proximal control, distal control, attack the injury ....
- Before prepping the arm, I would replace the paramedic tourniquet with a proper theatre tourniquet. I would change the tourniquet whilst someone reliable (i.e., me) was controlling the brachial artery above the injury with my fingers.
- The arm is prepped from the tourniquet downwards to the wrist.
- The hand goes in a see-through bag.
- Depending upon where the injury was would determine where I made my first incision.
- As the tourniquet has given me proximal control, I would perhaps extend the injury incision up and down (or even across), and get a suitable self-retainer in the wound.
- I would dissect down through the brachial aponeurosis and control the brachial artery in a standard fashion.
- If proximal control was challenging because of haematoma, I would make a longitudinal incision in between the biceps and triceps and identify the brachial artery in the upper arm, and then swing this incision downwards towards the antecubital fossa as a lazy S incision.
- At this point, one would hopefully have an idea of the nature of the injury.
- Any surrounding veins that had been additionally injured would no doubt be simply ligated using 3-0 vicryl sutures.

- If it were a simple laceration to the brachial artery, this may be amenable to a suture repair using something like 5-0 or 6-0 prolene.
- If it were a complete transection, I would be more inclined to do an interposition graft using either ipsilateral reversed arm vein (i.e., cephalic vein) or GSV harvested from either groin or ankle, as opposed to a direct repair of the two severed brachial artery ends (*I don't like tension on suture lines and I think in this case the brachial artery would require some trimming to get decent healthy vessels for the anastomosis, and all this could leave the two arterial ends a bit "stretched"*).
- In this context, I would do a Fogarty embolectomy of the outflow vessels and confirm decent inflow before doing my interposition grafting. I would also make sure to give the outflow a decent flush with heparinised saline as well, and then consider shunting the brachial artery to restore flow distally whilst I go hunting for vein. Finally, if there were no other competing injuries and I had achieved proximal and distal control, I would consider asking for heparin to be given whilst I was shunting the patient and doing the arterial repair …. the last thing I would want would be for everything to thrombose.
- If there were a concomitant median nerve or extensive tendon/muscular belly injury I would probably ask for plastic surgery assistance as well.
- Usually I would not consider an upper limb fasciotomy, but if there vascular injury was profound and I were dealing with a case of advanced ischaemia, I would consider an upper limb fasciotomy.

Other Considerations for Brachial Artery Injuries

- A high brachial artery injury may not be amenable to a tourniquet for proximal control. In this situation, you may need to do an axillary artery infra-clavicular cut-down to get proximal control.
- In damage control situations (and in particular if there are additional torso injuries), you should always consider shunting the brachial artery and repairing it at a later date when the patient is more stable.
- In worst-case scenarios with catastrophic haemorrhage, ligation is always an option. Just be aware of the ischaemic insult.

Machete Attack to Abdomen, Chest, Neck, and Arms: Unstable Patient

- For this scenario, the time is 1:30 am, and you are at home in bed.
- You get a telephone call from the vascular registrar who is waiting for the patient to arrive in A&E resus.
- The CODE RED trauma call has been put out because of the mechanism of injury, and because the patient is hypotensive, tachycardiac, and tachypnoeic.
- Put some clothes on and get in the car (again, don't speed).
- *On route to the hospital, you should be thinking of only two things:* Following the ATLS protocol (ABCDE or perhaps in this context CABCDE) and adhering to damage control surgical principles. If this patient is as bad as they sound, you are going to be making quick, pragmatic, and sensible decisions that stop major bleeding and control contamination ….
- You arrive in A&E resus around 13 minutes later.
- *Eyeball the patient →* You can see he is in a bad way. He has a tourniquet around his right arm with a big gash across his antecubital fossa that extends down his forearm.

He also has multiple stab wounds to the right side of his abdomen and chest, and a slash wound to his right neck.

- *Airway* → Patent. The patient is talking.
- *Breathing* → His oxygen saturations are 80% on room air, 92% on 15 l of oxygen via a non-rebreathe mask. His respiratory rate is 30. The doctor who did the primary survey said he has reduced air entry on the right side of his chest and it is hyper-resonant to percussion.
- *Circulation* → The blood pressure is 95/55 mmHg, heart rate is 120. There is blood dripping onto the floor from the wound in his right arm. There is blood around the patient's clothes. The neck wound does not seem to be actively bleeding and there is no expanding haematoma. It is a pretty nasty slash, but it does not appear to have breached platysma. The abdomen has two deep gashes in the right upper quadrant/right flank that are oozing blood. The abdomen is not distended and not obviously peritonitic. There is no bowel or omentum protruding from the abdominal wounds. There are no obvious injuries to the legs.
- *Disability* → GCS 15/15, no obvious head injury.
- *Exposure* → As already described.
- *Initial investigations* → All you have is a venous blood gas. The haemoglobin is 75, pH is 7.15, lactate is 8.0, base excess is −10.
- What is the working diagnosis right now? As per this scenario, the patient has a tension pneumothorax on the right, with a brachial artery injury on the right. The neck and abdominal wall injuries for the moment appear to be superficial.
- Plan at this stage? As far as I am concerned, the patient is getting an immediate finger thoracostomy in the right axilla. This releases a large hiss of air but no blood. The patient's haemodynamic status improves rapidly following this. Now he gets a formal chest drain insertion. I would make sure the major transfusion protocol has been instituted, and would make sure the patient is at least getting some O-negative blood. The ideal transfusion would be red cells, platelets, and fresh frozen plasma in a ratio of 1:1:1.
- Let's say that after giving the patient some blood and sorting out his chest drain, he is a bit more stable. We know he has a major vascular injury in the right arm, but currently this is controlled using a tourniquet. What do we do now? Straight to theatre, or would we go to CT?
- "By the book" as this patient is unstable and he has a vascular injury, it would not be incorrect to take the patient straight to theatre. However, I have to be pragmatic here and be honest in regards to what I think would happen in most trauma units. I think it would be fair to take the patient round for a very quick CT scan. In my unit, the CT scanner is literally 1 minute away from A&E resus, and we can get scans done and reported by a radiologist very quickly. I know that the patient is going to theatre anyways, but I still think a CT scan could be helpful even in this sort of setting. I am mainly interested in seeing what is going on inside this patient's abdomen and neck. A full trauma CT would hopefully be able to reassure me that his neck wound is superficial and there is no underlying carotid injury. Likewise, if the CT scan can tell me there is no obvious peritoneal breach, then again I don't have to worry about the abdomen. The chest will be scanned at the same time and at least it will be able to tell me if the chest drain is in the right place and if there is any other thoracic injury that needs urgent attention. Of note, I would only take the patient to CT if he had made an improvement following the initial primary survey life-saving measures. If the patient was in-extremis, he would bypass CT and just go straight to theatre, and I would do what needed to be done in theatre as I saw fit (i.e., if I was worried about the abdomen he would get a laparotomy, if I was worried about the chest he would get a thoracotomy, and if I was worried about the neck he would get a neck exploration). From my perspective, I do think CT, if used appropriately,

can help you to avoid unnecessary cavity explorations, and no doubt these sick trauma patients do benefit from unnecessary surgery ....

- The patient does go for a CT scan. The neck and abdomen are just superficial soft tissue injuries. The right chest shows that he has a moderate haemopneumothorax, but there is no active contrast extravasation. The chest drain is in the right place, and now it is swinging and bubbling and blood is collecting (you measure about 250 ml of blood in the drain and it is not filling very quickly).
- Now the patient goes to theatre, and the focus is on the right arm.
- The patient is still sick, and we are still in damage control mode ....
- The patient is positioned supine in the crucifix position, and he has a urinary catheter, arterial line, and central line inserted.
- The right arm tourniquet from A&E is removed whilst a responsible surgeon controls the brachial artery above the injury with a finger (i.e., you or me do this). At this point, you can see arterial spray coming from the wound which confirms a brachial artery injury. A theatre tourniquet is applied high up the arm and this achieves proximal control once again.
- He is draped from neck to knees to allow the neck, chest and abdomen to be operated on if necessary.
- The right arm is prepped below the tourniquet.
- Now you explore the right arm wound. You can see the brachial artery has been lacerated over a distance of 4 cm. It is not transected, but it is heavily damaged and definitely could not be repaired using a simple prolene suture. This would need an interposition graft repair. You extend your incision proximally and control the brachial artery a few centimetres above the injury. You can also see that the cephalic and antecubital vein have been transected.
- The distal brachial artery and origins of the radial and ulnar arteries are then exposed and controlled.
- The transacted veins do not get repaired. Stick clips on their ends and ligate them using 2-0 or 3-0 vicryl.
- You also notice there are some muscular belly/tendon injuries, and the median nerve appears to be transected ....
- At this point, I would speak to the anaesthetist and find out how the patient is doing. In this scenario, the anaesthetist is not happy. The patient is still acidotic (pH 7.20), his lactate is 5.5, his clotting is deranged, and he is hypothermic. We are still damage control mode.
- You perform a delicate distal thromboembolectomy of the radial and ulnar arteries, and a little bit of clot comes out followed by some reasonable backbleeding. You test the inflow and there is torrential spray from the proximal brachial artery.
- Ask for a shunt (dealer's choice).
- I would shunt this brachial artery injury. If the brachial artery was damaged at the brachial bifurcation, I would probably insert the distal end of the shunt into the radial artery.
- What about now? OK here are two options for the you the reader:
  1. Harvest vein from the leg, and do an interposition graft repair. Following this, ask the plastic surgeons to come in a repair all the muscle bellies, tendons, median nerve, etc. Let's spend the next 4 hours fixing this patient ....
  2. Leave the shunt in place (secure it of course so it doesn't get easily pulled out), do an upper limb fasciotomy, and then get the hell out of there. The wound is not closed. The patient goes to ICU, and as soon as he is metabolically improved, he comes back for a formal repair.

- No guesses as to what my answer is. I would manage this in the damage control setting, do the bare minimum to stop bleeding, control contamination, restore some degree of limb perfusion (via shunting), and then ship the patient off to ICU, in the hope we can come back later on when he is better.

Stab Wound to Left Chest and Upper Abdomen: Unstable Patient

- I was involved in this case a few months ago (i.e., for real) ….
- It is 1:30 am, you are called to A&E as a CODE RED major trauma call. You were on-site at the time, so go down straight away.
- You walk into A&E resus and immediately to your left you can see a young Caucasian male who looks to be about 25 years old. You can see two stab wounds to the left chest and upper abdomen. He looks pale and clammy.
- The A&E consultant is doing a FAST scan of his heart. There is clearly blood around the heart. She turns to you and says you should go and get ready to do a thoracotomy.
- Your emotional response is blunted because most trauma calls you attend are false alarms. Wait a second, am I going to do a clamshell on this guy? For real? I'm glad I just downed that energy drink ….
- You go and put a surgical gown and some gloves on, and ask the A&E nurses to open up the thoracotomy set.
- At this point, various other members of the major trauma team start appearing—anaesthetics, orthopaedics, the trauma coordinator, various nurses, some other A&E doctors show up, it becomes a bit of a mad house … heck even the cardiac surgical registrar shows up!
- **ATLS**

  Airway → Patent. Patient is communicating and actually fairly chilled out about all of this (at least for now he is).
  Breathing → Reduced air entry left side of chest, oxygen saturations 89% on room air.
  Circulation → Tachycardiac and borderline hypotensive.
  Disability → GCS 15/15.
  Exposure → Just 2× stab wounds as previously described.
- Patient gets large-bore IV access in both antecubital fossa, full set of bloods sent off (FBC, U&Es, coagulation, group and save).
- Heart rate is going up (130), blood pressure is now sinking (97 mmHg).
- Patient's ECG shows ST depression, and this is quickly followed by a transient episode of loss of consciousness associated with a ventricular pause …. What now? The A&E consultant does a rapid finger thoracostomy in the left chest and the patient rapidly improves and wakes up again.
- However, his blood pressure starts to plummet and his heart rate is increasing. The patient is looking more grey, pale, and clammy. He is more anxious. His GCS is dropping to around 13 now.
- What is the diagnosis? He probably had a tension pneumothorax that was just decompressed by way of the left finger thoracostomy. However, he also has cardiac injury and cardiac tamponade. He is now peri-arrest.
- What are you going to do? We all know this patient needs a thoracotomy, but where, when, and by whom? There is some discussion about transferring the patient upstairs for

a median sternotomy by the cardiac surgical team. I don't agree with this, neither does the A&E consultant. This patient looks like he is literally about to crash …. The other option is to do a clamshell thoracotomy right here and now. This is what we plan to do. This is how it was done ….

- Emergency theatre scrub nurse already has the whole thoracotomy tray open.
- I am scrubbed in and stood on the left of the patient.
- The cardiac surgical registrar scrubs in and stands on the right of the patient.
- I pour betadine over the chest and give it a good swathe using a white swab.
- The knife is ready to be given to me, the Gigli saw is ready to go, and we have already asked for some 3-0 and 4-0 prolene sutures—these are ready.
- I ask the anaesthetist to proceed, and once he is happy, the plan is for both arms to be lifted up above his head. The patient is anaesthetised, and once I get a thumbs up the arms are quickly lifted.
- I dive into the left side of the chest, and swing the blade across the manubrium.
- I run around to the right side of the patient and dive into the right chest.
- Finger sweep under the manubrium.
- Big clip goes under manubrium and is used to pull the Gigli saw through from one side to the other.
- Gigli saw divides sternum in about 15 seconds.
- Finochietto retractor is inserted into the right chest and cranked open.
- I use scissors to clear some adhesions/fibrous tissue between the sternum and the pericardium.
- The pericardium is tense; I cannot grab it with non-toothed forceps.
- I don't waste time, I ask for the skin knife and incise the pericardium.
- Blood shoots out under arterial pressure.
- The haemodynamic status improves rapidly.
- I use the scissors to make an inverted T cut in the pericardium, not straying too laterally to avoid damaging the phrenic nerves.
- I have a cardiac surgical registrar with me who I know to be practically at consultant level. I have just had a massive adrenaline dump, and think the burden of stress needs to be shared. He is the one who is going to stitch the cardiac injury …. I run around to the left side of the patient again and grab a sucker to assist.
- There is a 0.5-cm stab wound in the right ventricle. The heart is leaping around in the chest and blood shoots out with each heartbeat. A finger controls this. I suck the blood away, whilst the cardiac surgical registrar gets a 4-0 prolene suture in his hand. Over the next 60 seconds, this wound is stitched. We have control. Both of us breathe a sigh of relief. At this point we both remember to ligate / transfix the internal thoracic arteries.
- We know we now have to go up to theatre to formally explore, washout, and close the chest. However, he still has this left upper quadrant abdominal wound. We are worried it may have gone into the abdomen. Unlikely …. but we aren't sure. The patient is stable so we agree to take the patient to CT, and then straight up to theatres. This is what happens. There is no peritoneal breach, so we don't have to worry about the abdomen.
- The cardiac surgery on-call team arrive and myself and the cardiac surgery registrar confirm there are no other thoracic injuries, washout the chest, leave some drains, close the chest, and he goes back to cardiac ICU.

- The patient does very well. His post-op echocardiogram is normal. He goes home 6 days later. At outpatient follow-up 6 weeks later, he has no issues and is formally discharged.
- **BOOM POW!**
- By the way, in my A&E resus trauma thoracotomy operation note, I gave a shout-out to *Top Knife*—what a book!

High-Speed Road Traffic Accident. Aortic Transection/Pseudoaneurysm Just Distal to Left Subclavian Artery. You Are Called to A&E Resus as a Code Red Major Trauma Call

- It is 10 pm.
- You were on-site anyways.
- You go down to A&E immediately.
- There is a 26-year-old female patient who has been in a head-on collision with another car travelling at high speed.
- **ATLS**

  Airway → Patent. Patient is talking normally. She is complaining of severe pain in her chest and back and feeling slightly short of breath.

  Breathing → Oxygen saturations 93% on room air, 100% on a non-rebreathe mask, respiratory rate 26. Chest generally clear, but reduced air entry left base and dull to percussion.

  Circulation → Heart rate 100, blood pressure 100/80 mmHg. Can feel radial pulses and all lower limb pulses bilaterally. Abdomen soft and non-tender, non-distended. No obvious long bone fractures. Pelvis not tender. Patient can straight leg raise bilaterally.

  Disability → GCS 15/15. No obvious head injury.

  Exposure → Patient has open fracture of left wrist with bone protruding. However, the neurovascular status is intact. Patient also has a seatbelt mark across her chest.

- Large-bore IV access in both antecubital fossa.
- *Bloods sent:* FBC, U&Es, clotting, group and save.
- Options now:
  1. Allow orthopaedics to take patient to theatre to fix the wrist.
  2. Stick in a chest drain now.
  3. Arrange for immediate trauma CT (*which should automatically include a CT angiogram of the whole aorta*).
- I would arrange for an immediate CT scan in this setting. There is clearly something going on in this patient's thorax. She has had a high-speed RTA, she has a seat belt injury, she is complaining of chest and back pain, and there is a suggestion of blood in the left chest. Obviously we know the diagnosis because I have already told you, but you need to be recognising these cases on the spot (pattern recognition). I would not be sticking a chest drain in this patient at the moment because she sounds like she is reasonably stable, and given the possibility of an aortic injury if one were to stick a chest drain in, this might decompress any tamponade effect the patient currently may have .... Oh, and just as a matter of principle, orthopaedics should always come after ABC. I don't even care if it is an open fracture with neurovascular compromise, if there is a concern about the airway, breathing or circulation (i.e., torso/thoracic injuries), this needs to be ruled out first of all.
- The CTA shows a large 30-mm peri-aortic haematoma a few centimetres distal to the origin of the left subclavian artery, and there is a moderately sized left haemothorax.

- You contact the vascular interventional radiologist on-call and explain the situation. You both agree the patient needs an emergency thoracic aortic stent. The patient is counselled for this and goes immediately from A&E to interventional radiology for the procedure.
- Only after this would it be appropriate for orthopaedics to fix her left wrist.

A Little Bit More Information on Blunt Aortic Injury

- It often occurs after sudden deceleration as result of high-speed road traffic accidents or falls from great heights.
- The classic site of thoracic aortic injury is at the aortic isthmus in about 55–90% of patients admitted to hospital alive.
- The morbidity and mortality of this injury are high, causing sudden death in 80–90% of cases.
- You need to have a high index of suspicion for such cases. Particularly watch out for high-speed injuries, signs of chest wall injury, hypotension, and thoracic or interscapular pain.
- *A classification scheme for thoracic aortic injury has been proposed:* Type I (intimal tear), type II (intramural haematoma), type III (pseudoaneurysm), and type IV (rupture).
- There is some controversy around when and if to treat these patients, and ultimately you have to judge things on a case-by-case basis ....
- Thoracic aortic repair can be delayed if there are other extensive injuries requiring immediate stabilization. In such a context, the thoracic aortic repair would either be within 24 hours barring other serious injuries, or repair immediately after other injuries have been treated but prior to hospital discharge.
- Obviously however this depends upon the nature of the thoracic aortic injury and the nature of the competing non-aortic injuries. You have to use some common sense here. The ESVS guidelines on descending thoracic aortic injury recommend that patients with free rupture of a blunt traumatic thoracic aortic injury or a large peri-aortic haematoma (≥15 mm) should undergo emergency repair. The same guidelines also recommend that in cases of blunt traumatic thoracic aortic injury without large haematoma, delayed intervention should be considered to prioritise treatment of associated life threatening injuries.
- In contrast, "minimal aortic injuries" that present with an intimal tears or flaps can be managed conservatively with surveillance imaging.
- From a pragmatic perspective, this case demonstrates when you really should be getting on and fixing the thoracic aortic injury and not getting distracted by the non-life threatening orthopaedic injury.
- On the contrary, if this same patient came in with a grade 5 splenic rupture with a belly full of blood, and a CT angiogram showing a tiny intimal flap in the descending thoracic aorta, no guesses for what we are going to do here → she is going for a laparotomy and the "minimal aortic injury" isn't going to concern me in the present moment.
- It goes without saying that the "gold standard" management for a significant thoracic aortic injury is endovascular repair. This is your first option, and open surgery should be considered as a back-up.
- One final thing. A question I got asked in my FRCS Part B Examination was about an elderly woman with this very injury. However, she was a heavy smoker and she had no femoral pulses. I got shown a CT angiogram of the aortic injury just below the left

subclavian artery, and was shown another image that demonstrated her iliac arteries were both heavily diseased. The answer to give in this context is to say you would do a right axillary/subclavian cutdown to enable the thoracic stent to be delivered from above.

Climber Fallen from Height, Open Femur Fracture with Superficial Femoral Artery Injury, Stable Patient with Ischaemic Limb. You Are Called to A&E Resus as a Major Trauma Call

- It is 7 pm.
- You come in from home.
- This is a 46-year-old gentleman who was up a ladder installing some Christmas decorations on the roof of his house, and he slipped and fell landing onto his right foot.
- **ATLS**

  Airway → Patent. Patient is communicating normally. He is complaining of severe pain in his right heel and right thigh. He is not reporting any explicit blood loss on the scene.

  Breathing → Oxygen saturations 100% on room air, chest sounds completely clear.

  Circulation → Heart rate 100, blood pressure 100/80 mmHg. Abdomen is soft and non-tender, not distended. Patient has an obviously deformed right thigh. There is a 2-cm wound in the medial right thigh, and beneath this you can feel/see a bone spike. There is a large swelling in the medial right thigh that looks like a big underlying haematoma. The patient has a femoral pulse but nil distally. The right calcaneum is deformed, but there is no open wound. The right foot is cool with a capillary refill time of 4 seconds. The sensation and power in the right foot are reduced.

  Disability → GCS 15/15. No signs of head injury.

  Exposure → Apart from the right heel and thigh, there is no other obvious injury.

- Working diagnosis? Likely calcaneal fracture with open femur fracture and superficial femoral artery injury. The femoral artery may have bled into his thigh and thrombosed. In any case, the patient has an ischaemic limb (Rutherford 2B given the sensory and motor disturbance).
- Plan? Tricky one. Officially, and "by the book" any patient presenting with hard signs of vascular injury mandates immediate operative intervention.
- However, as I have alluded to before, I really think in the real world that this patient would go through the CT scanner first of all. He has had a significant fall, and there may be other things the CT could tell us, e.g., does he have a lumbar spine fracture? The CT could also tell us how bad the femur fracture is, what the injury to the SFA is like, where exactly is the injury etc. ....
- I know the patient is going to theatre anyways, but honestly I do think I would put this patient through the CT scanner and get some more information. After all, what is the point in having a CT scanner that can help your diagnostic work-up and aid your theatre plan, if you aren't go to use it? Maybe I will be criticised for saying this, but I would get a full trauma CT scan for this patient and extend the CT angio down his right leg.
- I also know that orthopaedics would want some imaging of his right calcaneum (X-ray or CT), and this seems fair.
- But in any case, let us say for simplicity sake that this patient does go through the CT scanner. It shows a fracture of the mid-femur and what looks like a transected SFA. The SFA appears to have thrombosed as there is no active contrast extravasation, although there is a large haematoma in the medial thigh adjacent to the vascular injury. There are no other thoracic or abdominal injuries, and no spinal injuries either.

- *Plan? Now let's get juicy* → This was actually a case scenario I was asked about in my consultant interview, so I am just going to get straight to the point and tell you what the right things to say are.
- The patient has hard signs of vascular injury and this mandates immediate surgical exploration.
- *Avoid large volume fluid resuscitation* → Adopt a "permissive hypotension" approach.
- The patient must be consented for vein harvest from the contralateral leg, and for fasciotomies, and also made aware of the possibility of amputation.
- The patient should get IV antibiotics.
- This is a joint ortho-vascular injury, so guess what, you are going to be doing the case with a consultant orthopaedic surgeon.
- *This is the surgical plan* →
  1. Prep from the umbilicus down and include both legs (with both feet in see-through bags).
  2. Gain proximal control first, followed by distal control. In this case, proximal control in my hands is going to be a standard vertical groin incision to allow me to clamp the proximal SFA. Distal control would ideally be a standard above-knee popliteal artery incision, but if there was haematoma here making dissection challenging, I would not hesitate to first control the below-knee popliteal artery.
  3. After this I would "attack the injury" and enter the haematoma. The transacted artery would be identified.
  4. Now I would do a Fogarty embolectomy of the distal SFA, confirm decent inflow from the proximal SFA, then shunt the vessels to restore perfusion. I would secure the shunt in place with some heavy ties to stop it getting pulled out. If there were no major bleeding, I would probably consider asking the anaesthetic for some intravenous heparin at this point to help maintain the patency of the shunt.
  5. At this point, I would do a fasciotomy.
  6. Now I would have a discussion with the orthopaedic surgeons. What do they want to do? Orthopaedics is not my area of expertise, but I would explain that the definitive management for this patient is to take great saphenous vein from his contralateral leg and do an interposition graft to repair the arterial defect. If we were in damage control mode, it may just be that this femur fracture gets an external fixation device and then he goes back to intensive care for optimization with the shunt in situ, with a view to coming back for a formal repair perhaps tomorrow …. If we were not in damage control mode, the orthopaedic surgeons may be able to fix the femur fracture in a more definitive manner, and after this, I would harvest some contralateral leg vein and then complete the arterial repair.
  7. *Whatever the case may be, just remember to stick to core principles*: ATLS and ABCDE, proximal control, distal control, then attack the injury, shunting, fasciotomy, interposition grafting using autologous vein from contralateral leg …. you can't really go wrong if this is your line of attack.

Fall from Roof, Middle-Aged Gentleman Impaled with Spike into Right Groin, Femoral Artery Bleeding, Unstable Patient. You Are Called to A&E Resus as Part of a Code Red Major Trauma Call

- This one is a bit scary.
- You arrive in A&E resus in the early afternoon (1:30 pm).

- The brief handover you get amongst all the commotion is that this is a 40-year-old male who fell of his roof at home and landed on his garden fence, impaling himself in his right groin. The patient pulled himself off the spike, and this was met with torrential haemorrhage from his right groin which he has struggled to control with direct pressure.
- The ambulance crew did a "scoop and run" and he has just rocked up in A&E.
- There is a trail of bright red blood across the floor and a paramedic is currently pressing down on the right groin.
- **ATLS**
  Airway → Patent. Patient is awake and talking normally. He is saying he is an idiot for falling off the roof.
  Breathing → Chest is clear, oxygen saturations 96% on room air, equal air entry bilaterally, tachypnoeic (respiratory rate = 30).
  Circulation → Pressure on groin has stopped active bleeding currently. Heart rate = 130. Blood pressure = 90/40 mmHg. Patient is pale and cool peripherally. He appears very anxious. His abdomen is soft and non-tender. When the paramedic lifts his hands, there is torrential haemorrhage from the right groin.
  Disability → GCS 15/15, no obvious head injury.
  Exposure → Blood all over the patient and trolley. No other obvious injuries. Legs do not appear to display any evidence of long bone fracture.
- *Venous blood gas:* Haemoglobin 70, lactate 7, pH 7.29, base excess −5.
- *Impression:* This is a femoral artery injury with catastrophic haemorrhage. The patient is in grade 4 haemorrhagic shock.
- This patient is not going for a CT scan.
- He needs to go to theatre immediately for surgical control of haemorrhage.
- However, one can think out of the box. There is the option to ask for a vascular interventional radiologist to insert a REBOA catheter into zone 3 to achieve temporary proximal control. This is what is done in A&E resus (obviously via the contralateral groin).
- The patient is then transferred immediately to theatre.
- The major transfusion protocol is activated, with a plan for the patient to be given red cells, platelets and fresh frozen plasma in a ratio of 1:1:1.
- The patient also gets some tranexamic acid.
- The patient is draped from xiphisternum all the way to include both legs.
- A large right vertical groin incision was made, and the inguinal ligament was identified quickly.
- A large self-retaining retractor was inserted and the common femoral artery was exposed, controlled, and then clamped just below the inguinal ligament.
- The SFA was identified and controlled from below the haematoma.
- The SFA was traced upwards and the profunda artery was identified and controlled.
- At this point, the REBOA catheter was deflated and the sheath was removed from the left groin.
- What you have before your eyes is what I can only describe as an obliterated common femoral artery. It is completely transected and about 2 cm of CFA are missing, leaving some ragged ends above and below. The SFA and profunda origins however appear to be intact. The groin is a war zone, and the dissection was challenging and confusing.

You ligated various superficial veins during the course of your dissection down onto the artery. En route you also discovered a deep and complex 3-cm laceration to the common femoral vein which was hosing dark blood up at you—this has been temporarily controlled by your assistant's fingers.

- What are your options now then?

  1. Repair the CFA with an interposition graft using contralateral GSV and consider a femoral vein patch repair also.

  2. Ligate the CFA and the common femoral vein and do a fasciotomy.

  3. Shunt the CFA, do a fasciotomy, and ligate the femoral vein.

  4. Repair the CFA with a short interposition graft (e.g., Dacron), repair the femoral vein with a prosthetic patch, create a sartorius flap, close the groin, don't do a fasciotomy but ensure the patient's legs are elevated post-op ....

- Your plan will be dictated by the nature of the injury and how sick the patient is. Talk to the anaesthetist. This patient already sounds pretty sick. Clarify what the lactate is, the pH, is there a clotting result, what is the patient's temperature? How many nasty vasoconstrictors are we on?

- My gut instinct for this patient is that he has almost exsanguinated on scene, and when he arrived, he was sick as a dog. Therefore, I would be inclined to veer towards a damage control approach. In this case, I would simply shunt the femoral artery, ligate the femoral vein (or shunt it also), do a fasciotomy, and then get the patient to intensive care.

- On the other hand, if the patient had responded well to the initial resuscitation measures, and the anaesthetist was giving me a more positive report (for example. the lactate had come down to 2, the pH had improved to 7.33, his haemoglobin was now 95, his body temperature was normal, his clotting was normal), I would be more inclined to try and to fix this problem. My choice for fixing this problem would be this: Short Dacron interposition graft to repair the CFA, being honest I probably would still ligate the femoral vein, I would do a sartorius flap, and I would do a fasciotomy.

- I know other people would advocate fixing the femoral vein. However, based upon my research, if I fix this vein with either a patch repair or an interposition graft, it will likely thrombose later on anyways .... Trying to fix this complex venous injury is also likely to lead to the patient bleeding more, and this may force me back into a damage control situation .... I try and remain pragmatic in these scenarios. However, I maintain an open mind. If I think I should fix the venous injury and pragmatically it seems appropriate, I would consider doing so.

- Other people would also advocate only using vein for an interposition graft. I see the value in this, but in my experience, the great saphenous vein is not usually a great size match for the common femoral artery, and it also involves a further cut in the other leg and further time operating .... what gets done is decided in the moment and based upon the variables you have in front of you at the moment.

- I would reassert this point in the close of this scenario → what you do does not really matter as long as you make some common sense decisions and adhere to solid vascular surgery/damage control principles. Various surgeons may have their own individual approaches, and after the fact they may pass comment that they would have done something different to you. But all this is of secondary importance. *Just remember that the patient came in bleeding to death, and your primary job is to stop the bleeding and save the patient's life. Do the best job you can and make decisions that you can justify if questioned about it later.*

Other Considerations

- To get proximal control of the hosing groin the Rutherford Morrison incision and external iliac artery control is always worth considering (classic approach).

- It is also worth considering an extended vertical groin incision that goes higher up than normal. You can dissect straight down onto the inguinal ligament and actually incise its lower border to allow you access to the external iliac artery in the lower retroperitoneum. This is useful if you are trying to control the CFA below the inguinal ligament, but there is a massive haematoma that is obscuring your dissection. You can also leave the lower edge of the inguinal ligament intact, and make a cut 1–2 cm above this point which will still allow you to enter the lower retroperitoneum.

- If you have hybrid theatre capabilities, I would consider trying to achieve temporary inflow control with a retrograde approach from the contralateral groin to allow balloon occlusion of the ipsilateral external iliac artery.

- If you are feeling fancy, but not that fancy, then REBOA into zone 3 is always worth a thought, as is what we did in this scenario.

Iatrogenic Injury to Radial Artery Related to Coronary Angiogram Access, Patient Has a Large Tense Pseudoaneurysm But the Hand Is Not Ischaemic. You Have Been Called to CCU to Assess the Patient

- This was a question I had in my FRCS Part B Examination (a Short Case).

- I will describe the case as it was described to me, and go through what information I had and what questions I was asked ….

- The history was as described above, and this patient had come in a few days ago with a non-ST segment myocardial infarction (NSTEMI).

- The patient had the coronary angiogram yesterday, had stenting of the right coronary artery, and has been commenced on dual antiplatelet therapy (aspirin and ticagrelor).

- I was shown a picture of a patient's left hand/wrist/forearm → a large swelling was visible (about 3–4 cm) on the volar aspect of the wrist overlying the radial artery puncture site. There was no active bleeding. The overlying skin looked to be under considerable tension (it was thin, shiny, and erythematous). The hand also looked well perfused, and I could see the patient had a good cephalic vein.

- The examiners asked me what the diagnosis was. I said the patient likely had a radial artery pseudoaneurysm secondary to the radial artery puncture. The examiners nodded (no brainer really), and then asked me what else I wanted to know in terms of examination findings.

- I asked about the pulse status. I was told that the ulnar pulse was palpable and the pseudoaneurysm was pulsatile. I asked if the radial artery was palpable beyond the pseudoaneurysm, and I was told it was.

- The examiner then asked if I wanted to do any other examinations. I said I would do an Allen's test. I had to explain what an Allen's test was. I must have said the right thing because the examiner nodded. It was fed back to me that Allen's test indicated that the perfusion to the hand via the ulnar artery alone was satisfactory.

- I was then asked what investigation I would like to do next. I said this: "Ideally I would start off with a non-invasive investigation like an upper limb arterial duplex." This was clearly the right answer because I was then handed some ultrasound images.

- The ultrasound report was that there was triphasic flow in the ulnar artery, there was a 3-cm radial artery pseudoaneurysm with a short narrow neck, there was colour flow in the pseudoaneurysm, and that the distal radial artery was patent (again with triphasic flow).

- The examiners then asked if I would like further investigations. I said in an ideal world I would get a diagnostic angiogram via the left brachial artery to confirm that the ulnar artery and palmar arch were both patent. The examiners then asked me about the result of the Allen's test I just did, and asked if this would change my management. I was then asked about potential complications of another diagnostic angiogram, and at this point, I felt like I should not have mentioned diagnostic angiogram and thus I backtracked a little bit ….

- The examiners then asked me what the options for management were. This is what I said:

  1. Conservative management alone is always an option. The examiners looked at me and asked if I thought this was appropriate. I said I did not think it was appropriate, but it was an option. I quickly moved on ….

  2. Ultrasound-guided thrombin injection. The examiners asked me about the pros and cons of this. The pros were that this was a minimally invasive procedure, and given that this patient has had a recent MI, it would avoid an anaesthetic so would perhaps be a reasonable approach. The disadvantages are that the thrombin may spill out and trash the hand, and the pseudoaneurysm was also quite big and if it was not decompressed it may lead to skin necrosis ….

  3. Expose the pseudoaneurysm (proximal and distal control) and then do a short interposition graft using the ipsilateral cephalic vein (*reversed*) that I can clearly see is of decent quality. The examiners asked how I would anaesthetise the patient. I said I could do this under local anaesthetic or block, and they seemed to think this was fair.

  4. Ligate the radial artery and decompress the pseudoaneurysm. The ulnar artery and palmar arch clinically seemed to be intact so the hand perfusion should be OK. Again, I would plan to do this under local anaesthetic or arm block.

  5. The examiners wanted to know what my definitive plan was. I said I would take the patient to theatre and aim to decompress the pseudoaneurysm and aim to do a short interposition graft repair using cephalic vein, but if there were any difficulties, I would not hesitate to ligate the radial artery. The examiners seemed to think this was a reasonable approach, but asked me about taking the patient to theatre when the patient had had a recent myocardial infarction. I said these cases are rarely straightforward, but if your hand is forced sometimes you have to operate and accept the risks. At this point I said I would make sure I had counselled the patient appropriately and given them an overview of the options available. I also said I would talk to the cardiology consultant looking after the patient and the anaesthetist, and come up with a sensible plan.

- At this point, the bell rang and I was thrust into another short case with very little time to think ….

Patient Stabbed in Neck with Expanding Haematoma. You Are Called Down to A&E Resus as Part of a Code Red Major Trauma Call

- It is 10:45 pm on a Friday night.
- The story is of a 30-year-old woman who was having an argument with her ex-boyfriend outside a bar, and he stabbed her in the left neck about 25 minutes ago.
- There was active bleeding on the scene, and this was controlled with pressure applied to the neck by a passer-by.

- The ambulance crew have done a familiar "scoop and run," and here she is in front of you in A&E.
- There is blood on the floor where she was wheeled in, and a junior A&E doctor is pressing on her left neck with a few green swabs.
- As per usual there is lots of commotion and panic.
- As you arrive, the rest of the trauma team are arriving (anaesthetic consultant, orthopaedic registrar, few more A&E clinicians, etc.).
- **ATLS**

  Airway → Patent. Patient is asking if she is going to die. Nobody answers this question. She is asked if she has any other injuries. The answer is no; she was stabbed in the neck once then her assailant ran away.

  Breathing → Chest clear on auscultation. Respiratory rate 40 (patient is hyperventilating), oxygen saturations 96% on room air.

  Circulation → Blood seeping out of neck. Haematoma currently obscured by green swabs that are being pressed down onto neck. You want some confirmatory information, so you put on a pair of gloves and take over control of the neck wound. You lift up the swab, and there is a 1.5-cm stab wound in the anterior triangle of the neck and arterial blood shoots out. You quickly re-apply pressure. Heart rate 100, blood pressure 95/60 mmHg. Abdomen soft and non-tender.

  Disability → GCS 15/15. No obvious head injury. You ask patient if she can move both her arms and her legs. She can do. There is no sign of stroke currently.

  Exposure → No other obvious injuries with rapid survey.

- **What is the diagnosis**? We have to assume here that this is a carotid artery injury resulting in exsanguinating haemorrhage. This looks like a zone 2 injury.
- **What are the priorities of management**?

  1. *The airway is the priority:* Bleeding is currently being controlled with direct pressure, but as far as I am concerned, there is a real risk the patient will lose her airway as a result of expanding haematoma. You talk to the anaesthetist and you both agree the patient should be intubated sooner rather than later. This takes place over the next few minutes in A&E resus (rapid sequence induction).

  2. *Do the basics down in A&E:* Good large-bore IV access in both antecubital fossa. Send off bloods for FBC, U&Es, coagulation, group and save. Make sure the major transfusion protocol is initiated. For the moment, I would still employ a "permissive hypotension" approach and avoid giving IV fluids. I would give the patient tranexamic acid.

  3. You decide not to take the patient for a CT scan. There is no point. You already know the diagnosis, and a CT is not going to alter your plan. This patient is going straight to theatre.

  4. Now we go to theatre ….

Principles of Operative Management of Vascular Injuries in the Neck

- You cannot sew what you cannot see. This means prep wide, and assume all zones of the neck are involved.
- I would position the patient in the supine position with both arms out (crucifix).
- I would actually prep the patient from the ear all the way down to both mid-thighs. This seems like a bit of an overkill, but you never know—you may need to open the chest, you may need to harvest some great saphenous vein from the groin etc. Better be safe than sorry.

- *Zone 1 injury* → Zone 1 injuries start in the thoracic outlet and extend from the clavicles to the cricoid cartilage. In a haemodynamically stable patient with a small contained haematoma here, you may consider endovascular intervention, i.e., a covered stent. However, getting proximal control here is extremely challenging, and frankly a neck dissection alone is not likely to be sufficient. Therefore, this sort of injury is probably going to force you to get proximal control in the chest. For this, your options are going to be ideally a median sternotomy, or a clamshell incision (*in desperate circumstances*). If you have to open the chest let's be honest—you are going to feel uncomfortable about doing it, and will question whether you should be doing it. Maybe a little voice inside your head says you should call interventional radiology to come from the groin and occlude the common carotid with a balloon. All I would say is if the patient has an injury trajectory that is going from the neck down into the superior mediastinum and the patient is dying in front of you, and time is not on your side, then you need to open the chest. So just do it.

- *Zone 1 injury management* → Whatever approach you have chosen, you will have to deal with what is in front of you (can't bail out now you have come too far). Let us assume you have done a median sternotomy for a zone 1 injury, and now you are confronted with a large red haematoma in the superior mediastinum. This seems a lot worse than what you were expecting. The anatomy is totally confusing and there is blood oozing all over the place. You know you have a major vascular injury sitting at the base of this haematoma. You know you now have to tackle this haematoma and somehow save the patient's life. I don't think anybody feels comfortable here, but these are some general points worth considering:

  1. I would recommend starting off at the bottom of your sternotomy wound and opening the pericardium. Open it in the middle by grasping it with your forceps then incising it vertically using your scissors. Avoid deviating laterally to preserve the phrenic nerves. From this point, you can advance upwards along the aortic arch into the haematoma to identify the thoracic outlet vessels ….

  2. However, I would first deal with the superficial layers of the superior mediastinum. If you encounter the thymus, divide it between clamps and ligate it using 2-0 or 3-0 vicryl. Don't indiscriminately slide your scissors upwards too prematurely. Look out for the left brachiocephalic vein. Isolate it, divide it between two clips, and ligate it using 2-0 or 3-0 vicryl ties.

  3. Now the superior mediastinum is starting to "open" up for you.

  4. Starting off at the aortic root, as you move upwards, you will come to the innominate artery bifurcation into the right subclavian and right common carotid arteries. Be careful not to injure the right vagus nerve as it passes in front of the right proximal subclavian artery. Also watch out for that sneaky anatomical variant where the left common carotid artery comes off the innominate artery (*if you clamp the innominate artery here the patient doesn't just stroke out, they will be dead as you are cutting off all the blood supply to the brain*).

  5. If you have normal anatomy, you will then trace along the aortic arch and find the left common carotid artery.

  6. Beyond this will be the left subclavian artery, but be careful here as the left vagus nerve passes down between the left carotid and left subclavian arteries to cross in front of the aortic arch and give off the left recurrent laryngeal nerve. The left subclavian artery is actually a posterior mediastinal structure in my opinion, as the aortic arch curves backwards. However, you should still be able to get proximal control here ….

7. Once you have gained at least some exposure and "pseudo-control" of these vessels, then you can consider "attacking the injury".

8. You can also extend your incision up into the neck to get distal control of the carotid artery, which is why a median sternotomy is ideal.

9. If you have a subclavian vessel injury, you may need to extend your incision laterally into the supraclavicular fossa to gain distal exposure of the subclavian arteries.

10. It goes without saying that the same principles of vascular injury repair apply in regards to the great vessels. If you have a big haematoma in the superior mediastinum, chances are you have a great vessel injury. If you unroof this haematoma prematurely, don't be surprised when things suddenly go "bang!" in your face. As such I recommend not diving into the superior mediastinal haematoma first of all, but instead going down to the pericardium and working your way upwards.

11. If you have an injury to the aorta, consider applying a side-biting clamp and doing a suture repair.

12. If you have an innominate or carotid artery injury, then if you are in damage control mode you can simply shunt them, get the patient off to intensive care, and then bring them back and do a venous interposition graft repair using reversed great saphenous vein once the patient is physiologically well.

13. For an innominate/carotid/subclavian artery injury you can also consider a patch repair or an interposition graft using Dacron or PTFE.

14. You may also need to ligate the vessel and do bypass (e.g., from the ascending aorta to the innominate artery just below the bifurcation).

15. If you have a venous injury, you can stick a side biting clamp on it and do a suture repair. If the venous injury doesn't look simple then simply ligate it.

16. Suffice to say if you are working in a unit with cardiac surgery availability, you should have called for their help way in advance ….

17. I would also make the vitally important point that these are lethal and complex injuries. Chances are your patient is not doing so well. So avoid doing fancy complex things if you can avoid it. Stick to core vascular surgery and damage control surgery principles and call for help early.

18. If there is a viable endovascular solution available, seriously consider this option!!!!!

- *Zone 2 injury* → Standard carotid exposure with a big incision running along the anterior border of sternocleidomastoid. Go through skin, subcutaneous tissue, ligate the external jugular vein, divide platysma, then retract the sternocleidomastoid muscle backwards. Expect there to be a juicy haematoma obscuring everything. Look out for the common facial vein and doubly ligate it. In this sort of case, I would be inclined to expose the common carotid as low down in the neck as possible, i.e., get a Langenbeck and pull the omohyoid down, and probably even consider exposing the common carotid in-between the two heads of the sternomastoid. Getting proximal control is the absolute first priority. Once you have achieved this the "textbook" advice is to get distal control and then attack the injury. Well, good luck with this. There is going to be a big haematoma probably, and getting distal control of the ICA and ECA is probably going to be difficult without first having to rummage through this haematoma …. But let's say you get the ICA and ECA sloped and controlled. Now we have to talk about the injury itself ….

1. *Zone 2 injury management* → You may have what appears to be a small injury to the carotid vessel. Perhaps you think you should just bang a few 5-0 prolene sutures in at this point. In the real world, perhaps this is what most vascular surgeons would do. However, at least from my own research, I don't think this is the correct answer

(officially). If a carotid injury is present, even though it may look innocuous, the interior of the vessel should be explored as simple perforations may hide a more extensive injury such as an intimal tear and thrombus. You would not want to do a super repair and then have your patient have a massive stroke in theatre recovery. I say if you have gotten to this point, you might as well do a proper job …. Do a longitudinal arteriotomy along the anterior vessel wall until normal vessel is reached. Now inspect the inside of the artery. Injured intima will either need to be repaired or resected. Thrombus should be removed and flushed out. Also don't forget that if you are going to insert a shunt or do a repair, don't forget to do a gentle thrombectomy of the inflow and outflow tracts with a Fogarty catheter first. Don't go too high into the internal carotid artery however, i.e., don't go beyond 2–3 cm from the carotid bifurcation to avoid damaging the intracranial ICA ….

- Here are your surgical options
  - Direct repair with end-to-end anastomosis, but only if you are confident, the suture line will not be under tension.
  - Interposition graft using a short prosthetic graft or non-reversed vein (ideally GSV harvested from groin).
  - If only the anterior wall is damaged, you can consider a patch repair.
  - If the operation is going to take a long time, you can shunt the vessel in the meantime.
  - If the patient is in extremis and you are in a pure damage control mode, you can shunt the carotid artery and then ship the patient off to intensive care to be stabilised.
  - If the patient is in extremis then the carotid can be ligated. Just remember that your patient is likely going to have an acute stroke.
  - Do bear in mind that endovascular manoeuvres are always theoretically possible, e.g., covered stents. However, I would just be very cautious about this. If someone has been stabbed in the neck, the platysma has been breached, the CT scan suggests a carotid injury (e.g., pseudoaneurysm) and the patient is stable, there may be a little voice saying you should treat it with a covered stent. However, if the knife has breached the platysma, you don't know where else has been injured. There may be an additional aerodigestive injury. My opinion is that if the platysma has been breached and you have a suspected carotid artery injury, the patient is going to theatre to be explored. I expect people will disagree with me, but I just think this is one of those times when open surgery is king.
  - On the subject of concomitant aerodigestive injury, if there is one present then if you have repaired the carotid artery make sure to cover your repair with an interposition muscle patch and drain the area as well.
- *Zone 3 injury* → Zone 3 extends from the angle of the mandible to the base of the skull. Access is limited by the mastoid and styloid bones. It is a tight and challenging area, and trying to get distal control of a carotid injury here is probably impractical.
- Zone 3 injury management →
- This would be a situation where I think interventional radiology would be ideal (i.e., I would consider this covered stent territory or angiographic occlusion territory).
- However, if you find yourself operating in this context, your incision and approach is again going to be the same as for a zone 2 injury; however, this time you would be extending your incision upwards behind the ear.
- For academic purposes, here are some things you can do to improve your exposure:
  1. Open mouth wide
  2. Dislocate mandible forwards

3. Mandibular osteotomy
4. Mastoidectomy
5. Excision of digastric muscle
6. Excision of styloid bone
7. Mobilise ear
8. Nasal intubation

- I say "for academic purposes" because I just cannot picture myself seriously entertaining many of the above fancy manoeuvres in an uncontrolled carotid trauma setting. Dividing the digastric muscle seems reasonable, but that would be about all I would probably consider in the real world setting. What I actually picture myself doing is making a big cut in a rather uncontrolled settling, getting proximal control, and then making some common sense decisions that result in me doing a simple procedure to stop bleeding ....

- As such, this is probably what I would be doing with a distal ICA injury that was bleeding in my face and I could not get proximal control:

1. Put my finger on the bleeding area.
2. Probably secretly panic and feel like I am not competent to deal with this sort of injury and think life is not fair.
3. Get my head back in gear and focus on the problem in front of me .... I need to stop bleeding and save the patient's life, what can I do? What did *Top Knife* say I should do?
4. *Oh yeah, I remember, I have these options:* I can ligate the vessel and leave it, or stick a Fogarty catheter in it, inflate the balloon, put some metal clips across the catheter, and leave the balloon in situ.

JMF's Reflections on This Type of Trauma

These are all scary traumas and I don't think any vascular surgeon would ever feel entirely comfortable in these settings. I also think it is really hard to write a book section like this. The possibilities of injury are vast, and every single scenario is going to be unique. On a good day, you are going to be confronted by a stable patient who maybe you can manage conservatively or maybe interventional radiology can come and save the day with a sneaky covered stent. However, there will come a time when you are going to be confronted by a patient who has some horrific injury and is dying in front of you. It may appear to be a carotid injury, but it may turn out to be something much worse .... You won't have much time to think and plan, and it will be something of a rollercoaster ride. You will have to think on your feet. You will have to have the heart of a king and the hands of a queen. You can choose all different types of incisions, approach from up, down, left, right, extend the incision here there and everywhere, shunt, patch, ligate, interposition graft, use vein, use plastic, use Dacron ... all these decisions you will have to make in the moment. However, remember that you did not cause this injury, and you are doing the best job you can to save the patient's life. Just stick to the core principles we have repeatedly discussed and go do some *Top Knife* work. **BOOM POW!**

Patient Fallen over at Barbecue, Landed on Left Side of Chest/Abdomen. Severe Pain with Hypotension. You Are Called to A&E Resus as a Major Trauma Call

- It is 2 pm.
- You rock up to A&E resus.
- You have a 54-year-old female in front of you.

- Apparently she was at a family barbecue having "a good time" (*which basically means she was walloped drunk*) when she fell over and landed on the barbecue itself.
- She landed onto her left ribs (this patient has a raised BMI so there was some kinetic energy involved here).
- She is complaining of left sided lower chest/upper abdominal pain.
- **ATLS**

  Airway → Patent. Patient is communicating normally.
  Breathing → Oxygen saturations 97% on room air. Chest sounds clear. Respiratory rate is 30. Tenderness over lower left ribs however.
  Circulation → Heart rate is 115, blood pressure is 100/70 mmHg. Abdomen is slightly distended and she has left sided guarding/peritonism. No obvious long bone fractures.
  Disability → GCS 15/15. No obvious head injury.
  Exposure → No other obvious injuries.
- *You have an arterial blood gas result:* pH 7.20, Hb 85, lactate 4.7, base excess −6.
- What is the diagnosis? This is a no brainer. This is a splenic injury until proven otherwise. By the book, she is bleeding and she is in at least grade 3 haemorrhagic shock.
- What do you do now? Do we need to elaborate? OK, yes we will as this is your FRCS examination … large-bore IV access in both antecubital fossa. Send of bloods urgently: FBC, U&Es, coagulation, group and save. Yes I would institute the major transfusion protocol as she is clearly bleeding. Give some tranexamic acid → A&E love it so why not.
- To CT or not to CT?
- I may be criticised at this point, but I honestly would not go for a CT scan if it were my choice. However, I can tell you hands down that I know with absolute certainty this sort of patient would go for a CT scan if I were not there at the initial primary survey ….
- As far as I am concerned, this patient is bleeding, and it is coming from her left upper quadrant. It is going to be her spleen. I am not entertaining the notion of "splenic preservation" in this setting. The patient is going for a laparotomy end of story ….
- However, if you have rocked up in A&E and the patient has already had a CT scan, now things get a bit awkward ….
- Let's talk about the grading of splenic injuries and when interventional radiology is relevant ….

  Grade 1 → Subcapsular haematoma <10% of surface area, parenchymal laceration <1 cm depth, capsular tear.
  Grade 2 → Subcapsular haematoma 10–50% of surface area, intraparenchymal haematoma <5 cm, parenchymal laceration 1–3 cm in depth.
  Grade 3 → Subcapsular haematoma >50% of surface area, ruptured subcapsular or intraparenchymal haematoma ≥5 cm, parenchymal laceration >3 cm in depth.
  Grade 4 → Any injury in the presence of a splenic vascular injury or active bleeding confined within splenic capsule, parenchymal laceration involving segmental or hilar vessels producing >25% devascularization.
  Grade 5 → Shattered spleen any injury in the presence of splenic vascular injury with active bleeding extending beyond the spleen into the peritoneum.
- Interventional radiology is rapidly becoming an accepted standard of care for the management of splenic trauma. However, this should only be considered in the case of haemodynamically stable patients. Also, as far as I am concerned, interventional

radiology is most suited to patients who are haemodynamically stable, but they display a definite contrast extravasation "blush" on their CT scan. This indicates an arterial bleed and, therefore, would be suitable for embolization.

- I am just going to be honest with you at this point, perhaps to my own detriment. I take the splenic grading system with a pinch of salt. What is more important to me is the haemodynamic status of the patient. This is my approach to splenic injury →

1. I eyeball the patient and I eyeball the CT scan.

2. If the patient is stable, isn't bleeding, the spleen isn't smashed to pieces, and the belly isn't full of blood, the plan is for conservative management. This means admit to a high observation bay or the trauma ward, serial abdominal examinations, and monitor the full blood count.

3. If the patient is bleeding on the CT scan but is haemodynamically stable, I will talk to interventional radiology about embolization.

4. If the patient is haemodynamically unstable and I strongly suspected a splenic injury given the mechanism and examination findings, I probably wouldn't even do a CT scan, I would just go for a laparotomy. If the spleen is injured, it is being removed end of story.

5. If the patient is haemodynamically "hovering" and there is a nasty splenic injury/ splenic haematoma/blush, I may be inclined to speak to interventional radiology. However, if I had any doubt, I would proceed to laparotomy.

6. I will have to be transparent at this point. Although I am a "new" vascular consultant, I have always identified with the "old school" mentality. I am a surgeon, and I think that an unstable patient with an obvious splenic injury needs to go for a laparotomy and have the spleen removed. Happy to be criticised, and more than willing to defend myself ….

Let's Get Juicy → How to Do an Emergency Splenectomy

- Stand on the right side of the patient.
- Midline laparotomy.
- DON'T YOU DARE USE THE MONOPOLAR DIATHERMY, I FORBID THIS— KNIFE ONLY!
- We are talking *Top Knife* here guys …. hey diddle diddle, right down the middle (preferably in less than 30 seconds).
- Don't twang the bladder, small bowel or liver please on your way in.
- Belly will be full of blood if the patient is in extremis → don't panic, suck some of the juice out, then pack in all 4 quadrants confidently and assertively.
- Stop the operation.
- Give the anaesthetist time to catch up.
- In the meantime ask for the omnitract.
- Seriously, this may seem like a faff, but do it. The omnitract really does help with your exposure, and it frees your assistant up to help you.
- Insert the omnitract and position all the pieces so that the abdominal cavity is nicely opened up.
- After a few minutes reconnect with the anaesthetist. Is she/he happy? I hope by now we don't need to reassert what they should be doing → massive blood transfusion protocol with red cells, platelets, and fresh frozen plasma is a ratio of 1:1:1.
- Place your right hand over the spleen and deep into the left upper quadrant—it is always higher and deeper than you think!

- The spleen may be in pieces or completely smashed to bits.
- In my experience, there will be some nuisance adhesions/ligaments that you need to deal with (lienophrenic, splenorenal, lienocolic, and splenophrenic attachments).
- These attachments may have already been obliterated. If they are not, my advice is this: Grab the damn spleen, pull it forwards with your left hand, take your scissors in your right hand, and just cut these attachments free. This is not a pretty dissection, just do what needs to be done to bring the spleen forwards (i.e., combination of sharp and blunt dissection).
- Your objective is to make the spleen a midline organ.
- *Word of warning* → Be careful not to injure the tail of the pancreas or the short gastric vessels (these are remarkably close).
- This is difficult to now describe, but use a combination of finger and scissor dissection to identify the splenic vessels at the splenic hilum .... You can use your left hand to actually cup the spleen and compress the hilum with your left fingers, and this liberates your right hand to do some scissor dissection.
- At the same time, ask your assistant to stuff some big packs into the left upper quadrant to tamponade any oozing areas.
- At this point, I will tell you what I would do. I would assertively identify the splenic hilum, ask for a big clip, and then put this right across the hilum. The spleen then gets cut free and handed out. I would then transfix the splenic artery and vein en masse using a heavy vicryl suture (i.e., 1-0 or 2-0 vicryl).
- Some people may individually ligate the splenic vessels, which is fair enough. As far as I am concerned, however, this is a life-saving manoeuvre, and this is trauma surgery, not elective breast surgery. I am not messing around, and I am not trying to impress anyone. The objective is to stop bleeding and save the patient's life ....
- At this point, I would speak to the anaesthetist and gauge how the patient is doing.
- If the patient were better than when I started, and this was an isolated splenic injury, I would probably close the abdomen.
- If the patient were displaying any elements of the lethal triad (acidosis, hypothermia, coagulopathy), I would just pack the abdomen, leave it as a laparostomy, and get the patient to intensive care ASAP (live to fight another day).

Patient Stabbed from Overhead (Ice-Pick Grip) in Left Supraclavicular Fossa, Haemodynamically Unstable. You Are Called Down to A&E Resus as a Code Red Major Trauma Call

- I hate these junctional injuries ....
- This is a 24-year-old male who has been involved in some drug deal gone wrong.
- It is 9 pm.
- You arrive in A&E.
- Blood is all over the place as usual.
- The patient is lying down, and you can see someone pressing a swab down over the left supraclavicular fossa.
- The primary survey is in progress.
- **ATLS**

    Airway → Patent. The patient is shouting at the healthcare assistant for sticking an orange cannula in his right arm.

Breathing → Respiratory rate of 36. Reduced air entry left side. Dull to percussion. Saturations of 89% on 15 litres non-rebreathe mask. Right side of chest is clear.

Circulation → Heart rate 120, blood pressure 97/63 mmHg.

Disability → GCS 15/15. No obvious head injury.

Exposure → No other obvious injury. Underneath the swab in the left supraclavicular fossa is a 2-cm stab wound. There is a big haematoma that is obscuring the clavicle and root of neck. The left hand is warm and seems reasonably well perfused, although it is difficult to feel a radial pulse.

- What is the working diagnosis? Proximal subclavian artery (+/− subclavian vein) injury with major haemorrhage into left chest. Patient is in either grade 3 or grade 4 haemorrhagic shock (4 more likely).

- What are your immediate steps?

- *Some basics* → High-flow oxygen, large-bore IV access (right arm), send off urgent bloods (FBC, U&Es, clotting, group and save), institute major haemorrhage protocol, tranexamic acid.

- *Step it up a gear* → What can you do right now to improve the situation?

- This is what I would do →

  1. Get a Foley catheter, stick in down the wound tract for a few centimetres, inflate the balloon, then withdraw it until it seems to be compressing something and won't come back any more (i.e., you hope you are compressing the subclavian vessels at this point). Get a heavy clip to close off the other end of the Foley catheter to stop any blood escaping.

  2. Get someone to lift the patient's left arm up. Bang some 1% lignocaine in the axilla (fifth intercostal space, mid-axillary line), give a quick clean of the area, grab the knife and proceed with finger thoracostomy. In this case, a load of blood comes out. Now a formal chest drain gets inserted. What a surprise the chest drain fills with about 1300 ml of blood in about 5 minutes.

- After this point, the patient is given two units of O negative blood, the oxygen saturations improve, the heart rate and blood pressure improve, and the chest drain stops filling.

- For a short period of time, everything seems to calm down, and you have time to think ….

- It looks like you have temporarily stopped whatever vessel was bleeding ….

- My initial thoughts are that this patient needs to go straight to theatre and not to the CT scanner.

- I'm thinking that the left subclavian artery has been injured quite close to the root of the neck. The knife may have caused some other mischief in the neck as well that I can only imagine right now …. I cannot just manage this injury with a Foley catheter as that was just a temporising measure. I need to fix this injury because the patient is bleeding, and that means I need to get proximal control, distal control, then attack the injury …. but the root of the neck is distorted by haematoma, and the supraclavicular area is all bruised and swollen there also. If I try to get proximal control by a standard supraclavicular incision, I will probably just dive right into the bleeding vessel. To get proximal control I need to be in the chest right? But that means I have to open the chest, and this feels a bit extreme! If I have to open the chest, how should I open the chest? Should I do a clamshell? The patient isn't crashing, so that doesn't feel right. Maybe I should go upstairs and do a median sternotomy … that seems more appropriate. But I know from my time studying anatomy that the left subclavian artery is (*pragmatically speaking*) a posterior mediastinal structure. Is getting proximal control of the left subclavian artery best achieved by way of median sternotomy? I'm pretty sure a median sternotomy would be better for a right subclavian artery injury, but not as good for the left. Maybe I can ask interventional radiology to come from the groin and do a diagnostic angiogram. Couldn't they help me achieve proximal control of this supposed left subclavian artery injury? Maybe they could stent the vessel. Well yes, theoretically IR could help me …. But wouldn't it be better therefore to get a CT angiogram first, and then I can decide if IR can help me or not …. oh wait, I had already decided against going for a CT angiogram …. Is there another incision I can use? Oh yes, I remember, I could consider a high third interspace left anterolateral thoracotomy incision and get proximal control this way …. Oh wait, I just remembered, there is yet another approach— I can actually make my incision directly onto the clavicle to expose the medial two-thirds of the bone, and then divide it with a power saw or bone cutters …. I could even disconnect the head of the clavicle from the sternum, and after removing the bone and underlying subclavian muscle, I would be brought straight into the scalene fat pad and phrenic nerve, and perhaps now I can get proximal control of the artery ….

- All these thoughts spin around in your head for about 30 seconds. At the end of this confusing thought process, you still don't know what the right thing to do and you start to second guess yourself ….

- **JUST PAUSE FOR A SECOND AND DON'T MAKE ANY DECISION.** The patient is temporarily stable and is not actively bleeding. Don't make any crazy decisions right now. Take a step back. Yes we know this is likely to be a major vascular injury, and yes perhaps it feels like there is overwhelming pressure on you to take this patient straight to theatre. However, fools rush in where angels fear to tread. If the primary survey manoeuvres had temporarily controlled the situation, I would try and gain more information to help me plan my attack. Seriously → for ruptured AAA patients, nobody now rushes these patients straight to theatre. We do CT scans for ruptured AAA patients because it helps us confirm what we are dealing with, and what is the most sensible strategy. We even get CT scans for unstable ruptured AAA patients routinely. So why not get a CT angiogram for this patient? *This is what I would do now in this setting.*

- The CT angiogram reveals a large haematoma at the root of the neck extending into the superior thoracic aperture. The left subclavian artery has been lacerated at the root of the neck, about 2-cm deep into the superior thoracic aperture. It is not transected nor is it thrombosed. The Foley catheter is sitting just next to it and tamponading the bleeding area, but there is still some minor contrast extravasation around this area. A small amount of contrast is still passing into the distal subclavian artery beyond the injury, and the distal subclavian still appears to be patent. There is a moderate haemopneumothorax of the left chest, but the chest drain appears to be in the correct position. The subclavian vein does not obviously appear to be injured or bleeding, but to be honest the large haematoma makes interpretation challenging.

- Options now? I would speak to interventional radiology and see if they are happy to stent this injury.

- My final remark at this juncture is this → before you embark on crazy adventures around the subclavian artery, take a few seconds to step back and pause. You may not need to dive into the chest or start sawing through the clavicle. You may be able to postpone the operation, leave the Foley catheter in, go for a CT scan, speak to interventional radiology …. Just remember this.

- At this point, we are going stop this case scenario, and move on to a very similar one that will expand our management options for subclavian/axillary artery injuries ….

Central Line Iatrogenic Injury to Right Subclavian Artery. Unstable Patient. You Are Called to Cardiac Intensive Care to Review This Patient at 2 AM

- You arrive on cardiac ICU.
- As you walk into the ward there are about 7 cardiac nurses, 2 cardiac anaesthetists, and a cardiac surgery registrar surrounding this patient.
- In front of you is a 64-year-old gentleman who is 4 days post-op following an elective aortic valve replacement and coronary artery bypass grafting for which he had a median sternotomy and right internal mammary artery to left anterior descending artery bypass.
- The patient's bed has been tilted so that he is head down and feet up to help improve his blood pressure (*this is not a good first impression*).
- The patient is intubated and ventilated.
- There is a very large swelling/haematoma in the right axilla/upper chest (size of a football).
- *The observations staring at you:* Heart rate 115, blood pressure 96/54 mmHg.
- The patient has had a slightly rocky post-operative course so far, and one of the cardiac anaesthetists attempted a right subclavian central line at around 7 pm last evening (i.e. about 6 hours ago). It is handed over to you that this was done under ultrasound, but was unsuccessful (i.e., the wire and sheath never advanced).
- After this attempt, the right axilla progressively swelled up over the past 6 hours and the patient became increasingly haemodynamically unstable.
- At the moment, his inotropic/vasoconstrictor requirements have significantly increased.
- The patient still has a decent right radial pulse and a warm well perfused hand.
- What is the diagnosis? Clearly there has been an iatrogenic injury to the right axillary or subclavian artery (i.e., it wasn't the vein that was being poked on ultrasound but the artery!). The patient is haemodynamically unstable.
- What is the immediate plan? Same as usual. In this case, there is already decent intravenous access, the bloods have just been sent, and the major transfusion protocol has been activated.
- What are your options? Conservative management ain't going to work. Take the patient straight to theatre? His chest has already been opened, and he has a bypass coming off a branch of the right subclavian artery. I am not so happy about making a supraclavicular incision, clamping the subclavian artery, or causing any mischief that might compromise his coronary artery bypass graft …. Maybe there is a minimally invasive endovascular option.
- You speak to the cardiac surgeon who did the operation, and you also speak to the vascular interventional radiologist on-call. All agree that proceeding to open surgery would preferably be avoided.
- The patient goes for an immediate CT scan.
- This reveals a small pseudoaneurysm in the right axillary artery about 2 cm below the clavicle with active contrast extravasation from the superior aspect of the artery. There is a massive haematoma surrounding this. The axillary artery is itself patent, and there is contrast passing distal to the injury.
- The interventional radiologist is happy to take this patient for an attempt at inserting a covered stent. This takes place, but emergency theatres are put on standby in case this attempt fails and the patient needs to go for open surgical repair.
- The interventional radiologist comes from the right common femoral artery and manages to insert a short covered stent over the injured area. This is below the clavicle. There is a good clinical and radiological result.

- The patient goes back to cardiac intensive care, and a few hours later, his haemodynamic status has improved, and he still has a warm well-perfused right hand and a decent radial pulse. The right groin access site is also satisfactory and his right leg perfusion is intact.

Gunshot Wound to Left Shoulder. Unstable Patient. You Are Called to A&E Resus as a Code Red Major Trauma Call

- It is 10:30 pm.
- A 33-year-old man has been shot in the left shoulder region 30 minutes ago.
- You don't know the details of the incident, apart from being told by the paramedics that he bled a lot on scene.
- This is a "scoop and run" case.
- As per usual there is a member of the A&E team pressing over a wound in the left upper chest/shoulder region.
- **ATLS**

    Airway → Patent. Patient shouting and swearing. You ask how many times he has been shot. The patient says he was shot once by his assailant.

    Breathing → Respiratory rate 30. Oxygen saturations 94% on room air. Chest sounds clear bilaterally.

    Circulation → Heart rate 120, blood pressure 100/60 mmHg. Abdomen soft and non-tender. No obvious long bone injuries. Just below the left clavicle near the coracoid process, there is a hole in the skin (i.e., this looks like the bullet hole). There is no torrential bleeding coming from the anterior wound, but there is a fairly sizeable haematoma underneath here that is protruding the skin forwards. The patient does not have a left brachial or radial pulse, the left hand is cool. The patient says his left hand feels weird and he has pins and needles at the tips of his fingers. He can still move his hand however.

    Disability → GCS 15/15, no obvious head injury.

    Exposure → You rapidly explore the whole body for any other bullet holes. The A&E team look at you like you are mad but you inspect the chest wall, abdominal wall, in the groins, both legs, and then ask for the patient to be logrolled so you can examine the back. You cannot find a second bullet hole.

- *Immediate management plan:* Large-bore intravenous access right antecubital fossa, send off urgent bloods (FBC, U&Es, clotting, group and save), activate major transfusion protocol, tranexamic acid, permissive hypotension approach currently (i.e., avoid giving blood or intravenous fluids right now). I would also stick a Foley catheter in the wound and inflate the balloon (same as previously discussed).

- What is the working diagnosis? The patient has been shot, and he probably has an axillary artery injury. It sounds like the artery bled a lot of scene, but the bleeding seems to have reduced now. The left arm looks ischaemic. As such I suspect the axillary artery may have been transected and gone into spasm (or completely thrombosed). I can only find one bullet wound, so the bullet must still be in the body.

- What do we do now? Here are your options:

    1. Take the patient straight to theatre.
    2. Get some X-rays (chest, abdomen, pelvis, left arm) and then go to theatre.
    3. Get a trauma CT and include a CT angiogram of the left arm. After this go to theatre.

- According to the respectable resources I use, the correct answer to get some X-rays first of all. Bullets do not respect anatomical boundaries, and we know this bullet has not left the body yet. As such, it may have traversed into another body cavity or region (e.g., into chest, abdomen or pelvis).

- In my particular unit, however, I would have to honest about what I think I would do in regards to asking for X-rays. My A&E department is literally right next door to the CT scanner, and I know it would be much quicker to get the patient a full body CT scan than it would to get X-rays of the chest/abdomen/pelvis. I also know that a CT scan starts off with a scout X-ray of the chest/abdomen/pelvis …. as such for pragmatic purposes if this patient were "stable" I would get an urgent CT scan (neck/chest/abdomen/pelvis, and I would also ask for the left arm to be included as a CT angio).

- For the sake of this scenario, the patient has a CT scan. This shows a bullet lodged just anterior to the left scapula. The axillary artery just below the clavicle has been transected and appears to have gone into spasm. There is no contrast extravasation currently. There is a sizeable haematoma around the lateral third of the clavicle and around the coracoid process. There are no other chest/abdominal/pelvic injuries. The angiogram shows there is still contrast getting down to the left arm via what must be collateral supply.

- What is your plan?

- Interventional radiology is not relevant here, conservative management isn't either. There may not be active bleeding, but the artery has been transected and the hand is ischaemic. As such, something has got to be done … Open the chest? I don't think so. This injury is quite distal and as such proximal control should be possible from outside the chest … let us go to theatre.

Let's Get Juicy → Trauma Surgery on the Axillosubclavian Artery Complex

- *Same principles as always:* Proximal control, distal control, then attack the injury.
- To get proximal control in the scenario in question, I would target the proximal left subclavian artery in the supraclavicular fossa first.
- The patient would be in the standard trauma crucifix position with the neck, chest, left arm, abdomen, and both legs (to mid-thighs) all prepped.
- These are the core steps to expose the proximal subclavian artery:
  1. This is a big transverse incision about 1-cm above and parallel to the clavicle starting over the head of sternocleidomastoid.
  2. The skin, fascia, and platysma are divided.
  3. Next the clavicular insertion of sternocleidomastoid is divided.
  4. The scalene fat pad must then be mobilised from medial to lateral but ideally preserved and reflected out of the surgical field.
  5. The subclavian vein should now come into view at the base of your wound.
  6. Now have a gentle feel with your finger for the anterior scalene muscle as it attaches to the first rib beneath. This is the part of the operation you must definitely not rush. You need to identify and preserve the phrenic nerve. The phrenic nerve passes downwards from a lateral-to-medial direction along the anterior surface of the anterior scale muscle (in fact there can be anatomical variations here, and the phrenic nerve may be inside the anterior scalene muscle). This nerve is very small and it is very easy to injure. Take your time to carefully identify it, then gently mobilise it. If you cannot first see the phrenic nerve, very carefully start to divide the anterior scalene muscle,

but do this with your scissors so that each muscle fibre you are dividing is happening as you look for the nerve …. you will probably be sweating at this point for fear you have already cut the nerve. The aim is to preserve this nerve and divide the anterior scalene muscle close to its insertion on the first rib.

7. Now the subclavian artery should be lying in front of you (in front of the middle scalene muscle and brachial plexus). Now the subclavian artery can be sloped and is ready to be clamped as required.

- Now your options are varied. This is dealer's choice, or horses for courses. As for me, in the trauma setting, I like a decent exposure and nice, long extensile incisions. I also do not mind dividing the clavicle. Therefore, I would extend the supraclavicular incision across the middle third of the clavicle and swing it down towards the infraclavicular fossa. I would extend it across the coracoid process, and I would have no hesitation to swing my incision down into the axilla (i.e., into proximal brachial artery territory).

- I would also have absolutely no hesitation to divide the pectoralis major muscle. This would be done by dividing its tendinous insertion into the humerus.

- However, in terms of exposing the axillary artery in the classical way, this is how it is done:

  1. Transverse incision about 8–10 cm in length, around 1 cm below the clavicle, starting at its medial third and running across towards the coracoid process (there is a natural dip in the infraclavicular fossa you can feel with your fingers).

  2. Dissect down through skin, subcutaneous tissue, and clavipectoral fascia.

  3. Now, split the pectoralis major muscle in the line of its fibres. You can use a big self-retaining retractor to improve exposure.

  4. You should see the pectoralis minor muscle with its insertion onto the coracoid process.

  5. There are a number of ways to divide the pectoralis minor muscle. One is to get underneath it with a swab, pull the swab up, and divide with monopolar diathermy. Another option is to use a Lahey and divide chunks of muscle at a time. Whatever you do, just be wary of the brachial plexus and neurovascular structures running underneath i.e. be gentle.

  6. The axillary artery should now be lying right in front of you.

- In the case we are discussing, we already know that there is a large haematoma just below the clavicle around the area of the coracoid process. Therefore, for pragmatic reasons, I would not start off with this "classical" axillary artery exposure. I would make my skin incision from the supraclavicular fossa, across the medial third of the clavicle, swing it down into the infraclavicular fossa, and then go even further across the shoulder and dive deep down into the axilla. I would divide the humeral connection of pectoralis major and identify the axillary artery here first in order to gain distal control away from haematoma. I would be very careful to avoid injuring in the brachial plexus and its branches however.

- Now I have proximal control of the proximal left subclavian artery (above the clavicle), and I have distal control of the distal axillary artery. The injury/haematoma is sitting just underneath the clavicle at around the region of the coracoid process, and I have not attacked this area yet.

- Now we have some options. We can go back to exposing the axillary artery in the classical way, or we can divide the clavicle. There is no right or wrong answer here, and the truth is you will do what you think is right in the moment (depending on the injury pattern). In the context of a bullet wound with a large haematoma underneath the clavicle, the high likelihood of an additional subclavian vein and brachial plexus injury, I think I would divide the clavicle ….

- To divide the clavicle, I would use a periosteal elevator to separate any surrounding tissue. I would cautiously use the periosteal elevator/knife/scissors to separate the underlying subclavius muscle as well. I would ask for a power saw and divide the clavicle at 45 degrees in the mid-point. This then allows me to retract the proximal clavicle upwards and the distal clavicle downwards (i.e., it opens up the wound nicely). There are other options of course. You can use the bonesaw or even a Gigli saw to remove a whole chunk of clavicle. Alternatively, you may not want to remove the clavicle at all. I know of trauma surgeons who are very against removing/cutting the clavicle, and they think that you can get away with fixing these sorts of injuries without removing it. Again, this is for you to decide. I like the idea of dividing the clavicle at 45 degrees because it does allow the wound to be opened up, and the two ends can also be drawn back together and it gives the upper limb orthopaedic surgeons an easier opportunity to fix it later down the line.
- In terms of dealing with the injury, here are some familiar points:
  1. If you are in damage control mode, you should probably shunt the vessel and do an upper limb fasciotomy.
  2. If you are in damage control mode, another option is to ligate the vessel and do an upper limb fasciotomy. For axillary artery ligation, the risk of distal ischaemia is about 20–30%, and for subclavian artery ligation, the risk of ligation is about 15–20%. For me, if I had managed to get proximal and distal control, I would rather shunt the vessel. In this case, the artery was already transected, not actively bleeding, and the arm was ischaemic, so if my plan is just to ligate the vessel then I really don't know why I bothered to take the patient to theatre in the first place. I took the patient to theatre to fix the problem, so I honestly would try and avoid ligation unless I really had no other choice (e.g., I encountered major bleeding that I could not control and the patient decompensates on table ….).
  3. Again, if in damage control mode, you can also consider primary amputation. However, I just don't think I would be doing this for this type of injury. This is a young man who is otherwise fit, and I think he deserves a chance at trying to salvage his arm. Fair enough my attempts at revascularization may not be successful, and he may ultimately require an upper limb amputation, and before taking him to theatre I would try to warn him of this possibility. However, I just don't think I would do a primary amputation in this setting, it feels too extreme and premature.
  4. On the other hand, if this was something like a close range catastrophic shotgun injury, the situation and my approach might be different. For example, if the left upper limb was a totally mangled mess with combined vascular/orthopaedic/plastic surgical injuries, and the arm was completely non-viable, a primary amputation might be considered in this context. I would never make this decision lightly or on my own however. I would get an orthopaedic consultant, plastic surgery consultant, probably a second vascular surgery consultant opinion, speak to the patient and family, and make a fair and balanced decision.
  5. If you are not in damage control mode, you can consider an end-to-end anastomosis (tension-free please), interposition grafting (preferably using reversed great saphenous vein, but possibility synthetic if you must), or do a bypass graft. Again, in any of the above contexts, it is still worth shunting the vessel whilst you are preparing for a vascular repair.
  6. If the vessel was not transected, you can consider a patch repair (vein or synthetic).
  7. It is also always worth considering a fasciotomy after your vascular repair. In this case with a major vascular injury and an ischaemic arm, I would probably do an upper limb fasciotomy.

8. Finally, if you encounter venous injuries, make some common sense decisions. If this a vein injury and you can do a simple suture repair, then do it. If it is a complex venous injury and you are in damage control mode, then ligate it. If you have a stable patient, time is on your side, and the arterial repair is not too overwhelming, then yes you can consider a more complex venous repair if you think this is appropriate ....

Final Comments on Vascular Trauma

I hope that these scenarios have given you a taste of reality, but also some grasp on how to answer questions for the FRCS examination. I have not covered every single possibility of trauma because this would require me to write an entire book on it, which is not my focus here. However, I have read a lot of books on trauma, I have worked in a major trauma unit for a few years, and I have tried to combine my academic knowledge with real world experience to give you what I hope will be a fairly balanced, pragmatic, and sensible approach to major vascular trauma.

I do not consider myself to be an expert in vascular trauma, nor would I consider myself to be highly experienced in this area. However, in my opinion dealing with vascular trauma is about keeping a cool head, having some courage, following core principles, being pragmatic, and making common sense decisions. If you are in the middle of one of these scenarios (for real or in the exam), and you feel like you are overwhelmed, just do what I do → ABCDE, remember damage control principles (stop bleeding, control contamination), remember vascular trauma principles (proximal control, distal control, attack the injury), and keep things as simple as possible.

GOOD LUCK.

CHAPTER 22

Vascular Graft and Endograft Infection

This is a very broad area. Basically anything can get infected. However, for pragmatic purposes, I have split it into four different areas: Carotid, thoracic aortic, abdominal aortic, and lower limb. These are the main "vascular infections" I am exposed to in the real world and what seem to be focused on in the FRCS examination. Obviously you can get upper limb infections, but frankly this is covered mainly by the vascular access chapters. In this chapter we will use some realistic case examples, and then walk through some FRCS-style examination stations.

Overall Baseline ESVS Guideline Recommendations

- When a vascular graft/endograft infection is suspected, it is recommended that every effort is made to obtain microbiological proof of infection.
- To obtain microbiological proof of vascular graft/endograft infection, the yield of at least three deep rather than superficial samples should be considered.
- For patients suspected of vascular graft/endograft infection, the use of ultrasound as the sole diagnostic modality is not recommended.
- For suspected vascular graft/endograft infection, CTA is recommended as the first-line diagnostic modality.
- For patients suspected of vascular graft/endograft infection, if CTA is contra-indicated, the use of MRA may be considered.
- For patients with a clinical suspicion of vascular graft/endograft infection and with non-convincing findings on CTA, the use of 18F-FDG-PET combined with low-dose CT is recommended as an additional imaging modality to improve diagnostic accuracy.
- Antimicrobial therapy is recommended in every patient with an infected graft/endograft.
- For the diagnosis and treatment of vascular graft/endograft infection it is recommended that the patient be transferred to specialised high volume centre with multidisciplinary experience in this pathology.

CASE 22.1: Infected Carotid Endarterectomy Patch

This patient presents to A&E and he is sitting outside the main department in the waiting area.

History

- This 87-year-old gentleman has come in because he has been having blood coming out of an ulcerated area of his right neck for 48 hours.
- This is at the site of a previous carotid endarterectomy he had done in 2018.
- He does not report any other neck operations.
- He feels fine in himself and the bleeding has been minimal and intermittent.
- He is not reporting fevers, sweats, or shakes.
- There are no other infective symptoms.
- His weight is steady, appetite is OK.

DOI: 10.1201/b22951-22

- He said that this ulcerated area has developed over a few weeks. It started as a very small lump, and the skin has only just started to break down and ulcerate.
- The original carotid endarterectomy was done for a mini-stroke and it was done under general anaesthesia. It started off as a local anaesthesia case, but when the carotid artery was clamped he became confused and was thrashing about, and had to be urgently converted to a GA.
- *Rapid assessment of risk factors*: Non-smoker, diet controlled diabetes, hypertension, and on treatment for raised cholesterol.
- *Other medical comorbidities*: Hypothyroidism.
- *Medication history*: Aspirin, atorvastatin, levothyroxine, and amlodipine.
- *Social history*: Is otherwise fit and well, independent, and self-caring. Lives at home with his wife. Good exercise tolerance.

Examination

- Patient is systemically well.
- Scar in anterior triangle of right neck along anterior border of sternocleidomastoid.
- In mid-point of neck (anterior triangle) centred on this scar is a 1 cm area of ulceration with a blood clot present. No active bleeding.
- No scars on other side of neck or over thyroid area.
- Upper and lower limb pulses normal.
- Chest clear.
- Abdomen soft and non-tender.
- Neurology grossly intact.
- Speech intact.
- GCS 15/15.

Your FRCS Short Case Begins

What is your working diagnosis?

- "I suspect this patient has a carotid patch infection with breakdown of the suture line. These are likely small herald bleeds, and thus my major concern is that there is a fistulous connection from the carotid patch to the skin and thus he is at imminent risk of catastrophic haemorrhage."

What is your immediate management plan?

- "First of all I would have alerted the A&E consultant and have the patient moved immediately from the waiting room to A&E resus. I would have warned the patient to not touch the area of ulceration and disturb the clotted blood. After this I would briefly counsel the patient on the suspected diagnosis, what I am worried about (torrential haemorrhage), and what I intended to do about it. I would explain that first of all we would need to do some investigations to assess the carotid artery to confirm/refute the diagnosis. In this case this would be either a CT angiogram arch of aorta and carotids, or a focused arterial duplex. I would also aim to keep the patient nil by mouth, gain large-bore IV access in the antecubital fossa, send off bloods for FBC, U&Es, clotting,

CRP, blood cultures, and crossmatch the patient a few units of blood. I would not start antibiotics at this stage. I would also phone another consultant vascular surgeon and alert the interventional radiology consultant on-call as this is a complex high risk case and getting support and second opinions is always a good idea. Finally, I would check the medical records and determine the details of the original carotid endarterectomy and clarify if this was a patch repair, and if so what type of patch was used."

The examiner hands you some images of a carotid duplex and its report.

- "There is evidence of suture line breakdown at the inferior aspect of the carotid endarterectomy patch. There is a small partially thrombosed pseudoaneurysm above this area that has a very small amount of contrast filling it. This is less than a centimetre below the skin at the site of the ulcerated area."

The examiner shows you some images of the patient's CT angiogram and asks you to comment on it.

- "The right carotid endarterectomy site is patent. The left carotid artery and internal carotid artery are also patent with minimal disease. The circle of Willis does not appear to be intact. There is an abnormality around the right common carotid artery, this appears to be a pseudoaneurysm that is very close to the skin. There is a small amount of contrast in this pseudoaneurysm. Based upon my clinical assessment and interpretation of these radiological studies, I strongly suspect that this patient has an infected right carotid endarterectomy patch and the inferior suture line is breaking down. There is a pseudoaneurysm at this site, and there appears to be a fistulous connection to the skin. I would assert that this patient is at extremely high risk of catastrophic bleed which would likely be fatal. This could happen at any minute."

What is your management plan?

- "There are three options here. One is to manage the case conservatively, which would essentially be a palliative approach. The second option is to explant all the infected material from the neck and repair the right carotid using autologous vein e.g. an interposition graft using non-reversed great saphenous vein. The third option is to arrange for an emergency covered stent insertion as a damage control procedure. I personally would support an emergency covered stent in this setting as it seems like the quickest simplest method to prevent catastrophic haemorrhage. I would of course discuss the case with my consultant colleagues and get their expert opinions, and also counsel the patient, and then reach a consensus view and proceed."

The patient has an emergency carotid stent with a good result. The external carotid artery also has an Amplatzer plug. What are you going to do now?

- "I would formally discuss the case in the vascular MDT, and involve the infectious diseases/ microbiology teams in the discussions. My provisional plan would be to get a CT PET scan to see whether the carotid endarterectomy site lights up, thus confirming (radiologically) that this is an infected patch. At this point we would then return to the two options as discussed before. A conservative management approach with life long suppressive antibiotics, or full explantation of the infected carotid artery and repair with autologous material."

If you were going to explant the infected carotid endarterectomy patch and stent, how would you approach this?

- "Before doing this operation I would first request a carotid balloon occlusion test to ensure the contralateral brain perfusion was intact in case I needed to ligate the carotid artery. In any case, the operation itself would be a 2 or 3 consultant vascular surgeon operation, with vascular surgeons more than senior and experienced than me. The priority would be proximal control, then distal control, removing all the infected tissue, and likely having to shunt the artery to maintain cerebral perfusion. The provisional plan would be to do an interposition graft using non-reversed GSV or alternatively a re-do GSV patch repair. I would debride all the infected tissues and send multiple samples for microbiology. If the anatomy was severely distorted and everything was falling apart, I would likely have to ligate the right carotid. The circle of Willis was however not intact on the CT angiogram, so it looks like this may not be a viable bail-out option."

The patient says he does not want surgery. What are your options in this context?

- "The plan would be either palliation, or lifelong suppressive antibiotics. In order to commence on antibiotics we would require microbiology samples to determine the likely culprit bacteria. This may come from a deep wound swab, blood cultures, or ultrasound-guided fine needle aspiration of the carotid patch."

The patient has a CT-PET. Everything lights up. The patient confirms he does not want explantation at this stage. He has a fine-needle aspiration of the neck. No culture results are available. In fact the blood tests are completely normal, blood cultures are normal, and the fine-needle aspiration comes back as negative. What would you do now?

- "I would get advice from microbiology on appropriate antibiotics."

The patient is started on co-trimoxazole. This causes renal failure. This is switched to oral ciprofloxacin and intravenous teicoplanin. The ciprofloxacin also gives the patient severe side-effects. This is stopped, and he continues on just IV teicoplanin via a midline. By this point (a few weeks later), the patient and microbiology think he should proceed with explantation. How would you plan the explantation?

- "As the circle of Willis is not patent, I would speak to neuroradiology about a carotid balloon occlusion test. My concern is that if we take him to theatre, and things turned ugly, we might have to ligate the right carotid artery. I would want to know if he would tolerate this. I also want to know if I needed to shunt the patient."

The neuroradiologist says that the cerebrovascular anatomy is abnormal. There is almost no connection from the left side of the brain to the right. The right internal carotid artery also supplies both the anterior and posterior circulation. The neuroradiologist is happy to do a balloon occlusion test, but he is certain the patient will fail it. What do you make of this?

- "Essentially we have no bail-out option. If we take him to theatre we cannot really ligate the right carotid artery. If we do so, the patient would likely have a massive total right-sided stroke. This cerebrovascular anatomy also explains why he did not tolerate carotid artery clamping under local anaesthesia with the original carotid endarterectomy."

Is there anything about this surgery that requires special planning?

- "I suspect the right ICA is also quite challenging to get control. How high does the stent reach? Can I see the angiogram from when the stent was inserted? Ah yes thank you.

The right ICA stent is above the angle of the mandible. Essentially we are in zone 3 of the neck. This means to get distal ICA control I would likely need help from a head neck surgeon or maxillofacial surgeon. We may need to dislocate the mandible or do similar procedures to gain suitable access."

Would you do this surgery?

- "I would not do it on my own. I would also not do it without discussing the case in the vascular MDT, and counselling the patient and family appropriately."

This is the outcome of the vascular MDT: "Surgery would be a high morbidity, highly complex procedure and would need careful discussion with the patient and family. If patient considers explant then to arrange US in presence of operating surgeon to assess possibility of explant without need for mandible division/dislocation."

- "This seems fair. I would speak to the patient and family and see what they wanted to do."

Are you aware of any other surgical options?

- "There is the EndoVac technique."

What is that?

- "The endovacuum-assisted closure (VAC) technique is a hybrid approach with three steps: (1) re-lining of the infected reconstruction with a stent, (2) removal of the infected vascular graft without clamping, (3) use of negative pressure wound therapy to permit granulation."

Would you consider this here?

- "I might consider it. However, the evidence base for this approach is limited. It is also still an operation that carries risks including wound healing problems, cranial nerve injury, bleeding etc. I could still picture trying to do this operation as a 'minimally invasive' compromise and perhaps still encountering significant complications. As per the vascular MDT, I would see what the patient thought."

Your FRCS Short Case Ends

JMF Reflections

This is a real case although suitably anonymised. It was a Dacron patch that was the culprit. My hand was eventually forced and I did proceed with the EndoVac technique after getting advice from an experienced vascular surgeon in Sweden (*thanks for your help Anders*). Currently, the patient is doing remarkably well and the neck wound is fully healed. The microbiology samples all came back as no growth. With vascular graft and endograft infection, this is not entirely unusual. An another explanation is that perhaps this was all a late inflammatory reaction to the Dacron patch. This isn't clear, but the management is not really any different in my opinion. I treated this as an infected Dacron patch. In any case the patient had a choice between palliation and the EndoVac technique, and the patient most certainly did not want to be palliated. Henceforth, EndoVac was what was done. I think if I encounter this sort of situation again, I will be very open to the EndoVac approach.

KEY REFERENCE

Thorbjørnsen K, Djavani Gidlund K, Björck M, Kragsterman B, Wanhainen A. Editor's Choice—Long Term Outcome after EndoVAC Hybrid Repair of Infected Vascular Reconstructions. Eur J Vasc Endovasc Surg, 2016, 51(5):724–32.

Relevant ESVS Guideline Recommendations

- For patients with supra-aortic trunk vascular graft/endograft infection, total removal of infected material followed by reconstruction with autologous material is recommended.
- In the emergency setting with active bleeding in patients with supra-aortic trunk vascular graft/endograft infection, a combined endovascular and surgical approach may be considered.
- Conservative treatment, including antimicrobial therapy without reconstruction, for supra-aortic trunk vascular graft/endograft infection may be considered for patients unfit for surgery.
- The EndoVac technique may be considered as a treatment option in selected patients with supra-aortic trunk vascular graft/endograft infection when neither total removal of infected material nor when usual conservative VAC therapy are considered feasible or safe.
- When patch corrugation is found on ultrasound follow-up after carotid endarterectomy, further investigations may be considered to exclude a vascular graft infection.

CASE 22.2: Infected Thoracic Aortic Stent (TEVAR)

This patient presents to A&E resus with frank haemoptysis.

History

- This patient has been coughing up bright red blood for the past 48 hours.
- It is not torrential bleeding, but he has been coughing up quite a lot of fresh bright red clots.
- This is coughing, not vomiting, according to the patient.
- He is not reporting any rectal bleeding or black motions.
- The patient feels slightly unsteady on his feet and almost collapsed on his way into A&E.
- He is not describing fevers/sweats/shakes, but a general malaise and whole body weakness.
- He is describing poor appetite and general weight loss.
- He says that he had a thoracic aortic stent inserted 2 years ago for an aortic dissection.
- *Rapid assessment of risk factors*: Ex-smoker, hypertension, and on treatment for raised cholesterol.
- *Other medical comorbidities*: Previous MI, angina, moderate chronic obstructive pulmonary disease, and moderate chronic kidney disease.
- *Medication history*: Aspirin, atorvastatin, ramipril, inhalers, GTN spray, and isosorbide mononitrate.
- *Social history*: Says he is otherwise fit and well, independent, and self-caring. Lives at home with his long term partner. Exercise tolerance of around 500 m limited by shortness of breath related to angina/COPD.

Your FRCS Short Case Begins

What is your working diagnosis?

- "Given the haemoptysis, systemic symptoms of malaise, poor appetite and weight loss, and the previous TEVAR, I am mainly worried that this TEVAR is infected and the patient has a life-threatening aorto-bronchial fistula."

What is your immediate management plan?

- "I would briefly counsel the patient on what I thought was going on, and highlight that these herald bleeds could be the preliminary to a massive torrential haemorrhage that would be life-threatening. I would make the patient nil by mouth. I would alert the A&E consultant and ask for their team's help in securing large-bore IV access and sending off urgent bloods (FBC, U&Es, coagulation, group and save, CRP, and multiple blood cultures). I would crossmatch 4 units of blood. I would alert the vascular interventional radiology consultant on-call and request an urgent CT angiogram of the whole aorta, arch vessels and intracranial vessels."

These are some images from the CT angiogram. Can you please interpret them?

- "There is some general haziness and evidence of inflammation around the top end of the thoracic aortic stent. There are also very small locules of gas around this area. There appears to be some native thoracic aortic damage just above the top end of the TEVAR, just distal to the left subclavian artery. I suspect this is a small mycotic pseudoaneurysm of the native aortic just at the top end of the stent. This would reinforce my suspected diagnosis of an infected TEVAR with erosion of the native aorta. Given the haemoptysis I would now proceed on the basis that this is an aorto-bronchial fistula."

Here are some blood results for you. Can you please interpret them?

- "These results indicate evidence of significant bleeding. The haemoglobin is 78. There is also evidence of probably chronic low-level sepsis with a white blood count of 13 and a CRP of 40. Again, this reinforces my suspected diagnosis."

What is your management plan now?

- "In the real world, I would avoid managing such a case in isolation. I would work collaboratively with more senior vascular surgery consultant colleagues, and additionally get expert input from my vascular interventional radiology colleagues. However, for pragmatic purposes this is what I consider to be an emergency case and it calls for quick thinking. I consider this patient to be at imminent risk of exsanguination, and I would therefore be aiming to do a quick and relatively simple procedure to prevent further bleeding. As a damage control procedure, I would request an emergency TEVAR extension. In this context we would likely have to plug the origin of the left subclavian artery, thus enabling us to extend the TEVAR beyond the area of native aortic wall damage."

What if the CT angiogram had shown that the patient had a dominant left vertebral artery?

- "By the book one should do a left carotid-subclavian artery bypass in this setting to prevent a posterior circulation stroke."

What if the CT angiogram had shown that the patient had a patent left internal mammary to coronary artery bypass?

- "If I block off this coronary bypass the patient will have a myocardial infarction and probably die. Therefore the patient would require a left carotid-subclavian bypass."

The patient gets his TEVAR extension with a good radiological result, and there are no more bleeding episodes. What is your management plan now?

- "The life-saving damage control procedure is completed. However, now we have to think about the long term picture. This patient has an infected TEVAR, and there are a number of ways to manage this. The overall management will be determined of course by patient fitness and patient choice. The first option to consider is a conservative or palliative approach with long term antibiotics (+/− irrigation and drainage of any collections). The second option is in situ reconstruction of the aorta using infection resistant material after removal of the infected graft with aggressive debridement."

What are your surgical repair options?

- "In this case, the prosthetic material is extending into the aortic arch (proximal to the left subclavian artery). Therefore, a median sternotomy or clamshell incision would likely be required. Total cardiopulmonary bypass, circulatory arrest and selective cerebral perfusion would need to be considered. Cerebrospinal fluid drainage may need to be considered in order to reduce the risk of spinal cord ischaemia. The infected material would need to be removed, and after this a thorough debridement of any necrotic/infected tissue from the arterial bed. Potential graft materials include: cryopreserved aortic allografts, rifampicin soaked and silver coated grafts, bovine pericardium, femoral vein grafts etc. It is also important to achieve coverage of these grafts with viable tissue e.g. intercostal muscle flap, omental flap, or pericardial flap. For the bronchial fistula, it is recommended to repair the bronchus surgically. The defect can be closed primarily or with an intercostal muscle or pericardial flap, but in most cases a bronchial resection and anastomosis or a lung resection is necessary. Naturally these are extremely complex and advanced cases, and in my practice I would refer such a patient to a specialist aortic centre if this type of surgery were being contemplated."

Are there other surgical repair options?

- "Yes. One could consider extra-anatomical bypass. To avoid reconstruction in a contaminated field and recurrent infection, an extra-anatomical bypass outside the infected field and secondary aortic ligation with removal of the infected graft or stent can be performed in one or two stages. To restore distal perfusion after aortic ligation, an axillo-bifemoral bypass can be performed, although retrograde blood flow to the visceral organs in this context may not be sufficient. The most commonly used extra-anatomical bypass is from the ventral aorta, i.e. from the ascending aorta to the supraceliac/infra-renal aorta. After this bypass the second stage of the operation would be to remove all the infected aortic material. The aortic stump needs to be oversewn and covered with an omental or muscular flap in order to reinforce the stump and diminish the risk of blow out. The other theoretical option is partial excision of the aortic graft, but for pragmatic purposes I am not so sure about this option. As I see it, if one part of the graft is infected, it is all infected. Therefore if I am going to take the trouble to open the chest and explant it, I might as well do a proper job. This feels like a half-hearted measure in my eyes, but I do recognise that it is discussed in the literature and there may well be a place for it in certain contexts."

Do you think this is a viable option for this patient?

- "Naturally these cases would be discussed in the MDT and the patient would be fully informed of their options. However, I am aware that the patient has ischaemic heart disease, chronic obstructive pulmonary disease, and chronic kidney disease. Surgery of this size and complexity carries significant risks of death, mainly related to cardiac, respiratory and renal impairment. As such the patient automatically would fit into the "high risk" category. I am aware of the ESVS guidelines on vascular graft and endograft infection, and that in patients with aortobronchial or aortopulmonary fistula closure of the airway defect and explantation of the infected material with in situ reconstruction should be considered as definitive treatment. However, in real world practice, it would be a joint decision between the patient and the vascular surgery team as to how the case is definitively managed."

The patient says he does not want surgery and wants to manage things conservatively. What would your conservative management approach be?

- "I would liaise with microbiology/infectious diseases about long term suppressive antibiotics. Hopefully we would have some positive blood cultures to achieve targeted antibiotics. I would also follow the patient up long term as these patients are at risk from recurrent infections and/or further fistulae."

Your FRCS Short Case Ends

Relevant ESVS Guideline Recommendations

- For fit patients with proven thoracic/thoracoabdominal vascular graft/endograft infection, total graft explantation is recommended.
- For patients with in situ reconstructions of thoracic/thoracoabdominal vascular graft/endograft infection, coverage of the newly inserted graft with autologous, and ideally vascularised, tissue is recommended.
- For patients with thoracic vascular graft/endograft infection that are at major risk of surgery, conservative treatment may be considered.
- For patients with suspected thoracic graft/endograft infection, in the absence of fistulisation to the oesophagus or airway or generalised sepsis, prolonged antimicrobial therapy combined with drainage of peri-graft fluid and/or irrigation may be considered.
- For patients with thoracic/thoracoabdominal vascular graft/endograft infection, partial explantation may be considered if infection is limited.
- For the reconstruction of thoracic/thoracoabdominal vascular graft/endograft infection, cryopreserved allografts may be considered the first choice graft material.
- After extra-anatomic reconstruction for thoracic/thoracoabdominal vascular graft/endograft infection, reinforcement of the aortic stump with autologous, and ideally vascularised, tissues should be considered.
- For patients with aorto-oesophageal fistula complicating thoracic/thoracoabdominal vascular graft/endograft infection, explantation of the infected material, repair of the oesophagus, and coverage with viable tissue is recommended as definitive treatment.
- In the emergency setting with active bleeding complicating thoracic/thoracoabdominal vascular graft/endograft infection with an aorto-oesophageal fistula, initial treatment with an aortic endograft, as a bridge to definitive treatment, should be considered.

- Conservative treatment of patients with an aorto-oesophageal fistula complicating thoracic/thoracoabdominal vascular graft/endograft infection is not recommended, except in a palliative setting.

- Treatment of aorto-oesophageal fistula complicating thoracic/thoracoabdominal vascular graft/endograft infection with an oesophageal endoprosthesis alone is not recommended.

- In patients with aortobronchial or aortopulmonary fistula complicating thoracic/ thoracoabdominal vascular graft/endograft infection, closure of the airway defect and explantation of the infected material with in situ reconstruction should be considered as definitive treatment.

- In the emergency setting of active bleeding complicating thoracic/thoracoabdominal vascular graft/endograft infection with an aortobronchial or aortopulmonary fistula, treatment with an aortic endograft should be considered.

- For patients with an aortobronchial or aortopulmonary fistula complicating thoracic/ thoracoabdominal vascular graft/endograft infection, preservation of the endograft may be considered after closure of the airway defect and coverage with viable tissue.

- For all patients treated for thoracic/thoracoabdominal vascular graft/endograft infection, lifelong follow up is recommended because of the risk of recurrent infections or fistulae.

CASE 22.3: Infected Abdominal Aortic Stent (EVAR)

This is a patient you see on the vascular ward.

History

- This is a 68-year-old gentleman who had an elective EVAR 3 years ago for an infra-renal abdominal aortic aneurysm.
- The procedure went smoothly and he was discharged home day 1 post-op.
- His surveillance scans so far have been unremarkable.
- However, over the past few months the patient has been getting night sweats and his appetite has reduced. He has lost a few kilograms in weight. He is also reporting a general fatigue and weakness.
- Specifically, the patient is not reporting vomiting up any blood, or any blood being passed from his rectum (fresh or black stools).
- Over the past 2 weeks he has developed a purulent, smelly discharge from the right side of his back where there is a small skin opening.
- *Rapid assessment of risk factors*: Ex-smoker, hypertension, on treatment for raised cholesterol, and type 2 diabetes.
- *Other medical comorbidities*: NAD.
- *Medication history*: Aspirin, atorvastatin, ramipril, amlodipine, and metformin.
- *Social history*: Is otherwise fit and well, independent, and self-caring. Lives at home with his wife. Good exercise tolerance can walk miles.

Examination

- *End of the bed test* → Patient looks like an open surgical candidate (i.e. looks fit).
- Patient is systemically well.
- Upper and lower limb pulses all present.

- Abdomen is soft and non-tender. Virgin abdomen. No scars.
- Sinus opening right paralumbar area that is discharging pus.

Your FRCS Short Case Begins

What is your working diagnosis?

- "This patient has an infected EVAR with a sinus connection from the retroperitoneum to the skin in the paralumbar area (until proven otherwise)."

What is your immediate management?

- "I would do some basic tests: FBC, U&Es, LFTS, coagulation screen, CRP, group & save, and multiple blood cultures. I would also take a deep wound swab from the sinus tract in the paralumbar area and send it off for microscopy, culture and sensitivity. I would request an urgent CT angiogram of the aorta. I would also request a vein scan of both lower limbs to assess the deep femoral veins."

Here are some relevant CT angiogram images. Can you please interpret?

- "The infra-renal EVAR is patent. There is fat stranding and inflammation around the entire graft. There are locules of gas around the top end. There is no contrast extravasation. I cannot see any direct connection to the duodenum to suggest an aortoduodenal fistula. There is clearly a fistulous tract in the retroperitoneum that is tracking towards the left paralumbar area. This confirms my suspected diagnosis. This is an infected EVAR."

What are your management options?

- "There are three broad management options: (1) conservative management/palliation, (2) full explantation and aortic repair, and (3) extra-anatomical bypass. In this case, I would be veering heavily in favour of full explantation with autologous aortic repair."

How would you approach this?

- "As a matter of principle this case would be discussed in the vascular MDT, and I would seek the expert opinions of senior and experienced vascular surgery and interventional radiology consultant colleagues. However, my approach would be this:
  1. 2 or preferably 3 consultant operation.
  2. This case would be done on a daytime elective theatre list with a dedicated vascular anaesthetist present.
  3. Midline laparotomy.
  4. Simultaneous harvest of superficial femoral vein(s).
  5. Supraceliac control (or alternatively an aortic occlusion balloon to achieve proximal control).
  6. Removal of aortic stent.
  7. Convert supraceliac control to infra-renal clamp.
  8. Debridement of native aortic tissue with multiple samples to be taken for microbiology, culture and sensitivity.

9. In situ aortic repair using superficial femoral vein.
10. Omental patch to cover the repair and any suture lines."

What other surgical options are available?

- "One could first do an extra-anatomical bypass i.e. an axillo-bifemoral bypass. After this one could proceed to do a laparotomy, remove the infected graft, and then close the aortic stump. I would cover the stump with an omental flap/wrap. There is also the theoretical option of partial graft excision."

What if the patient had an aorto-enteric fistula?

- "If the patient had an aorto-enteric fistula and presented with bleeding I would strongly consider a stent-graft as a "damage control" bridging procedure initially. After this I would proceed to surgery if the patient were deemed fit. The approach would be much the same, however, I would recruit an upper GI surgeon to help with the case. The type of the bowel repair would depend on the size and the location of the defect. A tension free duodenorrhaphy with direct suture of the duodenum can be performed if the bowel defect were minimal, however a complex duodenal reconstruction with resection and anastomosis may be required. Again, in this context, an omental flap would be used to cover the reconstruction and separate the new vascular reconstruction from the bowel."

What other graft options are available apart from autologous deep vein?

- "The other options include cryopreserved allografts, rifampicin-bonded grafts, silver-coated grafts, and xenogenous grafts."

The operation is performed with an in situ autologous repair using superficial femoral vein. The patient does well post-operatively. What would be your post-operative plan?

- "I would liaise closely with microbiology/infectious diseases. Hopefully the tissue samples from theatre would enable a targeted antimicrobial approach. The patient will require prolonged antibiotics and long term follow-up."

Your FRCS Short Case Ends

Relevant ESVS Guideline Recommendations

- Percutaneous drainage of peri-graft fluid with or without irrigation may be considered for microbiological identification and to reduce the bacteriological burden, but not as ultimate treatment in abdominal aortic graft/endograft infection.
- For fit patients with an abdominal aortic vascular graft/endograft infection, complete excision of all graft material and infected tissue is recommended for definitive treatment.
- For patients with an abdominal aortic vascular graft/endograft infection, in situ reconstruction with autologous vein should be considered as the preferred method.
- For patients with abdominal aortic vascular graft/endograft infection, cryopreserved allografts, silver coated grafts, rifampicin bonded polyester grafts, or bovine pericardium should be considered as alternative solutions.

- Partial excision of an infected aortic vascular graft/endograft may be considered when infection is documented as limited and the remaining material is well incorporated.
- For patients with abdominal aortic vascular graft/endograft infection and a large abscess or multi-resistant microorganisms, extra-anatomic reconstruction may be considered.
- Lifelong imaging follow up is recommended after in situ reconstruction with cryopreserved allografts for abdominal aortic vascular graft/endograft infection, in order to detect allograft degeneration.
- Securing a supra-coeliac clamp zone or using an aortic occlusion balloon may be considered as the first step before entering the aorto-enteric fistula area.
- In the emergency setting of active bleeding complicating abdominal aortic graft/endograft infection with or without aorto-enteric fistula, initial treatment with an endograft should be considered, but only as a temporary measure.
- In surgical repair of aortic abdominal graft/endograft infection with aorto-enteric fistula, omentoplasty or transfer of autologous vascularised tissue to cover the vascular reconstruction is recommended.
- In the emergency setting of active bleeding complicating abdominal aortic graft/endograft infection with an arterioureteral fistula, initial treatment with an endograft may be considered, but only as a temporary measure.
- For patients with an arterio-ureteral fistula and vascular graft/endograft infection, complete explantation of the graft combined with urological treatment with or without in situ arterial reconstruction should be considered.

CASE 22.4: Infected Prosthetic Femoral-Distal Bypass

You review this patient in the outpatient clinic 6 weeks following a right leg bypass for CLTI.

History

- This patient is 64-years-old.
- She says she had a right leg bypass 6 weeks ago for gangrene of her right foot.
- Since the operation the pain in her right foot has significantly improved and her gangrenous 5th toe has fallen off on its own last week.
- She is very happy with the progress so far.
- She is not reporting any fevers/sweats/shakes.
- Her appetite is good and her weight is steady.
- She has however noticed that the wound on her right anterior shin has broken down slightly and there has been some slight purulent discharge from this area.
- There has not been any frank bleeding.
- *Rapid assessment of risk factors*: Ex-smoker, hypertension, on treatment for raised cholesterol, and type 2 diabetes.
- *Other medical comorbidities*: NAD.
- *Medication history*: Aspirin, atorvastatin, amlodipine, metformin, and insulin.
- *Social history*: Is otherwise fit and well, independent, and self-caring. Lives at home with her husband. Exercise tolerance limited by claudication affecting the contralateral leg. Can walk about 300 m.

Examination

- *End of the bed test*: Looks well, looks like a surgical candidate (*no brainer really as she has just had a bypass*).
- Patient is generally quite thin with minimal muscle mass.
- There are no scars in the upper limbs or the contralateral leg.
- *Right leg pulse status*: Femoral pulse palpable, popliteal pulse palpable, and dorsalis pedis pulse palpable.
- Right groin looks well-healed.
- No vein harvest scars evident in the ipsilateral medial thigh/calf..
- Vertical incision over anterior tibial artery exposure site superficially dehisced.
- There is some purulent fluid seeping from anterior tibial exposure wound.
- There is also a "fullness" in this area that is pulsatile/expansile.

Your FRCS Short Case Begins

What is your working diagnosis?

- "I suspect this patient has had a femoral-anterior tibial bypass using prosthetic material. I believe this to be the case because there are no scars in the medial leg to suggest a great saphenous vein harvest. There are also no scars in the contralateral leg or arms to suggest vein harvest from these sites either. This may well be a femoral-distal bypass using a prosthetic bypass with a vein cuff. Given the distal wound dehiscence, pulsatile/expansile mass, and purulent discharge, I expect that this is a prosthetic bypass graft infection with a likely distal anastomotic site pseudoaneurysm."

What is your immediate management approach?

- "First of all I would counsel the patient on my suspected diagnosis, and what the potential implications are. I would explain that this could well be an infected prosthetic graft, and if this were confirmed to be the case, it very well may need explanting. This could compromise the perfusion to her right leg, and may well lead to worsening limb ischaemia and ultimately the requirement for a major amputation. I would make the patient nil by mouth, achieve large-bore intravenous access in the antecubital fossa, and send off urgent bloods for: FBC, U&Es, LFTs, CRP, coagulation, group and save, and multiple blood cultures. I would also very carefully send a wound swab from the anterior shin wound for microscopy, culture and sensitivity. I would arrange for an urgent CT angiogram of the lower limbs. I would also read through the previous medical notes and clarify the exact nature of the bypass operation, and ascertain what the vein mapping status of the contralateral limb/arms was. At this early stage I would not start antibiotics yet."

What do you mean when you say carefully send a wound swab from the anterior shin?

- "Aggressively jamming a wound swab into the anterior shin wound breakdown site is a recipe for disaster. There could well be anastomotic dehiscence and a pseudoaneurysm just underneath the skin. My sticking a wound swab into this area could very easily lead to the anastomosis rupturing, and an enormous amount of blood hitting me in the face at arterial pressure. This is something I would try to avoid. I would therefore take a wound swab of the purulent fluid and try to avoid opening Pandora's Box."

Here are some relevant CT angiogram images. Can you please interpret?

- "These coronal slices suggest there is indeed an anastomotic pseudoaneurysm at the distal anastomosis. There does appear to be a venous cuff given the prominence of the distal anastomosis. There is no contrast extravasation to suggest active bleeding. There is some haziness around the distal anastomosis and some gas in the tissues. This infective/inflammatory process appears to be very close to the overlying skin, and indeed I can see that this pseudoaneurysm is only around half a centimetres from the skin surface. I can see where the superficial tissues have dehisced, so yes indeed there is very well a direct fistulous connection from the anastomotic pseudoaneurysm to the skin surface. This is very concerning. In my professional opinion this patient is at very high risk of a catastrophic bleed from this distal anastomosis."

The original operation report confirms this is a femoral-anterior tibial bypass using ring-enforced PTFE and a Miller cuff. The patient does not have suitable vein in the ipsilateral leg or the contralateral leg. The upper limbs were not assessed. What is your management approach?

- "There are two broad options available in this specific context. The first option is to simply explant all the infected material and see how the right leg does. The second option is to explant all the infected material and consider a re-do bypass using autologous vein from the upper limb (s). As for my position, as this original bypass was performed for critical ischaemia, I would try and revascularise the limb with autologous vein if at all possible."

The patient has a bilateral upper limb vein map, and she does not have suitable upper limb vein for a femoral-distal bypass. How would you proceed in this context?

- "There are other bypass conduit options. Perhaps the patient has deep femoral vein. Alternatively, one might consider the following: cryopreserved allografts, prosthetic grafts, and xenogenous grafts. However, I must make it clear that my main worry at the moment is that the patient is at risk of a catastrophic bleed from the distal anastomosis. Preventing this is my main focus at the priority, with limb salvage coming in second (i.e. life before limb)."

So would you do a re-do prosthetic bypass in this context?

- "Honestly, I would be veering towards saying no. The advantages of prostheses are that they are readily available and operating time is shorter, but the re-infection rate is high when compared to autologous bypasses. I think if this patient has had a prosthetic bypass and it has gotten infected, the notion of doing a repeat prosthetic bypass in the setting of active infection seems impractical and unwise. Of course, if there was a large high quality randomised controlled trial that clearly demonstrated that re-do prosthetic bypass in the case of infection resulted in low morbidity, low mortality, and good limb salvage rates, I would be more than open to reconsider my current position."

So you would simply resign the patient to a major amputation? You would not even attempt limb salvage?

- "It depends on the clinical scenario, and my answer is not definitively no. The CT angiogram may show another target vessel such as the PT or peroneal artery. It looks like the original bypass was tunnelled laterally, so this time around there may be an option to position the bypass medially. Again, I would preferably use a vein cuff for the distal anastomosis if I was using prosthetic material. I would also consider using a cryopreserved allograft. If I were confident I could avoid the obviously infected areas, and if I were confident the groin was not infected, I would consider this. However, in this case I would most certainly do a sartorius flap."

You mentioned sartorius flap creation. What other muscle flaps are available for the groin?

- "Rectus femoris flap, gracilis muscle flap, rectus abdominis flap, and musculocutaneous anterolateral thigh flap."

Are there any other approaches to reduce infection in a re-do bypass setting?

- "One can consider antibiotic loaded beads, which often contain vancomycin, tobramycin, and gentamicin, or a combination thereof. The other important point is to thorough wound debridement and ensure copious washout with multiple litres of warmed normal saline (the solution to pollution is dilution)."

What if at the time of surgery the proximal groin site appeared to be infected? What are your bypass options now?

- "In this setting one would have to consider a lateral retro-sartorius bypass. This involves routing of the graft from the external iliac artery. One can perform the dissection lateral to the sartorius muscle a few centimetres away from the contaminated wound between healthy tissues. The new bypass conduit can be tunnelled laterally in the clean tissue, medial to the anterior superior iliac spine, and under the inguinal ligament through the psoas canal."

Your FRCS Short Case Ends

Relevant ESVS Guideline Recommendations

- For patients with peripheral vascular graft/endograft infection, in situ reconstruction with autologous vein is recommended if removal of the infected graft is likely to lead to limb ischaemia.

- For patients with peripheral vascular graft/endograft infection limited to only a part of the graft and in patients unfit for surgery, local irrigation and/or negative pressure wound therapy may be considered.

- For patients with a peripheral vascular graft/endograft infection and a large tissue defect, negative pressure wound therapy should be considered in order to promote wound healing following infected graft removal and debridement with or without vascular reconstruction.

- For patients with peripheral vascular graft/endograft infection, in situ reconstruction with cryopreserved allografts should be considered as an alternative after infected graft removal if it is likely to lead to limb ischaemia.

- For patients with a peripheral vascular graft/endograft infection and a large tissue defect, muscle or musculocutaneous flaps should be considered to promote groin healing following graft removal and debridement with or without vascular reconstruction.

JMF Reflections on Case 22.4

In the above mock examination station you (*the theoretical candidate*) are asked whether you would consider a redo prosthetic bypass in the context of a currently infected prosthetic bypass ....
The answers I have given above need to be taken with a pinch of salt because this is a theoretical scenario that is designed to test your resolve. Also recognise that this is something that you yourself may have said if put on the spot. However, once you commit to a certain pathway, you are then condemned to keep walking down that pathway. This is indeed a very difficult question to answer, and to be honest you are caught between a rock and a hard place. If you say you would do a redo prosthetic bypass, you then lay yourself wide open to be asked: "Isn't the risk of this bypass getting infected really high? Is this a safe approach?" If you go down this route you may answer by saying you would try to do an extra-anatomical approach, or use cryopreserved allografts if it is in situ reconstruction, do a flap, use antibiotic beads, copious washout, long term antibiotics, and you would survey this bypass very carefully. On the other hand, if you say you would not do a redo prosthetic bypass in an infected field, you then lay yourself wide open to be asked: "Are you just going to let the patient get an ischaemic limb and condemn them to a major amputation then?" Pragmatically, and between you and me, I don't think there is a right answer. I think you just have to weigh up the situation and make a decision that is reasonable. For me, a good way to answer these difficult questions is to say something like you would counsel the patient, get an expert second opinion, and discuss the case in the vascular MDT .... I would discuss both approaches i.e. doing a redo bypass and not doing a redo bypass, and I would emphasise the pros and cons of each approach. For me personally however I would make a decision and communicate what I thought the best course of action was. I don't like sitting on the fence. I would rather make a decision and be criticised, as opposed to avoid making a decision for fear of being criticised. When I was preparing for the FRCS Part B examination my trainers explained to me that I should always have *my plan*. This has stuck with me and I would similarly encourage you the reader to have *your plan* as well. After all, if you have no plan, then you will spend your entire consultant career feeling like you are stuck at a crossroads waiting for someone else to tell you what to do. This is not something I like the thought of .... You of course must make your own decision, however.

Open AAA Repair (Elective, Infra-Renal)

Pre-Operatively

- Review clinic letters, blood results, imaging, etc.
- Confirm fitness assessment is satisfactory (i.e. echocardiogram, pulmonary function tests or cardiopulmonary exercise testing, anaesthetic review).
- Confirm case has been approved by MDT.
- Confirm no nasty surprises, e.g. posterior left renal vein, left-sided IVC, duplicate IVC, porcelain aorta, and horrible aortic neck. *I know these cases should all go through the MDT and you would hope these things would have been picked up, but you never know ….*
- Measure out the size of the infra-renal aorta and iliac arteries. Have an idea in your mind what type and size of aortic graft you are going to use, and go and get some grafts and bring them to theatre.
- Go and see the patient yourself, examining their abdomen.
- Confirm lower limb pulse assessment.
- Counsel and consent the patient.
- Crossmatch 4 units.
- Make sure patient has had ECG done in past 7 days and confirm patient has not been getting any chest pain symptoms since pre-assessment (this is my practice anyways for any elective open aortic surgery based purely upon my own previous experiences).
- Make sure patient is already on best medical therapy (e.g., aspirin 75 mg OD and statin).
- Ask for cell-saver to be set up.
- Prophylactic antibiotics.
- Urinary catheter, arterial line, and central line +/− spinal/epidural.
- Shave abdomen and groins.

Intra-Operatively

- Dual consultant case.
- Supine position, break table to improve AAA exposure as required.
- I actually stand on the left side of the patient to begin with (*I have been told multiple times that this is an abnormal position but it feels correct to me. I am right handed and it feels appropriate to me*).
- Prep and drape abdomen and groins.
- Ioban drape.
- Supra-umbilical "inverse smile" incision (*I do midline for ruptures*).
- Monopolar diathermy to achieve haemostasis on the way down to sheath.
- Open up the sheath and identify the rectus muscles.
- Use your finger/big clip to get under each rectus abdominis muscle and pull a white swab through. You and your assistant then pull the white swab upwards to keep the muscle

DOI: 10.1201/b22951-23

under tension as your diathermy proceeds slowly through the muscles. Make sure you identify the epigastric arteries and buzz them.

- Once the rectus abdominis muscles are divided, both you and your assistant pull the abdominal wall upwards to lift it away from the abdominal viscera. Make a small incision into the posterior sheath just lateral to the midline and get into the abdomen with your fingers. Make another similar incision on the other side of the midline. Finger is swept under the midline to ensure no adhesions/bowels are present. Use 2× clips to divide the falciform ligament and ligate using 2-0 vicryl.

- Now use monopolar diathermy to fully open up the posterior rectus sheath/peritoneum medially and laterally. At the edge of the wounds, there will be the abdominal wall muscles that require division also.

- At this point, use some big wet packs to pack the omentum/transverse colon superiorly, small bowel to the right, and left colon to the left.

- Identify the fourth part of the duodenum and take the ligament of Treitz down.

- The inferior mesenteric vein often requires ligation.

- Once the fourth part of the duodenum has been liberated and drawn over towards the right side of the aorta, do a little bit of dissection around the aortic neck, and also start lifting the small bowel mesentery off the right side of the aneurysm. If convenient, you can also have a feel for where the iliac vessels are and do some gentle dissection around here.

- At this point when the AAA has been slightly exposed, I will insert the Omnitract.

- The Omnitract opens things up better, and you and your assistant are now in a better position to fully expose the aorta.

- In regard to the retroperitoneal tissues overlying the anterior surface of the AAA, I tend to use a Lahey, lift the tissues up and have my assistant diathermy in between.

- In regard to the aortic neck, me and my assistant grab the retroperitoneal tissues on top of the aortic neck with non-toothed forceps, and I use the monopolar diathermy to buzz in between. I would make a special point of dissecting slowly, methodically and purposefully around the aortic neck. There is a lot of vascular tissue around here, and if you go too quickly, it just bleeds and oozes and you cannot see anything and spend half your time-sucking blood as you dissect …. The objective is to get your finger down each side of the neck down to the vertebra.

- I would be very careful dividing the retroperitoneal tissues at the superior aspect of the aneurysm. The left renal vein will be here and it is easy to clobber. Deliberately and purposefully look for it, and carefully keep dissecting until you see a blue/purple horizontal structure. At this point, carefully dissect around it. Generally speaking, you can get a renal vein retractor underneath it and lift it out of the way. However, if it is genuinely hampering your operation, doubly ligate it using 2-0 vicryl. If you are going to doubly ligate it, however, don't ligate the other branches such as adrenal/gonadal veins.

- When dissecting around the iliac vessels, my only advice is this—watch out for the iliac veins. Just clear enough of the iliacs to get a clamp on them. I would not try and get round them with a Lahey to sloop the iliacs for fear of damaging to iliac veins. Avoid excessive dissection around the iliac bifurcation, particularly in men (i.e. sexual function).

- Also watch out around the left side of the AAA for the inferior mesenteric artery. It is easy to injure, and although this is not devastating and you would almost certainly ligate it anyways when you open the aneurysm, it just causes unnecessary stress having to stop it bleeding for 5 minutes.

- Ask for IV heparin and wait for 3 minutes.
- Use knife to puncture AAA, then straight scissors to open it up longitudinally.
- Scoop out the thrombus.
- At this point, take a pack and stick it in the aneurysm to control backbleeding.
- Do a T-shape at the aortic neck.
- Ask for a 2-0 prolene suture and deal with lumbars that are backbleeding.
- Word of wisdom → ask your assistant to press on obviously hosing lumbar backbleeders instead of just sucking the blood out.
- Now ask for an appropriately sized aortic graft (tube or bifurcated).
- Stick a self-retainer inside the aneurysm and open up the top end.
- *All I can say here is do a decent job with the top-end anastomosis and don't unnecessarily rush. I don't know why but I always feel a pressure on me to get this done as quickly as possible. However, as with any area of life, if you rush, you do a less decent job, and you end up spending more time correcting any mistakes you have made whilst rushing ….*
- I start off my anastomosis in the posterior midline. I do a parachute technique using 2-0 prolene. Again, as I have been told, you want to be doing BFBs (big friendly bites). Get a good grasp of "healthy" aortic neck tissue and take good bites of the graft, spacing them appropriately. If you can, particularly around the lateral aspects of the top-end anastomosis, use some of the redundant aortic neck tissue to provide extra buttressing (i.e. your suture goes from out-to-in on the graft, in-to-out of the aortic neck, out-to-in on some redundant aortic neck tissue, and then you continue your next bite of the graft out-to-in). I will also occasionally use pledgets to reinforce the superior / anterior suture line as well.
- Apply a clamp to the graft a few centimetres below the anastomosis and then warn the anaesthetist you are about to test the top end.
- **PRAY TO GOD THAT THE TOP-END ANASTOMOSIS IS SATISFACTORY.**
- Now move down to the iliacs and spend some time preparing them.
- Personally, if I am doing the bottom end, I will now walk around to the right side of the patient—again I find this much easier for me as I am right handed.
- If the table is broken, now flatten it out.
- Stretch the aortic graft out and cut it to size and shape using straight scissors.
- Again for the bottom end (or ends), I do a parachute technique.
- What I would say in regard to the bottom end is to continue to take it as seriously as the top end. The top end is the "big one," and I feel the bottom end doesn't get the respect it deserves. I have been doing bottom ends and noticed how people in theatre start to relax, start chatting, chilling out …. I have even found myself relaxing, and then when you test the bottom end, there is a big gap in the anastomosis. How the hell did that happen? Well, just a word of caution, maintain your focus throughout the entire operation. *It ain't over until it's over.*
- Give your anaesthetist advanced warning when you are close to completing the bottom end.
- Backbleed both iliacs, and use your fist to compress both femoral arteries in the groin and pump any clot backwards. Forward flush the top end. Now flush the graft and iliacs copiously (i.e. a couple of 20 ml syringes). I take this part really seriously. An old boss of mine who has now retired told me of a case he had when clot went down both legs of one of his elective AAA patients upon releasing the graft, and the patient ended up needing bilateral above-knee amputations ….

- Confirm the patient has bilateral femoral pulses restored.
- Ask someone to show you both feet (and ideally confirm foot pulses are present).
- If the anaesthetist is not happy with the blood pressure (i.e. hypotension), squeeze the graft and allow them time to catch up.
- If there is absolutely no pressure drop upon release of the legs, take this seriously. Clot may have gone down the iliac limbs.
- Ensure haemostasis (and when I say haemostasis, I don't just mean the anastomsoses. I mean as you are now entering the closing stages of the operation, don't switch off and leave obvious bleeding points here, there, and everywhere …. **Now** is the time to stop the bleeding).
- Confirm the left colon perfusion is satisfactory.
- Close the aortic sac using 2-0 vicryl.
- Close the retroperitoneum using 2-0 vicryl (cover the bottom and top-end anastomoses to reduce future risk of aorto-enteric fistula).
- Position the bowel in an appropriate anatomical position.
- Close the abdominal wall using looped PDS (two layers: Posterior and anterior rectus sheath).
- 3-0 monocryl to skin.
- Opsite dressing.

Post-Operatively

- Intensive care unit.
- Two post-operative doses of prophylactic antibiotics.
- VTE prophylaxis late that evening if no bleeding concerns (low-molecular-weight heparin).
- Flowtrons for both legs.
- Repeat blood tests that evening (FBC & U&Es are what I am interested in mainly).
- Best medical therapy to continue (i.e. aspirin and statin).
- Before discharge, have someone check a lipid screen to know what patient's LDL is.
- Oral fluids as soon as patient able, and work-up to soup and sweet, then sandwiches …. I don't want my patients starving for days on end. If they get an ileus, we can dial things back.
- Chest physiotherapy ASAP.
- Sit out from day 1 (ideally).
- Mobilise from day 2 (ideally).

Some Reflections on Open Aortic Surgery

These are things I have learned directly and indirectly. Most of these points come mainly from being trained by vascular surgeons who are 30 years older than me and vastly more experienced. They have passed on their wisdom to me, wisdom which has often been learned in a hard way by them years ago:

1. If upon release of the bottom end there is no femoral pulse (and there was one pre-operatively), even if the foot looks viable, don't leave this and "hope for the best." There are various surgical options, but the surgeon who gave me this advice recommended not taking the bottom-end anastomosis down, but instead doing an upstream femoral embolectomy from the groin, and if this is not successful, just do a jump graft down to the groin.

2. Always examine the pre-operative CT scan yourself and look out for the classic traps, e.g., posterior left renal vein, left-sided IVC, and duplicate IVC, etc.

3. If on the CT, the distance from the patient's abdominal wall skin to the supra-renal/ para-renal aorta is ≥20 cm, try to avoid open aortic surgery.

4. Avoid operating on a patient with a porcelain aorta. The top end is not going to be pleasant, and there is a very high chance your top-end anastomosis will be a disaster (not to mention bleeding from where you apply the clamp above the anastomosis).

5. Just because the MDT recommends open repair, it doesn't mean you are obliged to proceed. Don't ever do an operation that you are not happy doing.

6. Watch out for lumbar veins in the retroperitoneum (particularly the left lumbar vein). These veins can cause massive bleeding, they are very difficult to control, and patients can quite literally die on table. A really competent senior vascular surgeon (who trained me) advised me that if I encounter this, I should not underestimate this injury and think I can handle it on my own. He said call for senior help early. He learned this lesson in the most painful way as a new vascular consultant many, many years ago, and he has never forgotten this ….

7. Watch out for the iliac veins. I am aware of a patient who died because of an iatrogenic injury here. Again, the same story. Don't try and tackle this problem on your own, because chances are you will come off worse, and again patients can bleed out on table. Call for help early.

8. Remember that the big killer of open aortic surgery patients is **cardiac**. Make sure these patients are on best medical therapy and eyeball their pre-operative ECG yourself, etc. This is most certainly overkill I know, but I do routinely ask open aortic surgery patients about recent episodes of chest pain. I have quite literally cancelled open aortic surgery cases last minute (*and I mean literally last minute*) because a patient has had very recent episodes of chest pain, and when a new ECG had been completed it showed widespread ST-segment changes …. If this had not been spotted and I had proceeded with surgery, when I applied the aortic clamp no doubt the patient would have arrested on-table. I recognise I am pedantic, but if you are thorough and keep your eyes and ears open, you will spot important things that are easy to miss …. In this case the patient had previously been preassessed when an ECG was done and was clearly normal. Between being preassessed and coming in for the operation (short gap of just a few weeks), the patient had had a coronary event. There is of course an argument to do an ECG on the day of aortic surgery, which is my current practice. Again, this may be a bit pedantic, but if you do a fantastic open aortic aneurysm repair and the patient dies of a myocardial infarction post-operatively, you haven't actually achieved anything. By the way, I include all open aortic surgery in this context (especially aortic surgery for CLTI patients).

I think that exposure to open aortic surgery has taken a big hit with the EVAR revolution, and the modern-day vascular surgery consultant will not be as experienced as previous generations. This is just the nature of the beast. However, I think probably the pendulum will now start swinging back in favour of open aortic surgery. In any case, I think open aortic surgery will always be challenging. I think for the day one vascular surgery consultant, the main point is to *remain humble*. Don't do these cases on your own. Take them very seriously. Make sure the patient has been worked up correctly, counselled and consented appropriately, that the MDT supports you, that you have a good anaesthetist, some decent assistants, make sure you slept well and had a decent breakfast, etc. Above all else, if you run into trouble, don't be a hero, and call for help early. Pride comes before a fall.

CHAPTER 24

Carotid Endarterectomy

Pre-Operatively

- Go and see the patient yourself.
- Review the blood results, ECG, carotid duplex, and secondary imaging (i.e., CTA or MRA).
- Confirm the patient is on best medical therapy (I want my CEA patients on dual antiplatelet and high-dose statin therapy).
- Ask the patient if they have actually been taking their antiplatelet and statin tablets (this has caught me out big time in the past → you have been warned).
- If the patient says no, you can either postpone the case, or give the patient an antiplatelet right now. You may think this is insignificant and unimportant, but I can tell you that you won't find it funny when your carotid patch thromboses and you have to rush the patient back to theatre, only to then discover the patient hasn't been taking his aspirin and clopdiogrel as he was prescribed ….
- Counsel and consent the patient thoroughly.
- Mark correct side of neck.
- Speak to patient and anaesthetist about anaesthetic approach, i.e., general anaesthesia versus local anaesthesia.
- Ensure patient has prophylactic antibiotics.
- Shave the neck if required.

Intra-Operatively

- Position patient supine with body flexed to 20 degrees, and legs flexed to 20 degrees.
- Headrests in a head ring and bump rests horizontally under the shoulders.
- Break the table at the head end to extend and open up the neck further.
- Tilt the patient's head away from you.
- Prep and drape the neck from earlobe downwards.
- Use Ioban drape to provide further skin protection from infection.
- Long incision along the anterior border of the sternocleidomastoid, curving posteriorly away from the angle of the mandible to avoid damage to marginal mandibular nerve and parotid gland.
- Use monopolar diathermy to dissect through subcutaneous tissues and platysma.
- Ligate the external jugular vein using 3-0 vicryl ties.
- Identify the anterior border of sternocleidomastoid and dissect along this using monopolar diathermy.
- Once the sternocleidomastoid is sufficiently liberated, insert a self-retaining retractor.
- Identify the facial vein and doubly ligate it using 2-0 vicryl.

DOI: 10.1201/b22951-24

- Dissect along the anterior border of the internal jugular vein.
- As you dissect upwards along the anterior border of the internal jugular vein, look out for small tethering venous branches. Divide these using 3-0 vicryl ties.
- At the base of the neck identify the omohyoid muscle and use a Langenbeck retractor to gently pull it down.
- Identify the common carotid artery and dissect straight downwards onto its anterior surface.
- Dissect the patient off the carotid, i.e., minimal handling of the carotid artery.
- Doubly sloop the common carotid, being careful not to injure the vagus nerve.
- Advance upwards along the common carotid, but do not start to dissect around the carotid bulb yet.
- Identify the carotid bifurcation and work out where the internal carotid is.
- Carefully dissect out the internal carotid artery until you have a suitable length of "blue" internal carotid to clamp (obviously avoid injuring the hypoglossal nerve).
- *I really cannot emphasise this enough:* Get more distal blue ICA than you think you need. The more the better. If you have to then divide the digastric muscle. If you have to, divide the occipital artery to allow the hypoglossal nerve to be liberated upwards (the occipital artery tethers the hypoglossal nerve). Once everything is clamped and shunts are in place it is really difficult and irritating having to try to expose higher up the ICA….
- Be extremely careful not to injure the hypoglossal nerve, and consider gently slooping it and lifting it up as required.
- At this point single sloop the internal carotid with minimal disturbance of the vessel.
- Do not dissect the carotid bulb or the external carotid at this point.
- Ask the anaesthetist to give the patient IV heparin (70 units/kg).
- Wait 3 minutes.
- Clamp the internal carotid artery first, and proceed immediately to dissecting out and controlling the external carotid and superior thyroid artery.
- Now clamp the common carotid and external carotid arteries (superior thyroid artery sloop can be put on tension).
- Do a longitudinal arteriotomy into the ICA to until you reach healthy artery.
- At this point, if the patient is under a general anaesthetic I would shunt the patient. However, if the patient were under local anaesthetic, the anaesthetist would be speaking to the patient and having them squeeze on a squeaking rubber toy with their contralateral hand. If the patient were neurologically intact I would not need to shunt.
- Of note, I am flexible between GA and LA. I am also fairly flexible with shunts. For GA I think a Pruitt shunt is probably ideal. For LA I think Javid or Sundt shunts are better. I previously worked in a department where every CEA was done under GA, and the standard practice there was for everyone to use a Pruitt shunt. I actually think the Pruitt shunt is good for GA cases, but in my opinion, it is better inserted in a controlled manner, i.e., you are all set up for it because you are fully intending to use it. If you are doing a LA case and are hoping/expecting that the patient won't need a shunt, I find the Sundt shunt better because I can get it in quicker with less hassle. Again, shunts are dealer's choice. Just have your own plan.
- I insert the shunt into the common carotid first of all, flush it forwards, and then insert it gently into the internal carotid.
- Remember to apply the shunt clamps if you are using Javid or Sundt. Put the CCA sloop on tension if you are using the Pruitt shunt (or eventually the arterial pressure will force

the shunt out of the CCA and there will be a big explosion of blood in your face and 2 minutes spent getting the shunt back in).

- After about 10 minutes following giving IV heparin I would ask for an ACT to be checked. If required I would give more heparin.

- Use your Watson-Cheyne to complete the endarterectomy. I get across the plaque at the level of the CCA first and use Potts scissors to cut the plaque across over the Watson-Cheyne. Another neat trick is to get a Lahey across the posterior aspect of the plaque and then cut across the plaque.

- You can then use the Watson-Cheyne to liberate the plaque from the CCA into the ECA and then into the ICA.

- I try to feather the plaque at the ICA to avoid having to tack down any flaps.

- I very slowly and carefully lift the plaque upwards and gently use the Watson-Cheyne to caress the ICA backwards. When the bulk of the disease is lifted free, I use the Potts to make a tiny nick in the plaque at one edge.

- I will then use some non-toothed forceps to grab the ICA just above this cut plaque, and I pull the remaining plaque downwards and laterally.... On a good day the plaque just glides away leaving no flaps.

- If, however, it is a bad day, I will track down any flaps using 7-0 prolene.

- I suture in a bovine patch using 6-0 prolene.

- I suture the top part of the patch into the ICA using a parachute technique.

- I then suture one side down past the ECA, and use the other suture to come all the way down the other side, around the CCA, and back up to the ECA.

- As I am in the process of sewing in the bovine patch, I will regularly inspect the inner suture line to make sure no clot is building up, and I will flush the patch copiously and frequently using heparinised saline.

- If I am using a shunt, this will need to be removed as one comes to almost finishing the patch.

- Prior to completing the patch, it is vitally important to flush everything out thoroughly. I will first backbleed the ICA, then backbleed the ECA, then forward flush the CCA. Then I will flush everything out using heparinised saline.

- Now I complete the patch, being extra careful not to be too assertive and snap the delicate 6-0 prolene suture as I complete my knot.

- Once the patch is complete, this is how I release my clamps: (1) first temporarily backbleed the ICA, then reapply the clamp; (2) apply non-toothed forceps across the proximal ICA just at the level of the carotid bifurcation; (3) release the clamp on the ECA fully; (4) release the clamp on the CCA and allow the CCA to flush into the ECA; (5) After 10 seconds, release the non-toothed forceps on the ICA and then release the clamp on the ICA. Hopefully, this complicated manoeuvre has redirected any clot into the ECA and not the ICA.

- Spend 5–10 minutes on haemostasis.

- Insert a 14-French Robinson drain (when tunnelling it through the skin at the base of the wound avoid injuring the anterior jugular vein).

- Close the platysma using 2-0 vicryl.

- 3-0 monocryl to skin.

- Opsite dressing.

Post-Operatively

- Complete a detailed operation note.
- I like my CEA patients to be on dual antiplatelets for 7 days post-op. They can be stepped down to single antiplatelet after 7 days (i.e., just clopidogrel).
- Ensure patient is on high-dose statin.
- Prescribe 2× post-op doses of IV antibiotics.
- I don't routinely have my CEA patients go to intensive care/high dependency—only if there are blood pressure issues.
- I aim for a blood pressure from 100 to 160 mmHg.
- Don't send for your next theatre case before you have personally seen your CEA patient in recovery and are confident they are neurologically intact. I often wait for 30 minutes then go and see the patient in recovery unless I am called sooner.
- Complete the National Vascular Registry.

CHAPTER 25

Common Femoral Endarterectomy

Pre-Operatively

- Read through medical records, review relevant imaging and blood results.
- Confirm patient is on best medical therapy.
- Examine the patient's groin yourself
- Counsel and consent the patient.
- Prophylactic antibiotics.
- Make sure groin in shaved, also consider cleaning groin in anaesthetic room with chlorhexidine (belt and braces).

Intra-Operatively

- Position patient supine.
- Prep the groin with betadine.
- Ioban drape applied to groin.
- Vertical groin incision over CFA, extending a 2–3 cm above inguinal ligament.
- Dissect down through soft tissue directly onto CFA.
- Ensure inguinal ligament is sufficiently exposed medially and laterally.
- Dissect underneath inguinal ligament, deal with "vein of sod," and expose sufficient amount of soft external iliac artery that you can clamp.
- *Never dissect underneath inguinal ligament "blind"* → Get your assistant to retract upwards using a Langenbeck.
- Control inferior epigastric and circumflex iliac arteries using small vessel sloops.
- Expose and control SFA origin.
- *Exposure sufficient length of PFA* → Make sure to deal with overlying venous branches (get them before they get you).
- **THE PRIORITY IS OPENING UP THE PROFUNDA ARTERY.**
- Ensure you isolate and control all branches/collaterals before proceeding to do arteriotomy → this means looking medially, laterally, and underneath the CFA, and around the origins of the PFA and SFA.
- Give IV heparin.
- Do your arteriotomy from the CFA all the way into the PFA.
- Use your Watson-Cheyne to liberate the disease/plaque from the EIA all the way down to the PFA.
- Depending on the disease pattern, you may focus on opening the SFA. However, from my perspective, as a rule of thumb *you should always ensure the PFA is open*.
- Deal with the inflow first. I use the Watson-Cheyne to circumferentially go around the disease/plaque in the proximal CFA/distal EIA, and then after this I get a big clip and

DOI: 10.1201/b22951-25

grab the disease and pull it out. This often involves having to release the clamp on the EIA and get your assistant to use the sloop to control the iliac inflow. Whatever your technique, I want there to be torrential "audible" inflow achieved.

- Next deal with the PFA. I am gentler with this. I want to remove the burden of disease, but at the same time not leave a dissection flap. In essence this just means proceeding cautiously and using 6-0 or 7-0 prolene to tack down any potential flaps that might lift.

- Use some heparinised-saline flush to check there are no big flaps that are lifting, and remove any large areas of disease. However, remember this is not a carotid endarterecromy. You don't have to kill yourself removing every hint of disease from the artery for fear of causing a stroke. Remove the main bulk of disease, and otherwise get on with the operation ....

- Next thing is a patch repair. I don't mind what you use. I routinely use bovine patch, but on occasion I use reversed ipsilateral single layer GSV harvested from the groin incision. I think you should be flexible, but whatever the case may be, just have a plan.

- Start off your patch from the PFA using 6-0 prolene.

- I routinely use the parachute technique, but again if you want to tie down straight away then so be it ....

- When you are testing your anastomosis, make sure you have flushed the patch beforehand with heparinised-saline, and make sure you tell the anaesthetist before you release the leg.

- Ensure haemostasis.

- Insert a 14-French drain into wound if oozy +/− haemostatic agents if required (dealer's choice).

- Closure groin in 2 layers using 2-0 vicryl (3 layers if a very deep groin).

- 3-0 monocryl to skin.

- Opsite dressing (occasionally a PICO dressing if it is a high risk groin).

Post-Operatively

- Prescribe appropriate VTE prophylaxis.

- Prescribe 2 doses of post-op IV antibiotics (usually co-amoxiclav or teicoplanin if penicillin allergic).

- Write a decent operation note.

- Make sure you document the state of foot perfusion post-op, i.e., are there foot pulses, what is the capillary refill time.

- Complete the National Vascular Registry documentation.

- Make sure best medical therapy is instituted (as far as I am concerned all patients should be on VOYAGER regimen, i.e., aspirin 75 mg OD + rivaroxaban 2.5 mg BD plus high-dose statin, i.e., atorvastatin 80 mg OD).

If you want to open up the SFA origin this is also entirely acceptable. You can do a little remote endarterectomy or do a patch into the SFA. You can also create a Y-patch into both the PFA and the SFA. This is up to you. However, again to reassert my previous point, I still think the priority is to open up the profunda artery.

CHAPTER 26

Femoral Above-Knee Popliteal Bypass: Reversed Ipsilateral GSV

Pre-Operatively

- Read through medical records, review relevant imaging and blood results.
- Confirm patient is on best medical therapy.
- *Seriously → Always examine the patient's groin yourself!*
- Counsel and consent the patient.
- Make sure patient gets appropriate prophylactic antibiotics.
- Make sure groin in shaved, also consider cleaning groin in anaesthetic room with chlorhexidine (belt and braces).
- Mark the GSV yourself using ultrasound in the anaesthetic room.

Intra-Operatively

- Position patient supine.
- Prep the patient from umbilicus down to ankle.
- Ioban drape applied to abdomen, groin, and leg.
- Top end surgeon does vertical groin incision over CFA, extending a 2–3 cm above inguinal ligament.
- Bottom end surgeon makes incision directly over GSV marking.
- Both surgeons work towards each other, meeting in the middle.
- *Priority is the vein →* Do not damage it, ligate all tributaries carefully using 3-0 vicryl +/− ligaclips.
- Always harvest more vein than you think you will need.
- Top end surgeon will expose and control CFA/PFA/SFA in groin and disconnect saphenofemoral junction (SFJ).
- Never just "ligate" the SFJ. Seriously. I won't explicitly tell you why but just trust me. I routinely transfix it using 2-0 vicryl so it is **secure**.
- Bottom end surgeon can ligate the distal GSV using 3-0 vicryl, but I still routinely transfix it.
- Hand the vein out carefully to the scrub nurse to put it in a container with heparin-saline (*don't drop the vein on the floor*).
- The top end surgeon goes to a separate table and prepares the GSV (use a feeding tube to inflate it under pressure and 7-0 prolene to repair any small holes). I would recommend having 2× people do this because the vein tends to flap around like a sail in a gale (i.e., top end surgeon plus assistant).
- Bottom end surgeon dissects on superior border of sartorius, allowing them into the above-knee popliteal space.

DOI: 10.1201/b22951-26

- Insert ×2 self-retainers into this space to improve your access.
- *Take your time* finding the above-knee popliteal artery and don't panic if you are struggling to find it. On occasion, particularly in muscular patients, it can be tough to find. If you find yourself dissecting through a load of thick muscle, this is probably the vastus medialis muscle. You should go lower with your dissection so you are underneath this muscle. My advice is to take your time with this exposure, as it can be more challenging than you expect it to be! If you are really struggling to find the popliteal artery, go more proximally up the thigh and target the SFA in the adductor canal, then you can follow this down if necessary.
- There are often lots of veins surrounding the above-knee popliteal it and they are a pain to stop bleeding—go slow and steady.
- Control the above-knee popliteal artery over a suitable length.
- Insert tunnelling device from above-knee space up towards groin (anatomical, underneath the sartorius muscle).
- Give IV heparin.
- Wait 3 minutes.
- Do the top end first (end-to-side, using 6-0 prolene).
- Use blue marker pen to place dots on the superior aspect of the GSV graft.
- Tunnel the vein under arterial pressure into the above-knee space.
- Create bottom end anastomosis (end-to-side using 6-0 prolene).
- Ensure you flush the distal vessels with heparin-saline/flush graft downwards to remove any clot.
- Complete distal anastomosis.
- Warn anaesthetist before you give the leg back.
- Use handheld Doppler to ensure decent signal in popliteal artery below distal anastomosis.
- Eyeball the foot to see if perfusion improves.
- Ensure haemostasis.
- I don't routinely insert drains, but if oozy I will use 14-French Robinson drain.
- Top end closure—2-0 vicryl in 2 layers followed by monocryl to skin.
- Bottom end closure and GSV harvest sites—2-0 vicryl followed by monocryl to skin.
- Opsite dressings.

Post-Operatively

- Prescribe appropriate VTE prophylaxis.
- Prescribe 2 doses of post-op IV antibiotics.
- Write a decent operation note.
- Make sure you document the state of foot perfusion post-op, i.e., are there foot pulses, what are the handheld Doppler signals like, what is the capillary refill time.
- Complete the National Vascular Registry documentation.
- Make sure best medical therapy is instituted (as far as I am concerned all patients should be on VOYAGER regimen, i.e., aspirin 75 mg OD + rivaroxaban 2.5 mg BD plus high-dose statin, i.e., atorvastatin 80 mg OD).

CHAPTER 27

Femoral Below-Knee Popliteal Bypass: Reversed Ipsilateral GSV

Pre-Operatively

- Read through medical records, review relevant imaging and blood results.
- Confirm patient is on best medical therapy.
- *Seriously → Always examine the patient's groin yourself!*
- Counsel and consent the patient.
- Make sure patient gets appropriate prophylactic antibiotics.
- Make sure groin in shaved, also consider cleaning groin in anaesthetic room with chlorhexidine (belt and braces).
- Mark the GSV yourself using ultrasound in the anaesthetic room.

Intra-Operatively

- Position patient supine.
- Prep the patient from umbilicus down to ankle.
- Ioban drape applied to abdomen, groin, and leg.
- Bowel under thigh to abduct and lift knee upwards (this also relaxes the knee flexor tendons, thus making your arterial exposure easier).
- Top end surgeon does vertical groin incision over CFA, extending a 2–3 cm above inguinal ligament.
- Bottom end surgeon makes incision directly over GSV marking which will be around 1–2 cm posterior to tibia.
- Both surgeons work towards each other, meeting in the middle.
- *Priority is the vein →* Do not damage it, ligate all tributaries carefully using 3-0 vicryl +/− ligaclips.
- Always harvest more vein than you think you will need.
- Top end surgeon will expose and control CFA/PFA/SFA in groin and disconnect saphenofemoral junction (SFJ).
- Bottom end surgeon can ligate the distal GSV using 3-0 vicryl, but I routinely transfix it.
- Hand the vein out carefully to the scrub nurse (*don't drop it on the floor*).
- The top end surgeon goes to a separate table and prepares the GSV (use a feeding tube to inflate it under pressure and use 7-0 prolene to repair any small holes).
- Bottom end surgeon uses monopolar diathermy to divide fascia of superficial posterior compartment.
- This allows gastrocnemius to be pulled downwards with your fingers.
- Don't hesitate to divide proximal tendons around medial knee to improve your access.
- Insert ×2 self-retainers into this space to improve your access.

 DOI: 10.1201/b22951-27

- Your dissection should take you down onto a blue/purple structure → the popliteal vein.
- Dissect on top of this, up and down, thus enabling you to use non-toothed forceps to gently grab the vein and pull it down.
- Behind the popliteal vein will be the popliteal artery.
- Dissect on top of the popliteal artery so you enter the right vessel plane.
- I now dissect around the artery at this point, to enable me to get a Lahey around and sloop the vessel.
- Once your artery is slooped, you can pull it towards you and use your scissors to dissect up and down.
- Try and get as much length of popliteal artery as possible.
- Don't hesitate to take some of soleus down if you need to.
- Doubly sloop the popliteal artery.
- At this point I would turn my attention back to the above-knee popliteal space. I would dive deeper through the GSV harvest incision and take sartorius down.
- With my left index finger in the below-knee wound, I would cautiously enter the popliteal space behind the tibia and prepare an entry site for the tunneller (i.e., this is anatomical tunnelling to avoid creating an artificial popliteal entrapment by having the bypass compressed by the medial head of gastrocnemius).
- Now pass the tunneller from the below-knee space to the above-knee pocket you have just created (i.e., behind sartorius), and then continue it up to the groin.
- Alternatively you can tunnel from the groin down to the popliteal space.
- Give IV heparin.
- Wait for 3 minutes.
- Do the top end first (end-to-side, using 6-0 prolene).
- Use blue marker pen to place dots on the superior aspect of the GSV graft.
- Tunnel the graft under arterial pressure, avoiding kinking or twisting it.
- Create bottom end anastomosis (end-to-side using 6-0 prolene).
- Ensure you flush the distal vessels with heparinised-saline/flush graft downwards to remove any clot.
- Complete distal anastomosis.
- Warn anaesthetist before you give the leg back.
- Use handheld Doppler to ensure decent signal in popliteal artery below distal anastomosis.
- Eyeball the foot to see if perfusion improves.
- Ensure haemostasis.
- I don't routinely insert drains, but if oozy I will use 14-French Robinson drain.
- Top end closure—2-0 vicryl in 2 layers followed by monocryl to skin.
- Bottom end closure and GSV harvest sites—2-0 vicryl followed by monocryl to skin.
- Opsite dressings.

Post-Operatively

- Prescribe appropriate VTE prophylaxis.
- Prescribe 2 doses of post-op IV antibiotics.

- Write a decent operation note.
- Make sure you document the state of foot perfusion post-op, i.e., are there foot pulses, what are the handheld Doppler signals like, what is the capillary refill time.
- Complete the National Vascular Registry documentation.
- Make sure best medical therapy is instituted (as far as I am concerned all patients should be on VOYAGER regimen, i.e., aspirin 75 mg OD + rivaroxaban 2.5 mg BD plus high-dose statin, i.e., atorvastatin 80 mg OD).

Femoral Embolectomy

Pre-Operatively

- Go and see the patient yourself.
- Review the blood results and imaging (patient should have had a CT angiogram).
- If in doubt review CTA with interventional radiologist → don't want to get caught out by an iliac stenosis that needs stenting, etc.
- Make sure patient has had an ECG (i.e., is there atrial fibrillation?).
- Confirm the Rutherford status of the leg and how long the ischaemic insult has been.
- Counsel and consent the patient for operation (never forget to include fasciotomy on the consent form).
- Mark the leg.
- Have a meaningful discussion with the anaesthetist early on…. If the patient is very frail and does not need a fasciotomy, then a purely local anaesthetic approach is worth considering.
- IV heparin infusion should already be running, confirm this.
- Shave the groin.
- I would probably insert a urinary catheter in most cases to check urine output is ok, looking for myoglobinuria, etc.
- Alert theatre staff and radiology staff that you intend to do a diagnostic angiogram.

Intra-Operatively

- Position patient supine.
- Prep the patient from umbilicus down to ipsilateral ankle.
- Also prep the other groin (in case you need to do femoral-femoral crossover).
- Ioban drape applied to abdomen, groin, and leg.
- Vertical groin incision over the common femoral artery (CFA), extending a 2–3 cm above inguinal ligament (I do the operation with the heparin running, i.e., the patient should already have been given a bolus followed by infusion).
- Go straight down onto femoral vessels.
- Expose and control CFA below inguinal ligament, along with the superficial femoral artery (SFA) and profunda femoris artery (PFA) at their origins.
- *Important point* → Feel the vessels with your finger. Is it soft, or hard? If soft and you have a nice healthy femoral artery, then we are talking a horizontal arteriotomy. If it is a hard and diseased femoral artery, then we are talking a longitudinal arteriotomy and patch repair at end. If in doubt proceed as if you are going to have to do an endarterectomy.
- Clamp the vessels as required. If the embolus is upstream in the iliac artery, then use an appropriately sized Fogarty balloon and trawl until you achieve torrential inflow and all clot is removed. If it is downstream then trawl the SFA and PFA carefully → I say

carefully as in don't overinflate the embolectomy balloons and cause intimal damage to the vessels.

- If the clot is sat right at the origin of the common iliac artery on CTA (i.e., aortic bifurcation territory), be wary of sticking a balloon up there and forcing the clot down the other leg. If in doubt speak to interventional radiology about a contralateral iliac balloon occlusion as you do the embolectomy).
- Once you have cleared the vessels flush out copiously using heparinised saline.
- If I did a horizontal arteriotomy, I would close using 5-0 prolene. I do a double-layer continuous stitch, i.e., I start on one side of the arteriotomy and come to the other side with confident well placed bites that catch the distal intima to avoid a dissection plane, and then I use this same stitch to go back to the original starting point using more subtle bites of arterial wall in-between my previous bites. I then tie the 2× prolene strands together at the original starting point.
- If the artery is diseased and you did longitudinal arteriotomy then you will need to do an endarterectomy and patch repair.
- The diagnostic angiogram is dealer's choice, but "by the book" you should do one.
- Close the groin in 2 layers using 2-0 vicryl, followed by 3-0 monocryl to skin.
- Opsite dressing applied.

Post-Operatively

- Continue intravenous heparin for 24 hours.
- Prescribe 2 doses of post-op IV antibiotics.
- Write a decent operation note (this should include need to investigate source of embolism if this is not apparent, i.e., echocardiogram, 24–72-hour tape, make sure thoracic aorta has been visualised). Patient also needs formal anticoagulation plan prior to discharge. Also make sure you document the state of foot perfusion post-op, i.e., are there foot pulses, what are the handheld Doppler signals like, what is the capillary refill time).
- Make sure somebody hands over the patient to the on-call vascular surgery team for a review later. Make sure the on-call team specifically check for compartment syndrome if you elected not to do a fasciotomy.

Special Point

- As my old boss used to tell me, getting back bleeding from the SFA or PFA following an embolectomy does not mean a successful embolectomy. Back bleeding means that the vessel has a collateral circulation. It does not mean the SFA or PFA is properly cleared of embolus. You may have cleared some of the vessel and got some clot out, and this has enabled some proximal branches to back-bleed. However, the distal vessel may still be lodged with clot. This senior vascular surgeon remains unnamed, but he is actually one of my main role models. Many of his pearls of wisdom are scattered throughout this book. He insisted on doing an on-table angiogram after every embolectomy (femoral/popliteal/brachial). You can visually confirm that your embolectomy has been genuinely successful. An angiogram is good not just for the purposes of a successful operation, it is also good from a clinical governance perspective.

CHAPTER 29

Popliteal Embolectomy

Pre-Operatively

- Same as for femoral embolectomy.
- Mark out position of the great saphenous vein (GSV) in below-knee segment using ultrasound.
- Tell theatre and radiology that you are going to do a diagnostic angiogram.

Intra-Operatively

- Position patient supine with a bowl under the thigh to flex the knee and abduct the leg.
- Prep from groin to ankle.
- Ioban drape applied around leg.
- Make below-knee incision directly over GSV mark, but make your incision longer than standard below-knee incision (i.e., it goes down the leg further).
- Carefully expose the GSV to enable you to harvest some vein for use as a patch later on (I now cover the GSV with a wet swab to protect it as I continue with the below-knee exposure).
- Expose the below-knee popliteal artery in the standard fashion.
- Take a suitable length of soleus down from the back of the tibia.
- Follow the below-knee popliteal artery downwards, identify the anterior tibial vein, and divide it to allow you to expose and control the anterior tibial artery.
- Follow the below-knee vessels further down into the tibio-peroneal trunk. Ligate crossing venous tributaries as you go, and take your time.
- Ideally expose the posterior tibial (PT) and peroneal arteries.
- Make a longitudinal arteriotomy in the below-knee popliteal artery down towards the anterior tibial (AT) / tibioperoneal trunk (TPT).
- Use a Fogarty embolectomy balloon to clear inflow first.
- Once the inflow is sorted, take your time and clear the crural vessels. The AT can be a bit tricky given the acute angle, but if you use a small Lahey this can help. I would recommend trying to clear as many of the crural vessels as possible. I know some surgeons who are only interested in opening up one crural vessel, i.e., that old saying *"One crural vessel is enough"*. I completely agree with this notion in the trauma setting, and with a popliteal embolectomy you may have no choice but to open up one crural vessel. However, I think if you are there with the below-knee vessels exposed, you should at least try to open up as many as possible.
- After doing the crural embolectomy, at this point I will do a diagnostic angiogram. I do not close the arteriotomy yet. I ask for an infant feeding tube connected up to the contrast in a syringe. I will insert the feeding tube into the origin of the crural vessels (AT and TPT) and shoot separate runs as I inject. If the AT/PT/peroneal looks clear, then great. If not, I will do further balloon trawling. I may consider doing some on-table thrombolysis at this point down the culprit crural that I am struggling to clear.

- Once I am satisfied I will harvest a few centimetres of GSV (that I have already exposed and am lying at the base of my wound protected by a wet swab).
- I close the longitudinal arteriotomy using this GSV vein patch (reversed) using 6-0 prolene.
- If the ischaemic insult was advanced/prolonged then I would do a full fasciotomy (*if this is the case you probably should have started with the fasciotomy*).
- Take your time to achieve haemostasis. I don't mean spend 3 hours using the diathermy to create a kebab. I mean devote some time to dealing with obvious bleeders.
- Strongly consider using a 14-French Robinson drain in the below-knee wound.
- If you decide not to do a fasciotomy, close below-knee wound using 2-0 vicryl, 3-0 monocryl to skin, followed by an appropriate dressing.

Post-Operatively

- Same as for femoral embolectomy.

CHAPTER 30

Brachial Embolectomy

Pre-Operatively

- Go and see the patient yourself.
- Review the blood results and imaging (patient should have had a CT angiogram ideally from arch of aorta down the arm).
- If in doubt review CTA with a consultant interventional radiologist.
- Make sure patient has had an ECG (i.e. is there atrial fibrillation?).
- Confirm the Rutherford status of the arm.
- Counsel and consent the patient.
- Mark the arm.
- IV heparin infusion should already be running, confirm this.
- Alert theatre staff and radiology staff that you intend to do a diagnostic angiogram.
- I would routinely inject local anaesthetic around the brachial artery bifurcation using ultrasound in the anaesthetic room. I do this myself using a mixture of 10 ml 0.25% chirocaine and 10 ml 1% lignocaine. I inject this under vision using longitudinal ultrasound so I can visualise the needle tip injecting along the upper surface of the brachial artery.
- Alternatively, the patient can have an arm block or a general anaesthetic.
- I use the same ultrasound to help me mark out a "lazy S" so my incision will take me straight down onto the brachial bifurcation.
- I will also use the ultrasound to mark out where there is some decent cephalic/median cubital vein to use as a vein patch.

Intra-Operatively

- Patient is positioned supine with arm resting on an arm board.
- Prep the whole arm.
- Drape and keep hand in a see-through bag.
- Make your lazy S incision as per previous marking.
- Keep an eye out for some decent vein and don't damage it.
- Divide the brachial aponeurosis and get down onto the brachial artery.
- Expose and control brachial artery and the radial/ulnar arteries at the bifurcation.
- Be as gentle with the brachial artery as possible, i.e. don't poke or grab it with forceps. Treat it like a carotid. I find it very easily goes into spasm. Dissect the patient off the brachial artery and carefully sloop it.
- Horizontal or longitudinal arteriotomy depending on the setting (although I am more inclined to do longitudinal as I take these cases very seriously and treat them like a popliteal embolectomy).
- Careful Fogarty embolectomy trawl to restore inflow first, followed by separate passes down radial and ulnar arteries.

- At this point, I will pass an infant feeding tube into the origin of the radial and ulnar arteries, and do individual angiographic runs to ensure these vessels are clear. As with popliteal embolectomy, if needed, do some on-table thrombolysis down the culprit forearm vessel if you are struggling to clear it.
- Once satisfied, close the longitudinal arteriotomy using a reversed vein patch (i.e. some of the vein you saw on ultrasound or what you have identified in the antecubital fossa).
- If it is a big brachial artery, then it is ok to have done a horizontal arteriotomy and primary suture repair.
- Devote some time to achieving haemostasis.
- I routinely use a baby suction drain.
- Close the incision using 2-0 vicryl and 3-0 monocryl to skin.
- Opsite dressing.

Post-Operatively

- Continue intravenous heparin for 24 hours.
- Prescribe 2 doses of post-op IV antibiotics.
- Write a decent operation note (this should include the need to investigate the source of embolism if this is not apparent, i.e. echocardiogram, 24–72-hour tape, make sure thoracic aorta has been visualised). Patient also needs formal anticoagulation plan prior to discharge. Also make sure you document the state of hand perfusion post-op, i.e. are there wrist pulses, what are the handheld Doppler signals like, what is the capillary refill time etc.).
- Make sure somebody hands over the patient to the on-call vascular surgery team for a review later on.

Special Points

1. Don't treat brachial embolectomy as an "easy case". It is not a "smash and grab" operation to be done in 30 minutes. It is an operation that demands your focus and attention. Just be careful because these cases can be extremely unforgiving.
2. Be wary of frail, comorbid patients at the extremes of age with embolic upper-limb ischaemia. Often, at least in my experience, these limbs are actually Rutherford 1, and the patient does better with just anticoagulation. These patients often have severe underlying cardiac problems, and the ischaemic limb may be a "pseudo-terminal" event.
3. In the extremely rare event that a patient needs an additional upper-limb fasciotomy, ideally ask the plastic surgeons to come and do it. Don't get me wrong, I do know how to do an upper-limb fasciotomy, and vascular surgeons I am sure are fully capable of doing it. However, we don't do this very often, and I think if you work in a hospital where there are plastic surgeons available, from a clinical governance perspective, you are much safer asking them to help out. They are much more familiar operating in the forearm/hand, so the fasciotomy is better done by them probably.
4. If the brachial artery thrombosis following an endovascular access procedure, strongly consider a longitudinal arteriotomy and vein patch repair +/− interposition vein graft. If you are going to do an interposition graft, don't forget to do a gentle Fogarty balloon embolectomy of the inflow and outflow as well.
5. In the unfortunate situation where your embolectomy site repeatedly thromboses, make sure you check the ACT +/− give more heparin.

6. If you are struggling to clear the forearm vessels via the brachial artery, consider exposing the radial/ulnar arteries at the wrist and trawling upwards from here, with a vein patch repair of these small vessels at the end.

7. In the worse-case scenario, you may need to do a bypass from the brachial artery down to the radial/ulnar artery. If you are struggling to find vein in the arm for this bypass, go to the leg and harvest GSV.

8. Also be wary of "proximal disease" in the context of embolic upper limb ischaemia. I have had two recent cases of exactly this. One was a young gentleman with a Rutherford 2B upper limb ischaemia. He had embolus in his distal axillary artery, and also embolus around the very proximal subclavian artery. This was removed with the help of interventional radiology i.e. we did an over-the-wire embolectomy. A neurointerventional radiologist was also given the heads up in case any clot was dislodged and went into the carotid / vertebral system (*which never took place but we were ready for this*). The other case was a young woman with occlusion of the proximal brachiocephalic artery and further clot in the proximal axillary artery. Her hand was viable. The decision in this case was to manage conservatively with anticoagulation alone, with a plan to reassess in 6 weeks and then decide on further endovascular intervention. Just remember in these cases not to blindly rush into doing an embolectomy because of the genuine risk of causing a stroke.

CHAPTER 31

Lower-Limb Fasciotomy

For the sake of simplicity, let us assume that you are doing this for patient with compartment syndrome following an earlier revascularisation procedure. For example, the patient had a femoral embolectomy 5 hours ago and is now complaining of severe pain in the lower limb and/or with neurological compromise.

Pre-Operatively

- Go and see the patient yourself. Sometimes the signs are subtle, but if you are "on the fence" and have to make a decision, I would advise erring on the side of doing a fasciotomy.
- Personally, I don't waste much time trying to check the compartment pressures. Compartment syndrome is a clinical diagnosis in my opinion.
- Once you have made the diagnosis, you need to get moving quickly—consent the patient, mark the leg, and immediately go to emergency theatres to book the patient.

Intra-Operatively

- Supine position.
- Leg prepped and draped.
- Foot in a see-through bag.
- Two-incision approach.
- Lateral incision runs from 2 to 3 cm below fibula neck towards the lateral malleolus. Make your incision 1 fingerbreadth above the fibula.
- Incise the anterior compartment and open up along the whole length of your wound.
- I use my index finger to lift the anterior compartment muscle bellies upwards, enabling me to see the fascia that is enclosing the peroneal muscle compartment. I open this up again along the whole length of the wound. Be careful not to divide the superficial peroneal nerve that will be crossing in an oblique direction towards the foot in the lower part of the wound.
- I then make the medial incision 1 fingerbreadth posterior to the tibial border. It is basically a long extension of a standard below-knee popliteal artery.
- It runs all the way down to the medial malleolus. Try your best to avoid injuring the main body of the GSV.
- Open up the superficial posterior compartment so that the gastrocnemius can be seen.
- I open this layer all the way down towards the ankle, which will enable me to identify the Achilles tendon.
- From the lower part of the wound I then work back upwards, basically getting right onto the posterior border of the tibia, allowing me to open up the deep compartment. I take about 60–70% of soleus off the back of the tibia, but don't completely detach it.

DOI: 10.1201/b22951-31

- At this point, you have decompressed the 4× compartments: Anterior, lateral, superficial posterior, and deep posterior.
- Spend some time achieving haemostasis.
- I then routinely ask for a long 3-0 prolene suture with a straight needle that has a ball at the end of the sutures. I very loosely run this suture through the skin layers on each side to loosely approximate the skin—it can be drawn together over the next few days.
- Over this layer, I will apply Mepitel or Jelonet so the soft tissues are covered.
- This will be followed by blue gauze, and wool and crepe.

Post-Operatively

- Two post-op doses of IV antibiotics.
- Wound review in 48 hours.
- If wound is looking healthy, muscles viable, and not bulging too much, staff on ward can start to pull prolene sutures tighter to bring skin together.
- If muscle bellies not viable will need to return to theatre for further debridement.
- If muscle bellies too swollen to close skin, patient may require plastic surgical consultation for consideration of skin grafting.

CHAPTER 32

Hallux Amputation

Pre-Operatively

- Read through medical records, review relevant imaging and blood results.
- Is this being done for neuropathic sepsis/ischaemia? Are you going to close the wound or leave it open?
- Counsel and consent the patient (always mention risk of further debridement/adjacent toe amputation/more proximal amputation).
- Mark the patient.
- Do the team brief.
- Make sure patient gets appropriate prophylactic antibiotics.
- Discuss with anaesthetist in regards to appropriate anaesthetic approach, i.e. GA versus spinal/epidural, popliteal block, and ankle block.

Intra-Operatively

- Position the patient supine.
- Prep both the foot and go in-between the toes using a betadine-soaked swab.
- Use the knife to quickly make a tennis racket incision around the base of the hallux.
- Quickly disconnect the toe at the MTP joint.
- Use swab to apply pressure and help achieve haemostasis.
- Use either vicryl sutures of diathermy to control bleeding areas.
- Remove any necrotic tissue/devitalised tissue, redundant tendons/sesamoid bones as required.
- If infection/necrosis tracking proximally then proceed to ray amputation. Use periosteal elevator to expose proximal metatarsal shaft, then use bonesaw to divide metatarsal bone at 45 degrees.
- Washout wound with 1 litre of warmed normal saline.
- Change gloves and use clean bone nibblers to take clean proximal bone samples for histology and microbiology. At this point, leave wound open, pack with Kaltostat or Aquacell, apply Jelonet or Mepitel, blue gauze, and then wool and crepe.
- If no infection/necrosis tracking proximally then consider leaving the metatarsal head intact and closing the wound primarily using interrupted prolene sutures. Dress in similar fashion as if leaving wound open.
- *Core principles to remember* → Cut in smooth lines (no ragged edges) and never leave proud bone!
- Don't close infected wounds!

Post-Operatively

- Prescribe appropriate post-operative antibiotics.
- Write a decent operation note.

DOI: 10.1201/b22951-32

- Make sure you document the quality of foot perfusion, i.e. was there good bleeding/pulsatile bleeding/poor bleeding. If poor, the patient may require further imaging/revascularisation.
- Complete the National Vascular Registry documentation.
- Ensure patient is on best medical therapy if there is underlying peripheral arterial disease.
- Make sure you fill in the forms for the clean bone samples (for histology and microbiology).
- Plan for a wound review in 48 hours.

CHAPTER 33

Foot Debridement

Pre-Operatively

- Read through medical records, review relevant imaging and blood results.
- Examine the foot before you take the patient to theatre.
- Have a firm idea in your mind how sick the patient is and how bad the foot sepsis is.
- Counsel and consent the patient (mention need for radical debridement/amputate toes/proximal amputation etc.).
- Mark the patient.
- Do the team brief.
- Make sure patient gets appropriate prophylactic antibiotics.
- Discuss with anaesthetist in regards to appropriate anaesthetic approach, i.e. GA versus spinal/epidural, popliteal block, ankle block, ring block.

Intra-Operatively

- Position the patient supine.
- Prep both the foot and go in-between the toes using a betadine-soaked swab.
- **CLEAR THE SEPSIS!** If you have to choose between being conservative and being aggressive, **be aggressive**.
- If there is any dead or "dodgy" tissue, then excise it.
- If the bone needs to go, then remove it.
- Your objective here is primarily to save the patient's life (*I am not joking when I say that patients literally die from foot sepsis. You have to do a proper job first time around*).
- If toes are clearly involved in the septic/necrotic process, then remove them.
- If the infection/necrosis is spreading up the dorsal/plantar aspect of the foot, then open up the dorsal/plantar aspect of the foot.
- Use the Loeffler-Ballard incision as required.
- Remember that if you don't clear the sepsis, this means the patient will not get better and will simply have to come back to theatre again. Some people may think multiple trips to theatre is an acceptable plan → I don't.

Post-Operatively

- Prescribe appropriate post-operative antibiotics.
- Write a decent operation note.
- Make sure you document the quality of foot perfusion, i.e. was there good bleeding/pulsatile bleeding/poor bleeding. If poor, the patient may require further imaging/revascularisation.

DOI: 10.1201/b22951-33

- Complete the National Vascular Registry documentation.
- Ensure patient is on best medical therapy if there is underlying peripheral arterial disease.
- Make sure you fill in the forms for the clean bone samples (for histology and microbiology).
- Plan for a wound review in 48 hours.

CHAPTER 34

Transmetatarsal Amputation

Pre-Operatively

- Read through medical records, review relevant imaging and blood results.
- Examine the foot before you take the patient to theatre, and make sure you know what the vascularity is like!
- Counsel and consent the patient.
- Mark the patient.
- Do the team brief.
- Make sure patient gets appropriate prophylactic antibiotics.
- Discuss with anaesthetist in regards to appropriate anaesthetic approach, i.e. GA versus spinal/epidural, popliteal block, and ankle block.
- If this is a neuropathic foot with foot pulses, I would consider asking for a tourniquet.

Intra-Operatively

- Position the patient supine.
- Use a permanent marker pen and mark out your flaps before prepping. I don't measure out formally, but "eyeball it." I mark a horizontal line on the dorsal aspect of the foot where I intend to divide the metatarsal bones. I try to plan my level of bone division as distally as possible, knowing that I can always go more proximal if needed. I likewise try to mark the plantar flap to leave as much plantar tissue as possible. Some people use a "V" incision, but I actually prefer to make a long posterior flap in much the same way as a below-knee amputation flap.
- Prep both the foot and go in-between the toes using a betadine-soaked swab.
- I am flexible regarding the use of a tourniquet, but in my experience, these cases do bleed a lot more than you expect them to. Henceforth, if the foot has an intact blood supply I probably would elect to use a tourniquet.
- Make your skin incision and get down onto bone as soon as possible. I prefer to use the knife and work quickly. If there is an obvious arterial bleeder I will either ligate it or under-run it using 2-0 vicryl. If the tissues are generally just oozy I will just get a big swab and pack the wound tightly as I proceed.
- The priority is not to damage the posterior flap.
- Debride any non-viable tissues/excess tendons etc.
- Don't suture the flap in place if you know it is going to be under tension. In this case, consider liberating the flap further or using the bonesaw to amputate the metatarsal bones more proximally.
- Once I am down onto the metatarsal bones I will use a periosteal elevator to liberate the bones.
- I then come medially or laterally and use the bonesaw to divide the bones with a slightly curved incision.

302

DOI: 10.1201/b22951-34

- If this amputation is being done for infection, consider taking clean bone samples from the metatarsals to guide future microbiology decision-making.
- Once the forefoot is removed it is then much easier to achieve haemostasis.
- I generally put a corrugated drain inside the wound to allow any blood to escape (this drain is not sutured in place), and close the skin edges loosely using some interrupted 3-0 prolene vertical mattress sutures (obviously I leave a gap for the corrugated drain to escape).
- I then dress the wound with Mepitel or Jelonet, blue gauze, wool, and crepe (not too tightly though).

Post-Operatively

- Prescribe appropriate post-operative antibiotics (for me, 2 post-op doses of IV abx followed by completing 4 more days of oral antibiotics).
- Write a decent operation note.
- Make sure you document the quality of foot perfusion, i.e. was there good bleeding/pulsatile bleeding/poor bleeding. If poor, the patient may require further imaging/revascularisation.
- Complete the National Vascular Registry documentation.
- Ensure patient is on best medical therapy if there is underlying peripheral arterial disease.
- Plan for a wound review in 48 hours when if there is no bleeding concern the corrugated drain can be removed.
- Request a baseline foot X-ray now for future comparison.

CHAPTER 35

Above-Knee Amputation

Pre-Operatively

- Read through medical records, review relevant imaging and blood results.
- Specifically, check any X-rays or angiograms of the ipsilateral limb to make sure there is no metalwork in the femur **(THIS CATCHES A VASCULAR SURGEON OUT EVERY YEAR—DON'T LET IT BE YOU).**
- Counsel and consent the patient (*always mention risk of death, even in young patients who are not vasculopaths*).
- Mark the patient.
- Do the team brief.
- Make sure patient gets appropriate prophylactic antibiotics.
- Discuss with anaesthetist in regards to appropriate anaesthetic approach, i.e. GA versus spinal/epidural, femoral block, do they want a sciatic nerve catheter for local anaesthetic infusion etc.
- The patient will require a urinary catheter.
- I also routinely clean the thigh in the anaesthetic room with chlorhexidine (belt and braces).

Intra-Operatively

- Position the patient supine.
- Mark out the flaps carefully. I measure 10–12 cm above the upper border of the patella and use a permanent marker to identify the intended level of femoral transection. From this point, I use a piece of Nylon tape (or heavy vicryl suture) to measure the circumference of the thigh at this point. Then I divide this length by ×4. I then use this "quarter" length to measure out the flaps. From the area where I marked for femoral division, I use this "quarter" length to measure out an anterior flap and then a posterior flap (FISHMOUTH INCISION).
- I will then prep the thigh from the groin down to the mid-calf using betadine. I ask an assistant to lift the leg from the ankle as I do this. Once the leg is prepped I will apply the drapes underneath. At this point, I will apply a stockinet around the foot and calf. This stockinet is then very tightly wrapped up to the level of the knee using crepe bandage whilst the leg is still being elevated. This helps squeeze any blood out of the venous system/muscle bellies and limits blood loss during the operation. The crepe bandage is tightly secured in place and then the leg can be put down.
- I do most of the amputation using the knife.
- I make a swift and confident incision through the skin down through the underlying fascia all around the thigh at the level of my pre-marked flaps.
- The GSV will be identified, clipped, cut, and ligated using 3-0 vicryl ties.
- Once this is done, I used the knife to quickly cut through the bulk of the surrounding muscle (circumferential incision, deliberately cutting quite distally beyond the flaps in order to preserve as much muscle bulk as possible).

DOI: 10.1201/b22951-35

- On the medial aspect, I go slightly slowly through the medial muscle bulk. Once I am veering into the adductor canal, I will confidently swing my index finger medially, downwards and then swing it upwards and back towards myself in order to catch the femoral vessels. Once I have them in under my finger, I will sweep upwards and downwards to create some space. I then apply two large Robert's clips and cut the femoral vessels in between.
- I transfix the proximal SFA/SFV en masse using a heavy vicryl suture (i.e. 1-0 vicryl). I put a normal tie (2-0 vicryl) on the distal SFA/SFV.
- Once the femoral vessels are controlled, I again use the knife (or scissors) to completely free the femur from any soft tissue.
- I will use either the knife or heavy scissors to liberate the linera aspera, thus allowing me to use the perisoteal elevator and/or a white swab to clear the femur upwards to the level of intended bone transection.
- I will then ask for a guard to be applied around the femur, and use the powersaw to divide the femur at 90 degrees. I will also use the powersaw to file away any bone spurs at the end of the divided femur.
- The guard is removed and haemostasis is quickly achieved, preferably using 2-0 vicryl sutures to under-run bleeding areas.
- I will then wash the amputation stump wound with a litre of warmed normal saline.
- On closing, I will routinely leave a 14-French Robinson drain (tunnelled laterally), and I also routinely insert a sciatic nerve sheath catheter (again tunnelled laterally).
- I close the fascia using continuous 1-0 vicryl sutures (one surgeon starts in the middle and goes laterally, the other surgeon starts in the middle and goes medially).
- I use 3-0 monocryl for the skin (same principle, 2× surgeons each starting from the edges then meeting in the middle).
- I like to use honeycomb dressings for the skin.
- I also will conclude by saying that I think above-knee amputations should be done quickly and efficiently with minimal blood loss. These are often high-risk patients and I think they benefit the most from getting off the table as soon as possible. I think that using a knife and working quickly is the best way to minimise blood loss. However, I know there are vascular surgeons who disagree with me. One vascular surgeon I know thinks that amputations should be slow, methodical operations that should take a minimum of 2 hours, and I have seen people preferring to use the knife minimally and the diathermy maximally. Other surgeons believe in myodesis, i.e. attaching muscle to the femur to help maintain function. I don't do this because frankly the majority of above-knee amputations I am doing are in patients whom I don't think are ever going to mobilise again, and it just adds unnecessary complexity to an operation which I think should be quick and simple. Again, I write this just so you are aware of the fact that people have different approaches to the same operation. Whatever the case is, I am telling you that **YOU NEED TO HAVE YOUR OWN PLAN AND NEED TO BE ABLE TO JUSTIFY IT IF ASKED.**

Post-Operatively

- Prescribe appropriate post-operative antibiotics (I prefer 2 doses of IV abx, followed by 4 days of oral antibiotics).
- Write a decent operation note.
- Complete the National Vascular Registry documentation.
- Ensure patient is on best medical therapy if there is underlying peripheral arterial disease.
- I review my major amputation wounds in 72 hours.

CHAPTER 36

Below-Knee Amputation

Pre-Operatively

- Read through medical records, review relevant imaging and blood results.
- Specifically, check any X-rays or angiograms of the ipsilateral limb to make sure there is no metalwork in the tibia.
- Counsel and consent the patient (*always mention risk of death, even in young patients who are not vasculopaths*).
- Mark the patient.
- Do the team brief.
- Make sure patient gets appropriate prophylactic antibiotics.
- Discuss with anaesthetist in regards to appropriate anaesthetic approach, i.e. GA versus spinal/epidural, femoral block, and do they want a sciatic nerve catheter for local anaesthetic infusion….
- The patient will require a urinary catheter.
- I also routinely clean the lower limb in the anaesthetic room with Chlorhexidine (belt and braces).

Intra-Operatively

- Position the patient supine.
- Mark out the flaps carefully. I measure 4–5 finger-breadths below the tibial tuberosity and use a permanent marker to identify the intended level of tibial transection. From this point, I use a piece of Nylon tape (or heavy vicry suture) to measure the circumference of the calf at this point. Then I divide this length by ×3. I then use this "third" length to measure out the flaps. From the area where I marked for tibial division, I use this "third" length to measure out the flaps (this is the Burgess flap).
- I routinely use a thigh tourniquet to minimise blood loss → make sure you put wool underneath the tourniquet to protect the underlying skin.
- I will then prep from below the tourniquet down to the ankle using betadine. I ask an assistant to lift the leg from the ankle as I do this. Once the leg is prepped I will apply the drapes underneath. At this point, I will apply a stockinet (or foot bag) around the foot. I will then hold the leg up in the air at 45 degrees, wait for 30 seconds, and then apply the tourniquet 100 mmHg above the patient's systolic blood pressure.
- I cut through the skin and straight down to fascia using the knife, all around where the flaps are marked.
- The GSV will be identified, clipped, cut, and ligated using 3-0 vicryl ties.
- I continue to use the knife to divide the muscle bellies—I use a big clip to lift the anterolateral muscle bellies up and then run the knife across them.
- The AT vessels are transfixed using 2-0 vicryl.

DOI: 10.1201/b22951-36

- The periosteal elevator is used to liberate the fibula around 2 cm above the intended level of tibial transection. I then use the powersaw to divide the fibula at this level.

- I use a large clip to go behind the tibia, pull a gauze swab through to protect the tibial vessels, and use the powersaw to divide the tibia. I start off at an angle of 45 degrees, then once I am 1.5 cm into the tibia, I re-angle the powersaw at 90 degrees and go straight down to fully divide the tibia.

- Once the tibia is disconnected, I use the white gauze that was sitting behind the tibia to pull both the distal tibia and fibula forwards.

- This puts the tissues under tension, and I quickly remove the leg by confidently running the knife down the back of the tibia/fibula.

- At this point, I will fillet any excessive muscle. Ideally, one would preserve the gastrocnemius and soleus. However, if the muscle bulk is too much, the soleus will likely need to be trimmed / removed.

- The tibioperoneal trunk will be transfixed using 2-0 vicryl.

- The tibial nerve will be isolated and clipped.

- The SSV, if identified, is ligated using 3-0 vicryl.

- I use the powersaw (*in an unconventional manner*) to file away any sharp areas of bone on the tibial bone stump.

- At this point, the tourniquet is deflated and any bleeding areas will be oversewn using 2-0 vicryl stitches.

- A tibial nerve catheter will be inserted and tunnelled laterally.

- A 14-French Robinson drain will be inserted and tunnelled laterally.

- I close the fascia using continuous 1-0 vicryl sutures (one surgeon starts in the middle and goes laterally, the other surgeon starts in the middle and goes medially).

- I use 3-0 monocryl for the skin (same principle, 2× surgeons each starting from the edges then meeting in the middle).

- I like to use honeycomb dressings for the skin.

- Of note, I routinely use a tourniquet for my below-knee amputations. In my experience, these amputations tend to bleed more than above-knee amputations, and I therefore think using a tourniquet is better for the surgeon and for the patient. Not everyone agrees with my position, but I think my approach makes sense. No decent vascular surgeon would open an artery without getting proximal control first because there would be excessive bleeding … so why not apply it to be the below-knee amputation?

Post-Operatively

- Prescribe appropriate post-operative antibiotics (2 doses of IV antibiotics, followed by 4 days of oral antibiotics).

- Write a decent operation note.

- Complete the National Vascular Registry documentation.

- Ensure patient is on best medical therapy if there is underlying peripheral arterial disease.

- I review my major amputation wounds in 72 hours.

JMF Reflections

Below-knee amputations are tricky, and the margin between success and failure is slim and highly unpredictable. I take them very seriously. If you are doing a below-knee amputation, it is because you are likely thinking that the patient has rehabilitation potential, i.e. they might be able to use a prosthesis and walk again. Therefore, there is more pressure on you to get this operation done right!

For me, these are the key points:

1. Be confident that there is a good blood supply to get this stump to heal. In my book, I really want the patient to at least have a femoral pulse (*this is not a hard and fast rule, but generally speaking, I am not that keen on doing a BKA without a femoral pulse. Naturally one would prefer the patient to have a popliteal pulse also*).

2. Measure the level of tibial transection correctly (4–5 fingers below tibial tuberosity).

3. Measure out the flaps correctly (rule of 3s for the Burgess stump).

4. Don't leave the tibia "sticking out." I divide it at 45 degrees and trim off any sharp areas using the powersaw to make the bone stump smooth.

5. Divide the fibula 1.5 cm above the level of tibial transection.

6. Try and preserve decent muscle bellies to cover the bone ends.

7. However, don't leave too much muscle! If the muscle is too bulky, your wound closure is going to be tight and restrictive, and the muscle bellies may infarct. This can lead to the wound breaking down and getting infected. This is a fine balance, but if you can clearly see the muscle bellies bulging out as you are closing the skin, have a low threshold to stop and trim the muscle back a bit.

8. Really, focus on achieving haemostasis before you close, and leave a drain. If the patient gets a haematoma post-op, it can lead to pressure necrosis, then the wound starts to breakdown, then the patient has to go back to theatre, etc.

9. I am quite pedantic about infection. I clean the lower leg in the anaesthetic room with Chorhexidine, and then re-prep again formally in theatre using betadine. This is no doubt an overkill and I suspect many people will not agree with this. However, if these BKA stumps get infected it is really unpleasant. I also give a few days of antibiotics post-op. Microbiologists may not agree with this, but this is still my practice.

10. I know in vascular surgery open AAA and carotid endarterectomy and the other "fancy" procedures get most of the attention. However, in my eyes, vascular surgery wards are often populated with patients recovering from major amputations. This is my experience having worked in numerous vascular surgery units up and down the UK. I really do believe that major amputations are the "bread and butter" of vascular surgery. As such, I really do take major amputations very seriously. I want to devote them more attention, as I think they deserve it.

CHAPTER 37

Guillotine Amputation (Above Ankle)

Pre-Operatively

- *Let's be honest here* → The patient should have something like life-threatening diabetic foot sepsis if you are considering doing this.
- By the way, the chances are you will be doing this very late at night (*at least that is when I have done all of my guillotine amputations*).
- The infection in the foot should be pretty terrible, with necrosis/tracking sepsis/gas spreading up towards the malleoli.
- Make sure the patient has the appropriate medical treatment for sepsis, i.e. send off blood cultures, prescribe intravenous antibiotics, intravenous fluids, high-flow oxygen, check the lactate, and insert a urinary catheter ....
- Make sure the patient is counselled, consented, and marked.
- Include the possibility of needing to convert to a below-knee amputation ....
- I would let the family know what is going on.
- Get intensive care involved early.

Intra-Operatively

- Position the patient supine.
- Get a marker pen and draw a circumferential mark above the malleoli, superior to where you think the infection ends.
- If the patient has foot pulses, I probably would use a tourniquet.
- Liaise with your anaesthetist, but frankly I would rather the patient gets a quick general anaesthetic instead of messing around with popliteal blocks, etc. ....
- Grab the knife and make a confident cut all the way around the ankle.
- Horses for courses, but I go fast and deep, all the way around. I try to identify the anterior tibial and posterior tibial arteries, and the GSV and SSV, transfixing or ligating them as I go.
- Get down onto the bones quickly.
- Get the periosteal elevator and scrape upwards on the tibia and fibula.
- Grab the powersaw and go right through the tibia and fibula.
- If there is infection at this level, you either need to go higher with your amputation or preferably do a longitudinal (vertical) incision up the leg to open any infected tracts and excise any involved tendons etc.
- Ligate/transfix the peroneal artery (often you have to oversew it as it hides medially and superiorly to the divided fibula).
- Set the monopolar diathermy to "kill" and deal with any bleeding tissues.
- Remember that this is a true damage control procedure (not a fashion show).
- Take some Kaltostat or Aquacell and pack the distal stump, then cover with Mepitel or Jelonet, blue gauze, wool, and crepe.

DOI: 10.1201/b22951-37

- Try and get the whole case done within 15 minutes.
- *Worst-case scenario* → Convert to BKA.

Post-Operatively

- Prescribe appropriate VTE prophylaxis.
- Prescribe appropriate antibiotics, i.e. to treat life-threatening sepsis.
- Write a decent operation note.
- Complete the National Vascular Registry documentation.
- The patient may need to go to intensive care if this is septic shock.
- Have a plan for formal below-knee amputation once the sepsis/oedema has settled.

CHAPTER 38

GSV Endovenous Ablation

Pre-Operatively

- Read through the clinic letters, review any previous venous ultrasound assessments and check blood results.
- Go and see the patient and look at the leg yourself.
- Counsel, consent, and mark the patient.
- Clearly document in the medical records that the patient has been thoroughly counselled, i.e. mention indication, benefits of treatment, risks, and alternatives.
- *These are the risks I would mention:* Bleeding, infection, neurovascular injury, scarring, DVT/PE, thermal injury to skin, thrombophlebitis, bruising, swelling, itching, poor cosmesis, failed procedure, recurrence, need for further procedures, and local anaesthetic risks.
- *These are the alternatives I would mention:* Conservative management with compression stockings, open varicose vein surgery, foam sclerotherapy, and no intervention at all.
- Consider given single shot of prophylactic low-molecular-weight heparin depending on VTE risk assessment.
- I currently do these cases in a theatre setting, and I do a brief ultrasound assessment of the leg with the patient standing in the anaesthetic room before they come into theatre.
- If you were also doing multiple stab avulsions, mark these with the patient supine beforehand.

Intra-Operatively

- Patient's whole leg is prepped and draped from groin to ankle.
- Foot goes in a foot bag.
- I then tilt the patient into reverse Trendelenburg position (i.e. head up legs down).
- Sterile ultrasound probe used to identify the lowest point of reflux (I want to puncture vein as low as possible).
- I inject a small amount of 1% lignocaine where I intend to first puncture the skin.
- I use the ultrasound in transverse orientation and get the GSV in the centre of the screen.
- I use the needle and go through the anaesthetised area, slowly advancing downwards and forwards onto the top of the GSV. I take my time doing this to try and achieve puncture first time. In my opinion, this is the key to the whole operation—get this right and everything else should be easy.
- Once the needle is inside the vein on ultrasound, I will simultaneously check to confirm I have a flashback of blood.
- Now, I place the ultrasound down and secure the needle with my left hand.
- I will then carefully advance the laser fibre up towards the SFJ.
- I will use both transverse and longitudinal ultrasound orientations to settle the tip of the laser fibre 2–3 cm from the SFJ.
- Measure the length of laser fibre at this point and ask the theatre staff to record it.

DOI: 10.1201/b22951-38

- Now flatten the table out.
- I use the ultrasound predominantly in transverse orientation to inject tumescence around the GSV (get a nice HALO effect).
- As I get towards the upper thigh, I will switch to longitudinal ultrasound and inject tumescence in this manner. I like to see the tumescence needle getting good coverage around the tip of the laser fibre at the SFJ, and again confirm the laser fibre has not advanced too close to the junction or slipped into the common femoral vein.
- At this point, I will ask the theatre staff to lock the theatre doors and ensure everyone is wearing protective glasses.
- The laser procedure then takes place.
- If patient experiences pain, inject more tumescence.
- *Foam sclerotherapy or multiple stab avulsions under local anaesthetic can take place now depending upon your institution and practice.*

Post-Operatively

- Horses for courses, but I currently bandage the leg all the way up the thigh.
- This stays on for 2–3 days.
- I give the patient an above-knee compression stocking that they should wear for around 2 weeks afterwards.
- I follow-up patients in 6–8 weeks' time.
- If the patient has risk factors for VTE, I would prescribe a 1-week course of prophylactic enoxaparin.
- If very high risk for VTE, I would have discussed with haematology in advance (*and probably would have seriously questioned why I was doing the procedure in the first place if the risk of VTE was so high*).
- In your operation note make sure you say that you visualised the SFJ, that the laser fibre was positioned 2–3 cm away from the junction, the length of laser fibre that you used to do the procedure, the time of lasering, and the amount of energy delivered.

JMF Refections

Of note, I have worked in various units that do the above procedure in slightly different ways, using slightly different equipment from different manufacturers, some use a wire followed by the laser fibre etc. Others use radiofrequency ablation, some do avulsions, some don't. Some do foam sclerotherapy, some don't. Others have even done these cases under general anaesthetic because they think the patient needs a general anaesthetic for multiple stab avulsions. Everywhere is different. I came up with my technique and approach after reviewing lots of different approaches.

CHAPTER 39

Saphenofemoral Junction Ligation, Great Saphenous Vein Stripping, and Multiple Stab Avulsions

Pre-Operatively

- Read through the clinic letters, review any previous venous ultrasound assessments and check blood results.
- Go and see the patient and look at the leg yourself.
- Counsel and consent patient.
- Clearly document in the medical records that the patient has been thoroughly counselled, i.e. mention indication, benefits of treatment, risks, and alternatives.
- *These are the risks I would mention:* Bleeding, infection, neurovascular injury, scarring, wound healing problems, bruising, swelling, itching, poor cosmesis, recurrence, need for further procedures, anaesthetic risks, chest infection, and DVT/PE.
- *These are the alternatives I would mention:* Conservative management with compression stockings, endovenous treatment, foam sclerotherapy, no intervention at all, etc.
- Mark all the varicosities that you can see/feel with the patient standing.
- Confirm with the patient that all the varicosities that concern them have been marked.
- I then mark the exact position of the saphenofemoral junction using ultrasound.
- I routinely prescribe VTE prophylaxis for the patient to be given pre-procedure e.g., enoxaparin 40 mg.
- Clearly document that you have done all of the above in the medical notes.

Intra-Operatively

- General anaesthetic, prophylactic intravenous antibiotics, and patient supine.
- Prep and drape the groin and entire leg.
- Foot goes in a foot bag.
- Slightly abduct the leg / bend knee to improve exposure of the groin
- Small horizontal incision just medial-to-femoral pulse at site where SFJ was marked.
- I use monopolar diathermy to go through Camper's fascia followed by Scarpa's fascia.
- I then take a white swab and assertively sweep the tissues upwards and downwards.
- This almost always reveals the GSV as it is about to dive into the SFJ.
- At this point, I will insert a self-retainer.
- I then stay close to the GSV and follow it to the SFJ. I will isolate any tributaries and ligate them using 3-0 vicryl.
- Once the tributaries have been dealt with you will likely be able to see the SFJ quite clearly, however, this is not good enough.

- From my perspective, *you must identify the CFV above and below the SFJ*.
- I dive down from the SFJ and expose the CFV 1 cm above the SFJ.
- I then will carefully expose (and often have to ligate) the deep external pudendal artery that runs underneath the SFJ and on top of the CFV. This is an irritating little artery because you often cut it by accident. My position is this: Better for you to get it first before it gets you! I often end up ligating it, and this usually will enable me to confidently visualise the lower part of the CFV below the SFJ.
- Only after this I am certain which vein is the GSV and which is the CFV, and I am ready to disconnect the SFJ. I will transfix the SFJ using 2-0 vicryl.
- *The reason for this faff is this → I have been told stories about vascular surgeons who have stripped the CFV thinking it was the GSV. This is not going to be me!!!*
- I apply 2× clips to the open disconnected GSV and this allows me to more easily control the GSV and pass the stripper distally.
- With the stripper (that I use) I tie a 3-0 vicryl reel to the end of it. The stripper then advances down the GSV into the leg. Once it has reached the lower thigh it will inevitably poke at the skin, and I will make a stab incision in the medial thigh at this point and pull the stripped out more until the end of the stripper is at the level of the groin. I will use the 3-0 vicryl tie on the reel to tie the GSV to the stripper securely.
- Once this is done, I will pull the stripper out of the thigh, bringing the GSV with it. Once the stripper is out of the body, I can cut the 3-0 vicryl reel free.
- The reason to keep the reel attached to the stripper is just in case the stripper gets lost in the thigh, at least then you can pull the 3-0 vicryl tie and retrieve it!
- I will then use a 2-0 vicryl suture to close the cribriform fascia as a short single layer.
- I will then use 2-0 vicryl to close the groin fascia with 1× further layer, followed by 3-0 monocryl to skin.
- An opsite will be applied to the groin wound.
- After this multiple stab avulsions can proceed (the only thing I will say about the stab avulsions is to make sure you press on the areas after doing the avulsion as these patients can bleed a lot and don't do any avulsions around the ankle or fibula neck—you don't want to cause peroneal nerve injury or avulse the peroneal or anterior tibial/posterior tibial arteries. You might think this is unlikely but I have seen it happen!

Post-Operatively

- Steri-strips and low adherence dressings for stab avulsion areas, and bandage the leg all the way up the thigh.
- Find the right balance for how tightly you apply the bandage. Too tight and the patient's upper thigh ends up like a pork chop, too loose and the avulsion sites bleed more.
- This stays on for 2–3 days.
- I give the patient above-knee compression stocking they should wear for around 2 weeks afterwards.
- I follow-up patients in 6–8 weeks' time.
- If the patient has risk factors for VTE I would prescribe a 1-week course of low-molecular-weight heparin.
- If very high risk for VTE, I would have discussed with haematology in advance (*and probably would have seriously questioned why I was doing the procedure in the first place if the risk of VTE was so high*).

CHAPTER 40

Temporal Artery Biopsy

Pre-Operatively

- Read through the clinic letters, any ultrasound reports, check blood results, and make sure the patient is not on any anticoagulants.
- Palpate the temporal arteries and confirm you can feel them.
- Counsel and consent the patient (include facial nerve injury and scalp necrosis in consent).
- Put a mark on the correct side of face.
- When patient is in anaesthetic room, shave the hair around the temporal region.
- Use the handheld Doppler to mark out the exact position of the temporal artery.
- If there is lots of hair contaminating the field, use the ultrasound gel to direct it away.

Intra-Operatively

- Wear high-magnification surgical loupes for these cases.
- Prep and drape around the temporal area/ear.
- Have the bipolar diathermy available.
- Inject 1% lignocaine mixed with adrenaline along the line of the marked temporal artery.
- Give this 60 seconds to work, massaging the tissues using a swab.
- *Pop a small wet swab in this patient's ear* → This stops blood running down the ear canal and also reduces them being able to hear you complaining about how tricky these operations can be.
- Use the knife to incise the skin along the mark of the artery over at least 2 cm.
- After your skin incision, use a swab and apply gentle pressure over the incision for 2 minutes. This will help with haemostasis.
- After this, use the bipolar diathermy to deal with any residual bleeding areas.
- Use a very small self-retaining retractor to spread the tissues and expose the underlying fascia.
- Use your scissors to open up the fascia, hopefully revealing the pulsatile superficial temporal artery underneath. Always confirm the vessel is pulsatile, and ideally get your assistant or even the scrub nurse to doubly confirm this.
- If in doubt, ask for a sterile handheld Doppler to confirm what you think is the artery is indeed the artery.
- Dissect free at least 2 cm of artery and apply 2× small clips proximally and distally.
- Hand out the artery to be sent for histology.
- Use 3-0 vicryl to ligate both ends of the divided artery.
- Achieve haemostasis.
- 3-0 monocryl to skin.
- Opsite spray to skin +/− Opsite dressing.

DOI: 10.1201/b22951-40

Post-Operatively

- Label the histology specimen.
- Complete your operation note.
- Patient can go home the same day with outpatient follow-up by rheumatology.
- No stitches need removal.
- No need for vascular outpatient follow-up.

JMF Reflections

I would take these cases more seriously than you think you should. These are "little" cases that often get added onto your list without you really knowing much about them. However, they are not easy operations, and it is easy to encounter problems. Please do take them seriously. I am not going into details, but you can get easily burned. Be careful.

CHAPTER 41

Brachiocephalic Fistula Creation

Radiocephalic and brachiobasilic fistula creation follow the same principles.

Pre-Operatively

- Review any clinic letters, MDT outcomes, and/or fistula planning ultrasounds that have been done already.
- Go and examine both of the patient's arms, and look at their chest wall and neck as well.
- Ask the patient about previous central lines, tunnelled lines, pacemakers, etc.
- Confirm there is an ipsilateral radial pulse, and that there are no gross signs of central venous stenosis/obstruction.
- Use your eyes and fingers to check if there is a decent cephalic vein.
- Counsel the patient for brachiocephalic fistula creation.
- However, inform the patient that it is your routine practice to perform an ultrasound assessment in the anaesthetic room to confirm this is still the right plan.
- Consent the patient for brachiocephalic fistula creation.
- In the "other procedures," section of the consent form includes creating a different fistula in the same arm or creating a different fistula on the other arm.
- In the anaesthetic room, position the patient supine and put a tourniquet around the upper arm.
- Confirm that the brachial artery and cephalic vein are suitable (always scan the cephalic vein at the antecubital fossa and follow it up the arm).
- I mark out the course of both the brachial artery and cephalic vein using ultrasound, and I draw a horizontal line across the antecubital fossa 1 cm above where the vein and artery come closest together (this will be the line of my incision).
- I currently work in a unit where the anaesthetist does an arm block. However, previously I have done my own local anaesthetic administration in the anaesthetic room under ultrasound-guidance. As with the brachial embolectomy, I inject a mixture of 1% lignocaine and 0.25% chirocaine on top of the brachial artery and cephalic vein using the ultrasound in longitudinal orientation. I then anaesthetise the skin along the horizontal line where I intend to make my incision.

Intra-Operatively

- Patient positioned supine, arm out on board.
- Prep and drape arm, hand goes in see-through bag.
- Horizontal incision in antecubital fossa along pre-marked line.
- Use bipolar diathermy to control initial bleeding.
- Dissect through superficial layers, and target the cephalic vein first of all.

DOI: 10.1201/b22951-41

- Once you can see the vein, aim to dissect directly down onto it and get in the right-vessel plane.
- Avoid grabbing the vein with your forceps.
- Get a Lahey or Mixter around the vein as soon as you can and sloop it.
- Use the sloop to move the vein up/down/left/right to enable you to dissect it free.
- Have your assistant apply traction to the tissues surrounding the vein so you can divide them.
- Use a combination of cats-paws/mini-Langenbeck's and small self-retainers to aid your dissection.
- Dissect upwards and downwards to liberate a sufficient length of cephalic vein to enable you to swing it over towards the artery.
- Next turn your attention to the brachial artery.
- Dissect down to reveal the brachial aponeurosis.
- Divide the aponeurosis to reveal the brachial vessels underneath.
- Avoid injuring the brachial vein, identify the brachial artery, get in the right tissue plane, and expose the brachial artery so you have around 2 cm exposed.
- Use your Mixter to doubly sloop the brachial artery to get proximal and distal control.
- Now disconnect the cephalic vein and transfix the distal end using 2-0 vicryl.
- I get a blue cannula at this point and inject heparinised saline into the cephalic vein to both flush it and also dilate it (ask your assistant to press over the arm to compress the proximal cephalic vein).
- Once the vein is ready to go I apply a very gentle plastic bulldog to the proximal vein so it doesn't backbleed during the anastomosis.
- Ask for a beaver blade and make a small longitudinal arteriotomy in the brachial artery.
- Use 6-0 prolene to create an end-to-side anastomosis.
- I routinely parachute down to get things started off.
- Avoid grabbing the brachial artery or intimal layer of the vein.
- Before you complete your anastomosis, release the inflow and flush any clotted blood out. Then release the distal brachial artery and backbleed everything. Then backbleed the cephalic vein. Then use heparinised saline to flush everything out copiously.
- Do not tie your stitch yet. Instead, complete the final stitch, pull both sutures so they are under tension, and lock them together using a rubber shod.
- Release the fistula completely and confirm there is both a decent thrill and also a distal radial pulse.
- If the fistula is unsatisfactory, or there are concerns about the hand perfusion, you can loosen your anastomosis and address any issues.
- If the fistula and hand perfusion are intact, then you can simply release the rubber-shod and tie your 2× prolene sutures together.
- **TAKE DOWN THE CURTAIN.** This means the tissues that are abutting the medial aspect of the cephalic vein should be dissected free so that there is no tissue pressure compressing the fistula medially.
- Ensure haemostasis is achieved.
- Close the superficial layers with a single layer of 2-0 vicryl (don't stitch the fistula please).

- 3-0 monocryl to skin.
- Opsite dressing.

Post-Operatively

- Patient can go home the same day.
- No sutures need to be removed.
- Follow-up in vascular access clinic in 4–6 weeks.

CHAPTER 42

Peritoneal Dialysis Tube Insertion (Open)

Pre-Operatively

- Go and see the patient.
- Examine the abdomen yourself.
- Check blood results, any previous abdominal imaging, e.g. X-ray/CT/ultrasound results (don't want any surprises).
- Counsel and consent the patient.
- Make sure the renal access nurses have marked where the patient wants the PD tube to come out.
- In the anaesthetic room make sure the abdomen is shaved appropriately.
- Single dose of prophylactic IV antibiotic.

Intra-Operatively

- Supine position.
- Prep and drape abdomen.
- Vertical infra-umbilical skin incision.
- Dissect down to linea alba, staying in the midline.
- Use knife to score the midline over a few centimetres, and use 2× clips to grab the rectus sheath and pull up.
- Fully divide the rectus sheath using the knife.
- Use 2× further clips to grab the underlying peritoneum/fatty tissue and lift up.
- Feel with your fingers that there is no bowel underneath and then divide the peritoneum using dissecting scissors.
- Once you are into the peritoneal cavity, probe with your finger and sweep around to ensure no adherent bowel is lurking in your way.
- Use long non-toothed forceps to confirm there is a straight path into the pelvis.
- Curl the PD catheter up and grab it with a Rampley's forcep.
- Insert the Rampley's into the pelvis and then release the PD tube, carefully withdrawing the Rampley's from the pelvis to leave the PD tube in place.
- At this point, use 2-0 vicryl to secure the deepest PD tube cuff to the peritoneum.
- Following this, use a 10 ml syringe of normal saline to make sure that the PD tube easily flushes and aspirates.
- Now use looped PDS to close the rectus sheath—just be careful not to occlude the PD tube by being too aggressive with your closure.
- At this point, I will ask the theatre staff to connect a 500-ml bag of normal saline and run this through the PD tube into the pelvis (hang the bag on a drip stand above the patient). It should enter the pelvis quite quickly under gravity. Once the bag is empty I ask the

DOI: 10.1201/b22951-42

theatre staff to put the empty bag on the floor, and it should fill again. This reassures me that the PD tube is emptying and filling easily. If you have any doubt, then reopen the abdomen and correct any problems.

- Now tunnel the exterior limb of the PD tube from the infra-umbilical wound out towards the pre-marked spot.
- Avoid going too deep with this as you may hit the inferior epigastric artery and cause a big haematoma.
- Close the infra-umbilical wound using 2-0 vicryl and 3-0 monocryl to skin.
- Apply an Opsite dressing.

Post-Operatively

- In your operation note clearly document how many PD tube cuffs are present, and the position of the cuffs.
- Patient can use PD tube immediately.
- No further antibiotics needed.
- No sutures need removal.

CHAPTER 43

Peritoneal Dialysis Tube Removal

Pre-Operatively

- Review the medical notes, blood results, any relevant microbiology, observations, any previous abdominal imaging, and review the PD insertion operation note.
- Go and see the patient and examine the abdomen.
- Counsel and consent the patient.
- I would highlight to the patient that although the case is simple in principle, sometimes there are complications or you find sinister pathology, and in this case, you may need to make a bigger cut and/or do further procedures.
- *Indeed, you should always prepare for plan B. Most of these cases are straightforward but you never know what is in store for you. Most of these tubes are removed for PD peritonitis/ infection. I have seen a patient go to have his PD tube removed for PD peritonitis, and actually the diagnosis was peritonitis secondary to perforated diverticular disease. I have also removed a PD tube for PD peritonitis and at the time of the operation found the tube had been inserted straight through the small bowel. In both these cases, the patient required a laparotomy and bowel resection. On another occasion, I was removing a PD tube for PD peritonitis and I discovered a very strange, purplish/pink area of tissue that the PD tube was running right through as the tube entered the abdomen. I thought this was probably just granulation tissue but was worried it might be a small bowel injury. I called the general surgeons to come and have a look, and they also thought it was granulation tissue but could not confidently rule out a small bowel injury. They did a diagnostic laparoscopy and this confirmed there was no bowel stuck to the abdominal wall (and thus it was just granulation tissue). I mention these examples because these PD tube removals sound so simple, but in my experience, they can be full of surprises.*

Intra-Operatively

- Position the patient supine.
- Prep and drape the abdomen, leaving part of the exteriorised PD tube also prepped so you can tug on it to help identify its position during your dissection.
- Vertical infra-umbilical incision through old scar.
- Dissect downwards in midline.
- Tug on the PD tube to see where the tube is.
- Dissect directly onto the tube, and as soon as you can get a clip on it.
- Then use this clip to confidently pull the tube straight upwards.
- Use the monopolar diathermy to dissect down towards the linea alba so you can find the cuff.
- Once you at the level of the linea alba and onto the cuff proceed carefully.
- Use the diathermy to fully liberate the cuff.
- Once the inner cuff is free, you can pull the tube out of the abdomen.

DOI: 10.1201/b22951-43

- I cut the inner part of the tube and hand it out (asking for the tip to be sent for microbiology).
- The outer PD tube often has another cuff that will need to be dissected free as it holds the remaining tube in place, and once liberated, then you can remove the whole tube.
- *Be careful here. You may remove the inner tube after dissecting the inner cuff, and then find that the remaining outer tube pulls out very easily (i.e. no resistance). At this juncture you may assume that this is a PD tube with only one cuff. However, there may be a second cuff remaining that you are not aware of. In case of PD tube infection the second cuff can be eroded and as such it no longer holds on to the remaining PD tube. You may pull the remaining outer tube out, not realising you have left the second cuff inside the abdominal wall. A few months later, the patient may present with an abdominal wall infection / sinus, and an abdominal ultrasound may reveal this second cuff. This is why you should check the original operation note and confirm how many cuffs are present. This is also why I always write on my operation note (at the time of the original PD tube insertion) how many cuffs there are, and the position of the cuffs.*
- Liberating these tubes in my opinion is not really a science but an art. I don't know how best to describe it but you just have to be assertive with them. However, be cautious at the same time because there are abdominal structures close by and blood vessels in the abdominal wall. If you are overly confident or too assertive, the patient can end up with a visceral injury or something like an abdominal wall haematoma. On the other hand, if you are too cautious and timid this operation will end up taking as long as a fem-pop bypass. You just have to strike the right balance ….
- Close the midline using looped PDS.
- 2-0 vicryl to fascia and 3-0 monocryl to skin.
- Opsite dressing.
- I would not close PD tube exit site. It may in fact need some curettage and washout.

Post-Operatively

- Continue antibiotics if this was an infected case.
- Send catheter tip for microscopy, culture, and sensitivity if this was for PD peritonitis.

JMF Reflections

I have alluded to these points already. What you expect to be a simple PD tube removal may not be so straightforward. Just remember to stick to general surgical principles. If you remove the patient's PD tube and pus and/or bowel content start pouring out of the abdomen then don't just close the umbilical wound and bury your head in the sand. Do what needs to be done. If the patient needs a laparotomy then the patient needs a laparotomy. If the patient needs a laparoscopy then the patient needs a laparoscopy. If you are worried there might be a bowel injury then ask for a general surgeon to come and have a look with you. Perhaps you did not consent the patient specifically for a laparotomy or laparoscopy or bowel resection, and therefore you think that you are not allowed to do this. I have been in this situation and it is awkward because one of the basic principles of surgery is informed consent. However, another basic principle of surgery is patient care and proceeding in the best interests of the patient. I see absolutely no benefit in leaving a patient with a belly full of pus and faeces and perforated bowel, waking them up from a general anaesthetic, explaining that they have a belly full of pus and faeces and perforated bowel, getting permission to save their life, and then putting them back to sleep. If you think you have identified a serious life-threatening issue then make the right decision and act in the patient's best interests. *Oh and by the way, this is why at the start of this operation note I advised you to discuss these issues with patient beforehand ....You may think this is overkill and unnecessary, but when you find yourself in such a situation you won't regret it!!!!*

The other point worth mentioning is that some vascular surgeons tunnel PD tubes through the rectus abdominis muscle. I have no problem with this technique except for the fact it is a lot more difficult to remove. This is why you should review the original operation note. At least then you will have advanced warning that you are going to struggle a bit more getting the tube out.

CHAPTER 44

Questions

I have tried to design these questions so that they correlate to what one might expect to see in the FRCS Part A examination. I have also drawn a lot of this material from clinical scenarios I have experienced in real life. Some of the cases are from my direct experience, others are from indirect experience. At least therefore you can get some preparation for the exam, but also get a feel for real world vascular surgery. It is also important for you to understand that I (JMF) am setting these exam questions, and therefore I am also determining the answers. I will give you the answers and an explanation after you do the examination. However, some of the answers are open to interpretation. I am telling you what *I think* is the right answer. You may not agree with me.

1. A 68-year-old patient presents with a swollen right foot. There is necrotic skin over the dorsum of the foot with a large fluctuant collection under the skin. Pus is oozing from a break in the skin adjacent to this necrotic patch. There is an ulcer on the plantar aspect of the foot with purulent fluid discharging. The infection does not appear to have spread above the ankle; however, the right leg is oedematous from the knee down. The patient is pyrexial, tachycardic, and hypotensive. His WBC is 27, CRP 356, with acute renal failure and metabolic acidosis. An X-ray shows an obvious Charcot foot deformity with collapse of the midfoot, and severe osteomyelitis of the midfoot and hindfoot. There is also gas in the soft tissues of the foot. The patient has consented to go to theatre to definitively drain the sepsis and gives you permission to do what is necessary. What is your management plan?

   A. Incise and drain the abscess on the dorsum of the foot and do no more. The patient can be brought back to theatre on another occasion for further sepsis control if this drainage is insufficient.

   B. Proceed to a primary above-knee amputation.

   C. Proceed to a primary below-knee amputation.

   D. Explore the right foot and try to drain the sepsis. If the foot is non-viable because of gross sepsis proceed to an emergency guillotine amputation, with a view to below-knee amputation at a later date when the leg swelling has settled and the patient is systemically well.

   E. Perform a forefoot amputation and do not close the flaps primarily. This should allow any infection to drain and will enable the patient to keep his foot as he wanted.

2. A patient presents to A&E with a gunshot wound to the left chest. The patient has a patent airway, with reduced air entry at the left base with oxygen saturations of 85% on room air and a respiratory rate of 30. The haemodynamic parameters are stable currently. The patient has a CGS of 15/15. What is your management plan?

   A. Proceed to an immediate left anterolateral thoracotomy. This will enable you to decompress a likely tension pneumothorax and help achieve proximal control of any bleeding vessel.

   B. Ensure the patient is on high flow oxygen, performed a finger thoracostomy of the left chest followed by a formal chest drain insertion.

   C. Send the patient urgently to CT scan to find out what is going on in his left chest.

D. Telephone the thoracic surgeon on-call and say this patient has a chest injury that they need to come and sort out immediately.

E. Get a chest X-ray and only consider intervention now if it shows a tension pneumothorax.

3. A 62-year-old patient presents to your outpatient clinic with left calf pain on exercise. The patient thinks he can walk around half a mile before he has to stop. His symptoms are worse on an incline. He has no rest pain or night pain and sleeps with his legs flat in bed. He is a smoker. He is on medications for hypertension and raised cholesterol. He has an ipsilateral femoral pulse and nil distally. The left foot is warm and well perfused with no signs of tissue loss. He has an ABPI of 0.72. What is your management plan?

A. Arrange for an immediate diagnostic angiogram with the intention of treating a likely femoral artery occlusion with balloon angioplasty or stenting.

B. Request an urgent outpatient CT angiogram and ultrasound vein map. Tell the patient you are considering a bypass operation on him.

C. Advise the patient to stop smoking, commence on best medical therapy, and advise him to continue exercising. Offer a supervised exercise programme if one is available.

D. Commence the patient on naftidrofuryl and encourage him to stop smoking.

E. Advise the patient to avoid exercising if it causes him pain.

4. A 48-year-old right-handed female patient presents with left arm pain on exercise. She has no pain at rest. This happened 6 weeks ago and had an acute onset. These symptoms are significantly affecting her quality of life. She is a non-smoker and its otherwise fit and well. She has no pulses in the left arm, but normal pulses in the contralateral arm and both legs. There are no signs of critical ischaemia. How would you manage this patient?

A. Commence her on a suitable anticoagulant for a suspected embolic event. Request an ECG +/− 24–74-hour tape, echocardiogram, and CT angiogram of the arch of aorta and left arm.

B. Admit the patient urgently for consideration of a left brachial embolectomy.

C. Commence the patient on aspirin and high-dose statin therapy and encourage her to exercise. She does not require further investigation or treatment.

D. Request an urgent diagnostic angiogram via the femoral artery to visualise and treat a suspected proximal subclavian artery stenosis.

E. Commence the patient on high-dose steroids and refer the patient immediately to rheumatology for suspected Takayasu arteritis.

5. A patient is on the vascular ward 5-hour post-op following a right-carotid endarterectomy. You are called urgently to the ward because there is bleeding from the right neck. The patient's surgical drain is full and there is an expanding haematoma in the neck. The patient appears to be struggling to breathe. What is your immediate management plan?

A. Release the skin clips to decompress the likely large superficial haematoma and allow symptomatic relief.

B. Clamp the drain and reassure the patient and nursing staff that ooze following this operation is normal.

C. Immediately take the patient back to theatre.

D. Ask for an urgent senior anaesthetic review with a view to urgently securing the patient's airway.

E. Arrange for an urgent CT angiogram to see if there is contrast extravasation from the carotid patch before considering further surgery.

6. An 18-year-old male patient presents to A&E resus at 1 am in the morning having been stabbed in the left side of his abdomen. He is haemodynamically unstable with grade 4 haemorrhagic shock and a distended abdomen. The patient has a GCS of 15. What is your management plan?

   A. Arrange for an urgent CT angiogram.

   B. Resuscitate the patient with intravenous fluids and blood until normal blood pressure and heart rate are achieved, then arrange for a CT angiogram, and then consider surgery if there is a major vascular injury confirmed on CT.

   C. Permissive hypotension and immediate trip to theatre for a laparotomy +/− proceed.

   D. Insert a REBOA catheter into zone 3 and when the blood pressure normalises go to CT.

   E. Do a clamshell thoracotomy in A&E resus after the patient is intubated, clamp the descending thoracic aorta, and then take the patient to theatre for a laparotomy.

7. A frail elderly and comorbid patient has minor dry gangrene of the tip of the 4th toe. She has no rest pain or night pain and sleeps comfortably at night. There are no signs of infection. The patient only has a femoral pulse, with monophasic foot signals. The toe pressure is 47 mmHg. What is her WIfI stage, and what is the correct plan?

   A. WIfI stage 4. She is at high risk of a major amputation and requires urgent revascularisation.

   B. WIfI stage 1. She has a moderate risk of amputation and a moderate benefit from revascularisation. She should be considered for an urgent daycase diagnostic angiogram +/− endovascular treatment.

   C. WIfI stage 2. She has a low risk of amputation and high potential benefit from revascularisation. She should have an urgent outpatient MR angiogram to plan for a possible endovascular intervention.

   D. WIfI stage 1. She has a very low amputation risk and a low potential benefit from revascularisation. The patient and family should be counselled on the options, but there should be serious consideration of conservative management.

   E. WIfI stage 2. She has a low risk of amputation and moderate potential benefit from revascularisation. She requires an urgent outpatient CT angiogram and consideration of either bypass surgery or endovascular intervention.

8. A 79-year-old frail patient presents with a deep 6 × 6-cm ulcer with exposed tendon around the medial malleolus after being scratched by a dog 4 weeks ago. She has significant rest pain and night pain. She is known to have an occluded ipsilateral femoral-anterior bypass. This bypass was created last year using spliced vein from the same leg (great saphenous vein and anterior thigh vein) and lasted only a few weeks before it occluded. A previous CT angiogram demonstrates the AT was the only vessel supplying the ankle and the peroneal and posterior tibial arteries are occluded. The patient is systemically well. There are no gross signs of infection, but there is a lot of slough around the ulcer. The skin quality around the lower shin and calf is very poor. The old anterior tibial incision is around the mid-shin. She has a good ipsilateral femoral pulse. What is your management plan?

   A. Tell the patient that there are no further revascularisation options and advise either palliation or above-knee amputation.

   B. Advise the patient that re-do bypass surgery is unlikely to be a viable option. Warn her that she may ultimately require a major amputation in the future. However, request a CT angiogram and discuss the results in MDT to see if there are any further endovascular options available.

C. Advise the patient that she needs to be urgently admitted for an above-knee amputation as she is at risk of spreading infection that could threaten her life.

D. Ensure the patient is on best medical therapy, encourage her to exercise, and recommend wound care in the community.

E. Request a vein map of the contralateral leg to see if she has suitable GSV for a re-do femoral–posterior tibial bypass.

9. A 45-year-old gentleman presents to A&E with upper abdominal pain and vomiting. The pain radiates to his back. Erect chest X-ray shows no free gas and no signs of consolidation. The ECG is normal. What is your management plan?

A. Ensure the blood tests include LFTs and amylase to rule out acute pancreatitis.

B. Proceed to an immediate CT scan to rule out a perforation.

C. Diagnose this as gastroenteritis and send the patient home.

D. Arrange for a diagnostic laparoscopy to rule out acute appendicitis.

E. Commence the patient on oral lansoprazole or omeprazole and book an urgent outpatient upper GI endoscopy for likely gastritis.

10. A patient is 72-hour post-op following an elective open AAA repair with a tube graft. The patient was extubated quickly and was making a good recovery. He was stepped down from ICU to a normal ward very quickly. However, he does not feel very well. His renal function is deteriorating slightly. His inflammatory markers are increasing slightly. He has diffuse left-sided abdominal pain, but no frank peritonism. His lactate is normal. The patient looks systemically well. What is your management plan?

A. Take the patient immediately back to theatre to explore the abdomen.

B. Arrange for an urgent CT angiogram.

C. Discuss the case with the general surgery team on-call and ideally arrange for an urgent flexible sigmoidoscopy to examine the left colon for signs of ischaemia.

D. Plan for 24 hours of further clinical observation and if the patient deteriorates further request an urgent CT scan.

E. Increase the patient's analgesia and prescribe an enema for suspected constipation.

11. A patient is on the vascular ward following a below-knee amputation for non-salvageable critical ischaemia with advanced tissue loss. You are called to the ward because there is bleeding from the stump. The drain is full and there is frank arterial bleeding from the stump wound edges. There is a lot of blood around the patient's bed, and the patient is haemodynamically unstable. What is your management plan?

A. Take the patient immediately back to theatre.

B. Transfuse the patient blood to achieve a normal blood pressure, then transfer the patient to theatre for haemorrhage control.

C. Call for help. Press on the femoral artery in the groin to achieve proximal control. Transfer the patient to theatre as simultaneous resuscitation efforts take place.

D. Leave the patient on the ward with the nurse and foundation doctor and try and find a tourniquet from theatre, then rush back upstairs and apply it around the patient's thigh. After this resuscitate the patient en route to theatre.

E. Call for help. Delegate a trustworthy and sensible colleague to press down onto the ipsilateral femoral artery in groin to achieve proximal control. If there is a tourniquet readily available then use it. Resuscitate the patient and simultaneously arrange for a speedy return to theatre for definitive bleeding control.

12. A 98-year-old woman is admitted from a nursing home. She has advanced gangrenous changes to her left forefoot and heel. She has had two previous myocardial infarctions. She also has chronic kidney disease, diabetes, advanced dementia, and extremely poor mobility. She has no pulses in the left leg. There is a fixed flexion deformity of the left knee. What is the best management option?

    A. Urgent antegrade femoral angiogram with a view to endovascular treatment for limb salvage.

    B. Urgent MR angiogram and vein map with a view to femoral bypass.

    C. Primary left below-knee amputation.

    D. Conservative management/palliative care.

    E. Emergency guillotine amputation above the ankle.

13. A 29-year-old homeless patient is under your care at Christmas time with severe bilateral frostbite injuries to both feet. The left foot has extensive dry gangrene involving the toes, forefoot, midfoot, and hindfoot. The left heel is completely black. The right toes and forefoot are also gangrenous. The right heel however appears viable. There is pus coming out of the dorsal aspect of the right forefoot. The patient is pyrexial with CRP of 180. The orthopaedic and rehabilitation teams think the patient will have a better functional/rehabilitation outcome with bilateral below-knee amputations. What is the best management plan?

    A. Immediate bilateral below-knee amputations.

    B. Wait for another week for the gangrenous changes to fully declare themselves.

    C. Discuss the case with an international frostbite expert over the telephone and also ask for an urgent orthoplastic surgical review before committing to surgery.

    D. Do a guillotine amputation of the right foot above the ankle and a left below-knee amputation.

    E. Take to theatre for a radical right foot debridement alone.

14. A 49-year-old is 3-hour post-op in recovery following an elective below-knee amputation. A tibial nerve sheath catheter is in situ and infuses a low dose of local anaesthesia. This operation was done for chronic pain that developed following a previous Symes amputation for a traumatic foot injury 3 years ago. The patient, apart from being a smoker with raised cholesterol, is otherwise fit and well. The operation proceeded smoothly and a tourniquet was used with minimal blood loss. The patient starts complaining of chest pain radiating to his arm and suddenly has a cardiac arrest. The monitor shows ventricular fibrillation. Just before his cardiac arrest, the patient told the recovery nurse he had been getting chest pain episodes at home but never told his doctor. His pre-operative blood tests from this morning were entirely normal. What is the most likely diagnosis?

    A. Local anaesthetic toxicity from the tibial nerve catheter

    B. Pulmonary embolism

    C. Hypo/hyperkalaemia

    D. Myocardial infarction

    E. Hypovolaemic shock

15. A 72-year-old woman presents with vomiting, abdominal discomfort, and distension. She has not opened her bowels in 2 days and is not passing flatus. She says she has noticed a change in bowel habit recently, weight loss, and poor appetite. There is a fullness in her right iliac fossa. She also has a lower midline scar following a previous hysterectomy. What is the most likely diagnosis?

   A. Incarcerated/strangulated right femoral hernia causing small bowel obstruction

   B. Caecal cancer-causing bowel obstruction

   C. Adhesional bowel obstruction

   D. Sigmoid cancer causing bowel obstruction

   E. Caecal volvulus

16. An 80-year-old gentleman is 2 days post-op on the vascular surgery ward following a below-knee amputation for chronic limb-threatening ischaemia. He has atrial fibrillation and is usually on warfarin, but this has been held to do the amputation. He is now complaining of diffuse severe abdominal pain that started suddenly around 1 hour ago. His abdomen is soft and he does not have any guarding or peritonism. He looks well but appears to be in significant pain. What is the most likely diagnosis?

   A. Perforated abdominal viscus

   B. Acute diverticulitis

   C. Acute pancreatitis

   D. Acute mesenteric ischaemia

   E. Acute appendicitis

17. A 58-year-old woman is 3-weeks post-op following a right femoral to below-knee popliteal artery bypass using PTFE with a Miller cuff. This was done for chronic limb-threatening ischaemia with tissue loss/rest pain/night pain. The bypass is functioning and the patient has a warm well-perfused right foot. The groin site has broken down, prosthetic graft is visible, and there is visible purulent fluid surrounding the graft. What is the best management plan?

   A. Intravenous antibiotics, groin wound washout, and Sartorius flap coverage of the proximal graft.

   B. Subtotal explantation of the proximal part of the graft and no further revascularisation attempts.

   C. Explantation of the graft and repeat in situ bypass using prosthetic material.

   D. Explantation of the graft and replacement using autologous vein if available.

   E. Washout of right groin, debridement of devitalised tissue, and VAC application.

18. A 62-year-old female patient attends the renal access clinic for fistula planning. The patient is right handed. The radial and brachial pulses are palpable bilaterally. These are the results of her duplex assessment:

   Left radial artery triphasic, diameter 0.16 cm
   Left brachial artery triphasic, diameter 0.40 cm
   Left cephalic vein diameter at wrist 0.20 cm
   Left cephalic vein diameter at antecubital fossa 0.25 cm
   Left basilic vein diameter at antecubital fossa 0.31 cm
   Right radial artery triphasic, diameter 0.20 cm
   Right brachial artery triphasic, diameter 0.36 cm
   Right cephalic vein diameter at wrist 0.24 cm
   Right cephalic vein diameter at antecubital fossa 0.28 cm
   Right basilic vein diameter at antecubtial fossa 0.32 cm

What is the most appropriate fistula for her?

A. Right radiocephalic fistula

B. Right brachiocephalic fistula

C. Left radiocephalic fistula

D. Left brachiocephalic fistula

E. Left basilic vein transposition fistula

19. A 62-year-old gentleman presents with severe bilateral foot pain at rest and night time. He does not have to sleep with his legs hanging out of bed. Elevating his legs or lying on his side often eases his symptoms at night-time. He is able to walk around 400 yards before he gets intermittent claudication in both his calves. He is a heavy smoker, with moderate COPD, and is an alcoholic. He does not have diabetes. He is frail. He has no pulses in either leg. He has no tissue loss in either foot. The feet are warm. He has a toe pressure of 50 mmHg on the left and 60 mmHg on the right. He has significantly reduced sensation in both his legs to mid-calves. A CT angiogram shows bilateral severe external iliac disease, heavy common femoral artery disease, and a long SFA occlusion on the right. What is the most appropriate management plan for this patient?

A. Smoking cessation, best medical therapy, and regular exercise

B. Bilateral common femoral endarterectomies and iliac stents as a hybrid procedure

C. Aortio-bifemoral bypass and right femoral—popliteal bypass

D. Axillo-bifemoral bypass and right femoral—popliteal bypass

E. Axillo-bifemoral bypass alone

20. A 62-year-old gentleman is in intensive care in a hospital 1 hour away with biliary sepsis. He has bilateral pneumonia and acute renal failure. He also had chest pain the night before with a troponin rise to 4000, suggesting an additional myocardial infarction. The patient is also on noradrenaline. An 8-French central line was inserted via the right internal jugular vein so he could be filtered for his renal failure. However, the line has accidentally been inserted into the proximal subclavian artery, i.e. inside the chest. There is no active bleeding on his CT angiogram. What is the best management plan?

A. Advise the ICU team to pull the line out and give the patient tranexamic acid.

B. Advise referral to a cardiac surgery for a median sternotomy and direct removal of the line under vision with surgical repair.

C. Advise transferring the patient from ICU to ICU to the nearest tertiary vascular surgery centre with cardiac surgery, interventional radiology, and vascular surgery support on site. Plan to remove the line with a minimally invasive endovascular approach, with a backup plan to do a median sternotomy if required.

D. Plan to do a supraclavicular exposure and remove the line under direct vision with a Dacron patch repair of the defect.

E. Palliate the patient as there is no viable option to remove this safely.

21. A 65-year-old gentleman presents with a symptomatic 10-cm infra-renal AAA confirmed on CT angiogram. He is haemodynamically stable at the moment with a GCS of 15/15. He has a background of hypertension, gout, and diet-controlled diabetes. He is still working as a gardener and is fit with an exercise tolerance of miles. He has had no previous abdominal surgery. His CT angiogram demonstrates an 18 mm straight and disease-free infra-renal neck that is angulated by 30 degrees anteriorly. Iliac access appears suitable for an EVAR, and the aneurysm ends just before the iliac bifurcation. The femoral arteries are disease free and only 2 cm from the skin surface. What is the best management plan for this patient?

A. Standard infra-renal EVAR (percutaneous access under local anaesthetic)

B. Infra-renal EVAR with endoanchors

C. Open AAA repair with infra-renal clamp and tube graft

D. Open AAA repair with supra-renal clamp and bifurcated graft

E. Fenestrated EVAR

22. A 72-year-old gentleman has had a left brachio-axillary graft created this morning on an elective theatre list for end-stage renal failure. It is now 2-hour post-op and the patient is in recovery. The patient has pain in his left hand and forearm and "pins and needles" affecting his fingers. He also has reduced power in the hand. The graft is functioning and the patient otherwise has a warm well-perfused hand. He does not have a good radial pulse, but he has a strong biphasic radial artery signal using handheld Doppler. What is the most appropriate management plan?

A. Reassure the patient that the symptoms will settle.

B. Keep the patient in recovery with a plan to come back and reassess in 4 hours to see if his symptoms have improved.

C. Speak to the neurologist on-call and ask for urgent nerve conduction studies.

D. Take back to theatre immediately for graft ligation.

E. Arrange for an urgent diagnostic angiogram to confirm the run-off vessels to the hand have not been compromised, with a plan for brachial embolectomy.

23. You are assigned to a TAVI (transaortic valve insertion) list to help the cardiologists with vascular access for a re-do TAVI-in-TAVI valve replacement in a frail elderly gentleman. The patient has been set-up for a left axillary cut-down. The patient's INR this morning is 1.7. The patient also tells you he has had this operation before and you can see a scar in his left infra-clavicular space. The cardiologist has planned to do the procedure via the left axillosubclavian artery. The patient does not have femoral pulses. Please confirm your best management plan.

A. Cancel the procedure as his clotting is not corrected and a re-do axillary exposure is too difficult.

B. Continue without correcting the clotting and proceed to a left supra-clavicular subclavian cut-down.

C. Give 5 mg of intravenous vitamin K to correct the clotting and proceed to do a left re-do axillary cut-down. Ask for senior vascular surgery support. Proceed slowly and carefully.

D. Ask the cardiologists to do a percutaneous left axillary artery approach.

E. Change the operation last minute to a right axillosubclavian approach.

24. You have exposed the left axillary artery to allow access for a TAVI case. 9,000 units of heparin have been used throughout the case. A 14-French sheath is left in the artery at the end of the operation. Upon removal of the sheath you inspect the arteriotomy site. There is some minor atherosclerotic disease affecting the arterial wall. There is a minor dissection flap affecting the distal arteriotomy. The artery itself is quite small, and this is a fairly sizeable defect. What is your best management plan for repair of this vessel?

A. Primary repair using 7-0 prolene and give vitamin K

B. Primary repair using 5-0 prolene and give FFP

C. Patch repair using 5-0 prolene

D. Patch repair using 6-0 prolene and give protamine

E. Short Dacron or PTFE interposition graft and give tranexamic acid

25. A 79-year-old woman presents with a large aneurysm at the site of her left brachio-cephalic fistula. The aneurysm is pulsatile, is about 7 cm in size, and has a thrill in it. The overlying skin is thin, shiny, tight, and erythematous. There is a small ulcer over the top of the aneurysm and there is a tiny blood clot here. The patient says it has been oozing on and off for a few days. It is now 10 pm in the evening. What is the most appropriate management plan?

A. Refer the patient to the vascular access clinic on an urgent outpatient basis.
B. Admit the patient for fistula aneurysm repair in the next few days.
C. Admit the patient for an emergency covered stent insertion tomorrow morning.
D. Take the patient to theatre tonight for emergency fistula ligation and excision of aneurysm.
E. Reassure the patient and advise that she should continue dialysis, but avoid needling this area.

26. A 90-year-old frail and comorbid woman is referred to you by a stroke physician. She has a background of peripheral vascular disease and is known to have aorto-iliac occlusive disease. The patient has had a left hemisphere transient ischaemic attack (TIA) 4 weeks ago. Her carotid duplex shows she has a 50% left ICA stenosis. Her right ICA is occluded. The patient was not on best medical therapy at the time of her TIA, but she is now. She has not had any further neurological episodes. She has previously had a thyroidectomy for thyroid cancer 10 years ago. What is the most appropriate management plan?

A. Urgent left carotid endarterectomy
B. Urgent right carotid endarterectomy
C. Urgent left carotid stent
D. Best medical therapy alone
E. Urgent right carotid stent

27. A 74-year-old gentleman presents with a left hemisphere TIA 3 days ago. He is reasonably fit and independent. He has not had any previous neck surgery. His carotid duplex reveals an 80% left ICA stenosis. His right ICA has a <50% stenosis. A CT angiogram confirms these findings. The left carotid bifurcation is below the mandible. What is the most appropriate management plan?

A. Urgent left carotid endarterectomy
B. Urgent left carotid stent
C. Best medical therapy alone
D. Best medical therapy and urgent left carotid endarterectomy
E. Best medical therapy and urgent left carotid stent

28. A 58-year-old gentleman with hypertension presents with sudden onset chest and back pain. A CT angiogram demonstrates an uncomplicated type B aortic dissection. What is the most appropriate management plan?

A. Urgent TEVAR.
B. Best medical therapy and admit to vascular ward for close monitoring.
C. Analgesia, arterial line for blood pressure monitoring, intravenous beta-blockade, and admit to intensive care for close monitoring. Aim for systolic blood pressure <150 mmHg and heart rate <100.
D. Analgesia, oxygen, arterial line for blood pressure monitoring, intravenous beta-blockade, and admit to intensive care for closing monitoring. Aim for systolic blood pressure 100–120 mmHg and heart rate <60.
E. Refer the patient to cardiology.

29. A 64-year-old gentleman presents with a complicated type B dissection. He is complaining of a painful right leg. He does not have a right femoral pulse and you conclude he has a Rutherford 2B ischaemic limb. His left leg has a full complement of easily palpable pulses. He also has normal upper limb pulses. His CT angiogram does not show any visceral/renal malperfusion. What is the most appropriate management plan?

   A. Ask interventional radiology to insert an emergency TEVAR and to try and recannalise his right iliac artery
   B. Left axillary-bifemoral bypass
   C. Right to left femoral-femoral crossover
   D. Left to right femoral-femoral crossover with right leg fasciotomies
   E. Right axillary to right femoral bypass with right leg fasciotomies

30. A 24-year-old gentleman presents to A&E as a code red major trauma call. He has been involved in a high-speed road traffic accident (he came off his motorbike). His CT brain also shows a left-sided extra-dural haematoma with midline shift. He has sustained bilateral open femur fractures and bilateral open ankle fractures. He also has multiple rib fractures. Finally, his CT angiogram reports a small intimal tear in the descending thoracic aorta just beyond the left subclavian artery (but with no pseudoaneurysm or haematoma). What is the most appropriate management plan?

   A. This patient needs an emergency TEVAR to prevent catastrophic aortic rupture. This takes priority over all other injuries.
   B. For the moment this patient does not require urgent intervention for this aortic injury.
   C. The patient needs emergency neurosurgical and orthopaedic intervention, and once this is completed the patient will require an emergency TEVAR.
   D. The patient requires a clamshell thoracotomy and suture repair of the descending thoracic aorta in A&E resus.
   E. The patient should have a REBOA catheter inserted in A&E to optimise his cerebral perfusion.

31. A 78-year-old patient is rushed to cardiac theatres following a TAVI complication. Essentially, during the TAVI insertion, the valve slipped into the left ventricle and now needs to be surgically removed, followed by open aortic valve replacement. This procedure was being done via bilateral percutaneous femoral access using 16-French sheaths. The right femoral sheath has been removed and repaired successfully using proglides. The left femoral sheath proglide closure failed after multiple attempts, so has been left in situ. It will need surgical removal. The patient is pretty unstable and the cardiac surgeons want to open the chest as soon as possible and will need to put the patient on bypass. There is currently a lot of oozing from around the left femoral sheath. It is now 4 pm and your on-call shift finishes in 2 hours when another vascular consultant will start his on-call. What is the most appropriate management plan?

   A. Advise the cardiac surgeons to proceed with their median sternotomy, put the patient on bypass, and wait for the cardiac surgeons to fix the cardiac problem. When they are finished you will remove the left femoral sheath and repair the arterial defect.
   B. Advise the cardiac surgeons to proceed with their surgery first, and once they are finished you can hand the job over to your evening on-call vascular surgery consultant colleague.

C. Ask for another vascular surgery consultant to come and help you. Plan to remove the left femoral sheath and repair the femoral artery swiftly and efficiently, and then allow the cardiac surgeons to proceed.

D. Pull the left femoral sheath out and press on the groin for 20 minute whilst the cardiac surgeons proceed.

E. Wish you had a simpler case to deal with during your first ever week on-call as a vascular consultant. Life does not seem fair to me.

32. You have just done a right carotid endarterectomy on a patient. The case was difficult as the carotid bifurcation was high, the neck was "deep" with limited mobility due to cervical spondylosis, and you were operating right underneath the hypoglossal nerve which was slouped to help with access. It was done under general anaesthetic using a Javid shunt. You were reasonably happy with the result as there was a good handheld Doppler signal in the ICA upon completion of the patch. When the patient is waking up in theatre he is not moving his left arm or left leg very much. The right side movements are much more impressive. Pre-operatively the patient's neurology was completely normal as this case was performed for a TIA. What is the most appropriate management plan?

A. Call for senior vascular surgery assistance and plan to immediately re-explore the carotid patch for suspected patch thrombosis.

B. Take the patient for an urgent CT angiogram to see if he has had an embolic event during the surgery.

C. Wait for an hour to allow the patient to fully wake up following his general anaesthetic. If the neurology does not improve then arrange for a CT angiogram.

D. Commence the patient on an intravenous infusion of heparin and discuss the case with the stroke physician on-call.

E. Run down to the vascular MDT and ask for everyone's opinion on the case.

33. You are doing an elective open AAA repair with a foundation doctor as your assistant. You are trying to sloupe the right common iliac artery when suddenly there is a large gush of dark venous blood. What is the most appropriate management plan?

A. Ask for two larger suckers to enable you to visualise the area whilst you try to stitch the venous injury.

B. Put a load of haemostatic agents around the bleeding point and carry on with the operation.

C. Press over the bleeding point with your finger, stop the operation, update the anaesthetist and the theatre team, and call for senior vascular surgery consultant assistance.

D. Resect the overlying iliac artery to enable you to ligate the underlying iliac vein.

E. Ask your assistant to stitch the bleeding point as this is a good training opportunity.

34. You are referred a 90-year-old female patient from a district general hospital 30 minutes away for bilateral lower limb ischaemia. This patient is known to have metastatic bowel cancer. She has presents profoundly unwell with mottled legs. The mottling extends up to the lower abdomen. This is fixed mottling. She has no lower limb pulses. A CT angiogram is reported as "aortic thrombus that extends from the infra-renal aorta to the common iliac origins." What is the most appropriate management plan?

A. Accept the patient for immediate transfer with a view to bilateral femoral embolectomies followed by bilateral above-knee amputations.

B. Advise that this is a terminal event and the patient should be kept in the current hospital and palliated.

C. Accept the patient for immediate transfer with a view to an axillo-bifemoral bypass and bilateral lower limb fasciotomies.

D. Advise intravenous heparin for 24 hours and then for formal oral anticoagulation, and you will ask a consultant colleague to come and review the patient in next 24–48 hours.

E. Ask for the referring doctor to discuss the case with interventional radiology with a view to thrombolysis.

35. A 69-year-old gentleman presents to A&E with right iliac fossa pain, fevers, and vomiting. A CT scan has revealed acute appendicitis and an 8-cm infra-renal AAA with no concerning features. You are referred the case by the A&E consultant. What is the most appropriate plan?

A. Admit the patient under your care. Take the patient first for a laparoscopic appendicectomy. After this arrange for an emergency EVAR on the same admission.

B. Admit the patient under your care. Take the patient for a laparotomy. Perform an open appendicectomy followed by an open AAA repair.

C. Advise referral to the general surgical team for them to manage the appendicitis which is the current priority. You will discuss the case in the vascular MDT with a view to determining if this is suitable for EVAR and when vascular intervention is recommended.

D. Accept the patient for an emergency EVAR. Once the AAA is treated you will refer the patient to general surgery for consideration of appendicectomy.

E. Take the patient for an open appendicectomy yourself via a short incision over McBurney's point. Wait 1 week then take the patient for a midline laparotomy and do an open AAA repair.

36. A 62-year-old gentleman presents to A&E at midnight with sudden onset chest pain, back pain, and abdominal pain. He is shocked with a systolic blood pressure of 90 mmHg and a heart rate of 100. His GCS is 15/15. He has a palpable abdominal aortic aneurysm, and FAST scan confirms the aneurysm is about 8 cm in diameter. What is the most appropriate management plan?

A. Take the patient immediately to theatre for an open AAA repair via a midline laparotomy.

B. Give the patient lots of intravenous fluids and blood products to achieve normal haemodynamic parameters, then go for an urgent CT angiogram of just the abdomen.

C. Aim for permissive hypotension and take the patient for an urgent CT angiogram from the arch of the aorta down to both groins to visualise the femoral artery bifurcations.

D. Insert an aortic balloon via the femoral artery to optimise the haemodynamic parameters and then take the patient for an urgent CT angiogram.

E. Do a left anterolateral thoracotomy in A&E resus and clamp the descending thoracic aorta and then take the patient to theatre for a midline laparotomy.

37. A 24-year-old female presents with a self-inflicted stab wound to her right medial thigh. She has a large haematoma in the inner thigh that is expanding. She has a femoral pulse in the groin but nil distally. She is currently haemodynamically stable. What is the most appropriate management plan?

A. Refer the patient to interventional radiology for a right femoral diagnostic angiogram +/− covered stent insertion for suspected femoral artery injury.

B. Aggressive intravenous fluid resuscitation followed by urgent CT angiogram.

C. Take to theatre, attack the injury, shunt the injured artery, and then consider interposition graft repair using ipsilateral great saphenous vein.

D. Take to theatre, gain proximal and distal control, shunt the injured artery, consider interposition graft repair using contralateral great saphenous vein, and do a lower limb fasciotomy.

E. Take to theatre, gain proximal and distal control, and repair the injured artery using a prosthetic graft, followed by a lower limb fasciotomy.

38. A 72-year-old gentleman presents with advanced Rutherford 2B right leg ischaemia. An urgent CT angiogram shows a thrombosed 3-cm popliteal aneurysm. The patient has patent 3 vessel run-off below the knee. It is 8 pm now and you are starting your night shift as the vascular consultant on-call. What is the most appropriate management plan?

A. Ask interventional radiology to proceed to thrombolysis of the popliteal aneurysm, followed by a covered stent insertion.

B. Commence the patient on intravenous heparin and plan to take to theatre in the morning for a popliteal embolectomy.

C. Take the patient to theatre for a posterior approach popliteal aneurysm repair using PTFE.

D. Take the patient to theatre for a medial approach exclusion and bypass using ipsilateral great saphenous vein.

E. Take the patient to theatre for a medial approach exclusion and bypass using ipsilateral great saphenous vein, followed by a lower limb fasciotomy.

39. A 49-year-old patient presents to your diabetic foot clinic with gangrenous changes to the tip of his right hallux. His toe pressure is 29 mmHg with a WIfI stage of 3. He has a femoral and popliteal pulse only. The patient has had a vein map which shows good quality ipsilateral great saphenous vein from groin to ankle. The patient has also had a diagnostic angiogram. Endovascular intervention has already been attempted and was unsuccessful. There is diffuse severe infra-popliteal disease, but there is a medial plantar artery and the foot arch appears intact. What is the most appropriate management plan?

A. Plan for a repeat endovascular attempt.

B. Counsel the patient for a right below-knee amputation.

C. Plan for a right popliteal—plantar artery bypass using ipsilateral great saphenous vein.

D. Plan for a right femoral to posterior tibial bypass using ipsilateral great saphenous vein.

E. Perform a hallux amputation with no plans for further revascularisation.

40. A 59-year-old gentleman presents to A&E resus in an adjacent hospital at 3 am with profound grade 4 haemorrhagic shock. He has been bleeding profusely from a sinus in his right groin. An initial venous blood gas reveals a haemoglobin of 65, a pH of 7.12, and a lactate of 11. The A&E registrar over the phone is panicking. He says the patient has told him he has had a bypass 5 years ago by a vascular surgeon. The patient has a laparotomy scar and vertical scars in both his groins. There is no active bleeding, but the right leg also looks ischaemic. Based upon this limited information, please choose the most appropriate management plan.

A. Advise the A&E registrar to get an urgent CT angiogram and to review the patient's medical records and then call you back with the results.

B. Advise the A&E registrar to blue light the patient over to your hospital's A&E resus department immediately, with O negative blood in the ambulance to maintain the patient's conscious level (i.e. permissive hypotension). Aim for simultaneous resuscitation as you plan to take the patient to theatre for right groin exploration and ligation of a likely dehisced right limb of an infected aorto-bifemoral bypass graft.

C. Advise aggressive resuscitation using intravenous fluids and blood first, and when the patient's haemodynamic parameters are improved, then transfer the patient over to your A&E department. On arrival arrange for an urgent CT angiogram and liaise with interventional radiology about covered stent insertion.

D. Aim for permissive hypotension and transfer the patient over to you urgently. Take the patient to theatre with a plan to ligate the right limb of a suspected infected aorto-bifemoral bypass, followed by a right axillo-femoral bypass to reperfuse the right leg.

E. Aim for aggressive fluid resuscitation and transfer the patient to your hospital once the patient is stabilised. Plan to take him to theatre for emergency ligation of his right infected/dehisced aorto-bifemoral limb, followed by left to right femoral-femoral bypass.

41. A 40-year-old homeless gentleman presents with bleeding from his right groin. He is an active intravenous drug user. As you arrive in A&E resus, there is blood all over the floor. A paramedic is pressing down over the right groin to stop what has been described as torrential haemorrhage. What is the most appropriate management plan?

A. Arrange for an urgent CT angiogram to confirm the diagnosis.

B. Ask interventional radiology to insert a plug in the right external iliac artery and then take the patient to theatre for a right above-knee amputation.

C. Take the patient to theatre and do a vertical groin incision with a plan to do a suture repair of the underlying arterial defect.

D. Take the patient to theatre and plan to gain proximal control via a Rutherford Morrison incision and then proceed to repair the femoral vessels using a bovine patch.

E. Take the patient to theatre and plan to gain proximal control via a Rutherford Morrison incision and then proceed to ligate the femoral vessels.

42. A 74-year-old female patient with a known 4.9-cm AAA on surveillance presents with sudden onset back pain and collapse. She is currently haemodynamically stable. She is otherwise reasonably fit for her age with no previous abdominal surgery. Her CT angiogram shows that she now has a ruptured 5.3-cm infra-renal AAA that is suitable for a standard percutaneous EVAR. What is the most appropriate management plan?

A. Urgent open AAA repair via a midline laparotomy

B. Urgent percutaneous EVAR under local anaesthesia

C. Urgent percutaneous EVAR under general anaesthesia

D. Urgent aorto-unifemoral EVAR followed by a femoral-femoral crossover graft

E. Urgent open AAA repair via a retroperitoneal approach

43. An 82-year-old frail gentleman with multiple medical comorbidities presents with chronic limb-threatening ischaemia of the right leg. He has wet gangrene of his hallux with severe rest pain and night pain. He only has a femoral pulse. He has scars on his right medial leg from vein harvesting for a previous coronary artery bypass. His WIfI stage is 4. An MRA reveals diffuse stenotic disease of his right SFA. His below-knee

popliteal artery looks healthy and he has 2-vessel run-off down to the foot. What is the most appropriate management plan?

A. Plan for a right below-knee amputation.

B. Plan for a right femoral below-knee popliteal artery bypass using PTFE with a Miller cuff.

C. Plan for a right SFA angioplasty +/− stenting followed by hallux amputation.

D. Plan to amputate the right hallux and only revascularise if there are signs of poor wound healing.

E. Plan for palliative care only.

44. A 74-year-old patient is discussed in the vascular MDT. The patient had an infra-renal EVAR last year and the most recent surveillance imaging has reconfirmed a type 2 endoleak. The aortic sac has increased in size by 9 mm since the last scan. What is the most appropriate management plan?

A. Continue to monitor the patient with no current plans for intervention.

B. Plan for embolisation of relevant feeding vessels (e.g., inferior mesenteric artery/ lumbar vessels).

C. Plan for midline laparotomy and oversewing of the inferior mesenteric artery and any back bleeding lumbar vessels.

D. Plan for laparoscopic clipping of the inferior mesenteric artery +/− any lumbar vessels.

E. Advise the patient that type 2 endoleak is completely benign and no intervention will ever be required.

45. A 64-year-old patient presents to the diabetic foot clinic with a large "sausage" left hallux. The entire hallux is massively swollen and hot to the touch. There is a large ulcer at the tip of the hallux that is discharging pus, and the underlying hallux bone is visible at the base of the ulcer. An X-ray and an MRI confirm advanced osteomyelitic destruction of the distal phalanx. The patient has foot pulses and is systemically well. However, the hallux has an awful smell. What is the most appropriate management plan?

A. Long term intravenous antibiotics (i.e. 6 weeks) and outpatient follow-up once the antibiotic course is completed.

B. Hallux amputation.

C. Local debridement of the hallux tip in the foot clinic treatment room and plan for repeat clinical review after the weekend.

D. Amputation of the distal phalanx of the toe and primary closure.

E. Refer to the orthopaedic team on-call to see if the hallux can be salvaged.

46. A 34-year-old woman post-partum has an ultrasound-confirmed left femoral-popliteal DVT. She has a moderately swollen left leg but no signs of phlegmasia. She is not in pain. She is systemically well. She is 3 days post-partum following an emergency caesarean section. The patient is not known to have any bleeding problems and her caesarean section wound seems to be healing well. The obstetric team are happy for her to have therapeutic anticoagulation. What is the most appropriate management plan?

A. Plan for catheter-directed thrombolysis +/− iliac vein stenting

B. Plan for limb elevation alone

C. Plan for a femoral vein thrombectomy and IVC filter insertion

D. Plan for systemic intravenous thrombolysis

E. Plan for limb elevation and therapeutic anticoagulation +/− compression stockings

47. A 47-year-old gentleman presents with superficial thrombophlebitis of his right great saphenous vein. There is inflammation and erythema around the medial aspect of the mid-calf and lower thigh. An ultrasound confirms no underlying DVT, and there is a 10-cm length of thrombophlebitic GSV from the mid-calf to the lower thigh. The whole GSV is confirmed to have underlying reflux. What is the most appropriate management plan?

    A. Commence the patient on 45 days of fondaparinux 2.5 mg OD +/− NSAID treatment, with a plan for outpatient follow-up in a few weeks' time to consider intervention.

    B. Take the patient to theatre for emergency ligation of the right saphenofemoral junction and GSV stripping.

    C. Reassure the patient and recommend limb elevation and paracetamol.

    D. Commence the patient on lifelong warfarin.

    E. Do a local anaesthetic cut-down of the GSV in the mid thigh and ligate it to prevent the inflammatory process from spreading upwards.

48. A patient is 8-hour post-op following an emergency open AAA repair which was performed for a ruptured 9-cm infra-renal AAA. The patient had a tube graft repair and the abdomen was closed. The patient is now in intensive care. You are called to see the patient because his renal function is deteriorating, his ventilation requirements are increasing, his noradrenaline requirements are increasing, his lactate is climbing, and his abdomen is more distended and tense. The haemoglobin is around 100 and is not dropping. The abdominal compartment pressure is 32 mmHg. What is the most appropriate management plan?

    A. Optimise analgesia, nasogastric tube insertion, neuromuscular blockade, furosemide, and optimise ventilation.

    B. Transfuse more blood, aiming for a haemoglobin of 120.

    C. Arrange for an urgent flexible sigmoidoscopy to diagnose suspected left colonic ischaemia.

    D. Arrange for an urgent CT angiogram to check there is no intra-abdominal bleeding.

    E. Urgent decompressive laparotomy.

49. A 68-year-old gentleman is in the coronary care unit following an emergency PCI for an ST-segment elevation myocardial infarction. The cardiologists gained access via the right femoral artery under ultrasound. You have been asked to see the patient because of hypotension. You examine the patient and the groin looks unremarkable. However, the patient is complaining of back pain. His blood pressure is 80/40 mmHg with a heart rate of 110. What is the most appropriate plan?

    A. Rush the patient to theatre for a laparotomy.

    B. Resuscitate the patient and arrange for an urgent CT angiogram.

    C. Insert a REBOA catheter via the left groin and inflate in the infra-renal aorta, and then transfer the patient to interventional radiology for a covered stent insertion of a presumed left iliac artery retroperitoneal bleed.

    D. Transfer the patient immediately to theatre for a Rutherford Morrison incision and repair of a presumed external iliac artery bleed.

    E. Tell the cardiologists that the groin looks reassuring so this hypotension must be cardiac re-related.

50. A 68-year-old gentleman is admitted to the surgical assessment unit 2-week post-op following a right femoral endarterectomy for chronic limb-threatening ischaemia. The patient had a bovine patch repair. The patient is systemically unwell with fevers and sweats. He has a WBC of 20 and a CRP of 300. The right groin wound is erythematous and there is purulent fluid pouring from a sinus in the centre of the wound. What is the most appropriate management plan?

   A. Take a wound swab and confidently stick it right into the heart of the wound and give it a good "shake and stir."

   B. Do not probe the wound at all, and arrange for an urgent CT angiogram.

   C. Ask the vascular surgery core trainee to take the patient to theatre for wound exploration/incision and drainage of abscess.

   D. Refer the patient to interventional radiology for ultrasound-guided aspiration of a suspected superficial wound collection.

   E. Reassure the patient, commence him on oral antibiotics, and bring him for outpatient review in 1 week.

END OF EXAMINATION

CHAPTER 45

Answers

1. D – This patient required a guillotine amputation. Around a week later, this was converted to a BKA.

2. B – Do the basic first aid measures first of all in the resus bay. That is the point of the primary survey.

3. C – In this book, claudication equals conservative management.

4. A – This is a delayed presentation of what is likely an embolic event. I would anticoagulate her and investigate why this happened.

5. D – The airway is the first priority in my opinion.

6. C – This chap just needs to go to theatre for a laparotomy.

7. D – Low WIfI score in a frail comorbid elderly patient means sensible decision time in my book.

8. B – No doubt she is heading for an amputation. But don't rush into this unless you have to.

9. A – Think pancreatitis.

10. C – Sounds like left-sided ischaemic colitis. Do a flexi sigmoidoscopy.

11. E – Don't panic. Get some help, proximal control, resuscitate, and theatre.

12. D – The best surgeons know when not to operate.

13. C – This was a difficult case and there was some pressure on me to proceed straight to bilateral BKAs. In the medical notes I documented that I thought the patient would ultimately require bilateral BKAs, and that I thought this should be the definitive plan from the outset. However, I resisted the temptation to go straight for bilateral BKAs, and got further input from orthoplastics after discussion with an international expert in frostbite injury (thanks Chris). The patient got a left BKA and guillotine right Chopart amputation, followed by various plastic surgery attempts to salvage the right foot. These attempts were unsuccessful. The patient ultimately did require bilateral BKAs. I still think in this case, however, it was wise to give the orthoplastic surgeons a chance to try and achieve limb salvage on the right. If I had proceeded straight to bilateral BKAs in a young man with a possible limb salvage option, and not included orthoplastics in the discussion, I would likely have been open to significant criticism.

14. D – Very bad luck but myocardial infarction was the cause.

15. B – This has right colonic malignancy written all over it.

16. D – This is why patients with atrial fibrillation are anticoagulated. This patient clearly has an embolus in his SMA.

17. D – This needs explanting, and repair would ideally be autologous.

18. D – Looks perfect for left brachiocephalic fistula.

19. A – Claudication in my book means conservative management. This patient's severe rest pain and night pain was actually due to painful alcoholic neuropathy.

20. C – Managed to deal with this using Angioseal device and various balloons and wires (IR did it with me and my "buddy" waiting to do median sternotomy if required).

DOI: 10.1201/b22951-45

21. C – This is a trick. I am setting you up for an EVAR but want you to say open. He clearly doesn't need a suprarenal clamp.
22. D – Come on, this is ischaemic monomelic neuropathy. Ligate the graft.
23. C – Gave vitamin k, took my time, and went through old scar. Great result!
24. D – Come on, it is begging for a patch repair. Heparin = protamine.
25. D – If you sit on this, it is going to go bang!
26. D – How much easier can I make it for you?
27. D – Watch out for the trap. Left CEA and BMT!
28. D – C is a trap. Moral of the story is read the whole question and all the available answers properly!
29. D – Come on, we know this now.
30. B – This is a minimal aortic injury.
31. C – This was a difficult one, but if you go on cardiac bypass first, the femoral access site will just bleed, and the leg will probably end up ischaemic. You go first, cardiac surgery second.
32. A – Trust me, if you find yourself in this exact situation, just go back to theatre not for CT. The ESVS guidelines are correct.
33. C – Why are you doing this case on your own in the first place? Just stop before you make the situation worse and call for help.
34. B – This is non-salvageable and terminal. You should not be revascularising dead legs anyways.
35. C – Common sense. The appendicitis is the acute issue that needs to be addressed, so let general surgery take some ownership here. The AAA can be dealt with afterwards.
36. C – In this case, the patient has a ruptured thoracoabdominal aortic aneurysm. If you go straight to theatre, prepare for a nasty surprise when you try to get proximal control. My advice with ruptured AAAs is this: **DON'T FLY BLIND**.
37. D – Read chapter on vascular trauma.
38. E – If you do thrombolysis for this, you will trash the run-off. Just go to theatre, do a bypass via medial approach, and do a fasciotomy.
39. C – This angiogram was screaming out for a pop-plantar bypass and this was what was done. Great result!
40. B – This was an intimidating case. No messing around. Permissive hypotension, get over to this A&E right now. Groin exploration revealed suture line erosion with right graft limb thrombosed. Ligation and no reconstruction. Patient required right AKA shortly afterwards. Microbiology samples confirmed it was infected. CT showed entire aortic graft was infected and patient ultimately went for explant.
41. E – Good luck getting proximal control in the groin. Please don't reconstruct.
42. B – As per IMPROVE trial, generally EVAR is better for ruptures, and more so in women.
43. C – This is begging for endovascular intervention.
44. B – Type 2 endoleak may be benign, but if associated with sac expansion, it is more sinister.
45. B – I have told you the entire hallux is involved. The patient needs a hallux amputation.
46. E – Femoral-popliteal DVTs don't get thrombolysis in my book.

47. A – ESVS and NICE would support option A.

48. E – This is advanced abdominal compartment syndrome. Open the abdomen urgently.

49. B – Watch out for these cases. Chances are this is a retroperitoneal haematoma, but it could be something else like cardiogenic shock. Take a step back and think of the differential diagnosis before rushing into a potentially unnecessary and risky intervention. Maybe people think otherwise but I say CT first.

50. B – If you play "shake and stir" with Club Tropicana playing in the background, be prepared for a big party with a load of bright red blood in your face (talk about ordering a Bloody Mary). You may think this is a joke, but it isn't. I know of cases when this has happened. Moral of the story is this → don't poke skunks.

Key References for Book

These are the key references/resources that I have mainly used for the creation of this book. When I did my FRCS Examination, particularly Part B, these were the main resources for my revision efforts. When I was actually in the Part B Examination I would frequently quote recommendations and conclusions from these guidelines and papers by name. I heavily use these guidelines and papers throughout this book not because I am plagiarising, but because I want to bring authority and credibility to this work. Otherwise, without these papers and guideline recommendations, this would just be a book of me expressing my opinions (*and frankly who cares about my opinions without authoritative justification*). Indeed, this was my exact approach for the examination, and for my current day-to-day clinical practice. These guidelines and key papers in my opinion represent a compass for your vascular surgery practice, and they should help you to remain facing true north. They do not answer every question, and one must remember that they are only guidelines and papers, so don't blindly adhere to them if the clinical scenario does not correlate. They are useful, however, and have been written by highly credible authors with a lot of knowledge and experience. I have also included some great books and podcasts that I have found really helpful.

Instead of referencing these resources hundreds of times, I am just going to do it once and for all here.

KEY GUIDELINES

Abdominal aortic aneurysm: Diagnosis and management [Internet]. Nice.org.uk. 2020 [cited 19 January 2022]. Available from: https://www.nice.org.uk/guidance/ng156

Björck M, Earnshaw JJ, Acosta S et al. Editor's Choice—European Society for Vascular Surgery (ESVS) 2020 Clinical Practice Guidelines on the Management of Acute Limb Ischaemia. Eur J Vasc Endovasc Surg (2020) 59(2), 173–218.

Björck M, Koelemay M, Acosta S et al. Editor's Choice—Management of the Diseases of Mesenteric Arteries and Veins: Clinical Practice Guidelines of the European Society of Vascular Surgery (ESVS). Eur J Vasc Endovasc Surg (2017) 53(4), 460–510.

Chakfé N, Diener H, Lejay A et al. Editor's Choice—European Society for Vascular Surgery (ESVS) 2020 Clinical Practice Guidelines on the Management of Vascular Graft and Endograft Infections. Eur J Vasc Endovasc Surg (2020) 59(3), 339–384.

Conte MS, Bradbury AW, Kolh P et al. Global Vascular Guidelines on the Management of Chronic Limb-Threatening Ischemia. Eur J Vasc Endovasc Surg (2019) 58, S1–S109.

De Maeseneer MG, Kakkos SK, Aherne T et al. European Society for Vascular Surgery (ESVS) 2022 Clinical Practice Guidelines on the Management of Chronic Venous Disease of the Lower Limbs. Eur J Vasc Endovasc Surg (2022) 63(2), 184–267

Good medical practice [Internet]. Gmc-uk.org. 2019 [cited 19 January 2022]. Available from: https://www.gmc-uk.org/ethical-guidance/ethical-guidance-for-doctors/good-medical-practice

Good Surgical Practice—Royal College of Surgeons [Internet]. Royal College of Surgeons. 2014 [cited 19 January 2022]. Available from: https://www.rcseng.ac.uk/standards-and-research/gsp/

Kakkos SK, Gohel M, Baekgaard N et al. Editor's Choice—European Society for Vascular Surgery (ESVS) 2021 Clinical Practice Guidelines on the Management of Venous Thrombosis. Eur J Vasc Endovasc Surg (2021) 61, 9–82.

Lower limb peripheral arterial disease—NICE Pathways [Internet]. Pathways.nice.org.uk. 2021 [cited 19 January 2022]. Available from: https://pathways.nice.org.uk/pathways/lower-limb-peripheral-arterial-disease

Naylor AR, Ricco JB, de Borst GJ et al. Editor's Choice—Management of Atherosclerotic Carotid and Vertebral Artery Disease: 2017 Clinical Practice Guidelines of the European Society for Vascular Surgery (ESVS). Eur J Vasc Endovasc Surg (2018) 55(1), 3–81.

Riambau V, Böckler D, Brunkwall J et al. Editor's Choice—Management of Descending Thoracic Aorta Diseases: Clinical Practice Guidelines of the European Society for Vascular Surgery (ESVS). Eur J Vasc Endovasc Surg (2017) 53(1), 4–52.

Schmidli J, Widmer MK, Basile C et al. Editor's Choice—Vascular Access: 2018 Clinical Practice Guidelines of the European Society for Vascular Surgery (ESVS). Eur J Vasc Endovasc Surg (2018) 55(6), 757–818.

Wanhainen A, Verzini F, Van Herzeele I et al. Editor's Choice—European Society for Vascular Surgery (ESVS) 2019 Clinical Practice Guidelines on the Management of Abdominal Aorto-iliac Artery Aneurysms. Eur J Vasc Endovasc Surg (2019) 57(1), 8–93.

Varicose veins in the legs—NICE Pathways [Internet]. Pathways.nice.org.uk. 2020 [cited 19 January 2022]. Available from: https://pathways.nice.org.uk/pathways/varicose-veins-in-the-legs

KEY PAPERS

Adam DJ, Beard JD, Cleveland T et al. Bypass versus Angioplasty in Severe Ischaemia of the Leg (BASIL): Multicentre, Randomised Controlled Trial. Lancet (2005) 366(9501), 1925–1934.

Ahmad N, Thomas GN, Gill P et al. Lower Limb Amputation in England: Prevalence, Regional Variation and Relationship with Revascularisation, Deprivation and Risk Factors. A Retrospective Review of Hospital Data. J R Soc Med (2014) 107(12), 483–489.

Anand SS, Bosch J, Eikelboom JW et al. Rivaroxaban with or without Aspirin in Patients with Stable Peripheral or Carotid Artery Disease: An International, Randomised, Double-Blind, Placebo-Controlled Trial. Lancet (2018) 391(10117), 219–229.

Antithrombotic Trialists' Collaboration. Collaborative Meta-Analysis of Randomised Trials of Antiplatelet Therapy for Prevention of Death, Myocardial Infarction, and Stroke in High-Risk Patients. BMJ (2002) 324(7329), 71–86.

Belch JJ, Dormandy J, Biasi GM et al. Results of the Randomized, Placebo-Controlled Clopidogrel and Acetylsalicylic Acid in Bypass Surgery for Peripheral Arterial Disease (CASPAR) Trial. J Vasc Surg (2010) 52(4), 825–833.

Bonaca MP, Bauersachs RM, Anand SS et al. Rivaroxaban in Peripheral Artery Disease after Revascularization. N Engl J Med (2020) 382(21), 1994–2004.

Bradbury AW, Adam DJ, Bell J et al. Bypass versus Angioplasty in Severe Ischaemia of the Leg (BASIL) Trial: Analysis of Amputation Free and Overall Survival by Treatment Received. J Vasc Surg (2010) 51(5), 18S–31S.

Brittenden J, Cotton SC, Elders A et al. A Randomized Trial Comparing Treatments for Varicose Veins. N Engl J Med (2014) 371(13), 1218–1227.

Brittenden J, Cooper D, Dimitrova M et al. Five-Year Outcomes of a Randomized Trial of Treatments for Varicose Veins. N Engl J Med (2019) 381(10), 912–922.

Broderick C, Watson L, Armon MP. Thrombolytic Strategies versus Standard Anticoagulation for Acute Deep Vein Thrombosis of the Lower Limb. Cochrane Database Syst Rev (2021) 1(1), CD002783.

Brunkwall J, Kasprzak P, Verhoeven E et al. Endovascular Repair of Acute Uncomplicated Aortic Type B Dissection Promotes Aortic Remodelling: 1-Year Results of the ADSORB Trial. Eur J Vasc Endovasc Surg (2014) 48(3), 285–291.

CAPRIE Steering Committee. A Randomised, Blinded, Trial of Clopidogrel versus Aspirin in Patients at Risk of Ischaemic Events (CAPRIE). Lancet (1996) 348(9038), 1329–1339.

Comerota AJ, Kearon C, Gu CS et al (ATTRACT Trial Investigators). Endovascular Thrombus Removal for Acute Iliofemoral Deep Vein Thrombosis. Circulation (2019) 139(9), 1162–1173.

Dutch Bypass Oral anticoagulants or Aspirin (BOA) Study Group. Efficacy of Oral Anticoagulants Compared with Aspirin after Infrainguinal Bypass Surgery (The Dutch Bypass Oral Anticoagulants or Aspirin Study): A Randomised Trial. Lancet (2000) 355(9201), 346–351.

GALA Trial Collaborative Group. General Anaesthesia versus Local Anaesthesia for Carotid Surgery (GALA): A Multicentre, Randomised Controlled Trial. Lancet (2008) 372(9656), 2132–2142.

Gohel MS, Barwell JR, Taylor M et al. Long Term Results of Compression Therapy Alone versus Compression Plus Surgery in Chronic Venous Ulceration (ESCHAR): Randomised Controlled Trial. BMJ (2007) 335(7610), 83.

Gohel MS, Heatley F, Liu X et al (EVRA Trial Investigators). A Randomized Trial of Early Endovenous Ablation in Venous Ulceration. N Engl J Med (2018) 378(22), 2105–2114.

Gohel MS, Mora MSc J, Szigeti M et al. Long term Clinical and Cost-Effectiveness of Early Endovenous Ablation in Venous Ulceration: A Randomized Clinical Trial. JAMA Surg (2020) 155(12), 1113–1121.

Golledge J, Moxon JV, Rowbotham S et al. Risk of Major Amputation in Patients with Intermittent Claudication Undergoing Early Revascularization. Br J Surg (2018) 105(6), 699–708.

Harrison SC, Winterbottom AJ, Coughlin PA et al. Editor's Choice—Mid-Term Migration and Device Failure Following Endovascular Aneurysm Sealing with the Nellix Stent Graft System—A Single Centre Experience. Eur J Vasc Endovasc Surg (2018) 56(3), 342–348.

Heart Protection Study Collaborative Group. MRC/BHF Heart Protection Study of Cholesterol Lowering with Simvastatin in 20,536 High-Risk Individuals: A Randomised Placebo-Controlled Trial. Lancet (2002) 360(9326), 7–22.

IMPROVE Trial Investigators. Comparative Clinical Effectiveness and Cost Effectiveness of Endovascular Strategy v Open Repair for Ruptured Abdominal Aortic Aneurysm: Three-Year Results of the IMPROVE Randomised Trial. BMJ (2017) 359, j4859.

Jones AD, Waduud MA, Walker P et al. Meta-Analysis of Fenestrated Endovascular Aneurysm Repair versus Open Surgical Repair of Juxtarenal Abdominal Aortic Aneurysms over the Last 10 Years. BJS Open (2019) 3(5), 572–584.

Liu Y, Yang Y, Zhao J et al. Systematic Review and Meta-Analysis of Sex Differences in Outcomes after Endovascular Aneurysm Repair for Infrarenal Abdominal Aortic Aneurysm. J Vasc Surg (2020) 71(1), 283–296.

Mills JL Sr, Conte MS, Armstrong DG et al. The Society for Vascular Surgery Lower Extremity Threatened Limb Classification System: Risk Stratification Based on Wound, Ischemia, and Foot Infection (WIfI). J Vasc Surg (2014) 59(1), 220–234.

Multicentre Aneurysm Screening Study Group. Multicentre Aneurysm Screening Study (MASS): Cost Effectiveness Analysis of Screening for Abdominal Aortic Aneurysms Based on Four-Year Results from Randomised Controlled Trial. BMJ (2002) 325(7373), 1135.

Nienaber CA, Rousseau H, Eggebrecht H et al. Randomized Comparison of Strategies for Type B Aortic Dissection: The INvestigation of STEnt Grafts in Aortic Dissection (INSTEAD) Trial. Circulation (2009) 120(25), 2519–2528.

Nienaber CA, Kische S, Rousseau H et al. Endovascular Repair of Type B Aortic Dissection: Long Term Results of the Randomized Investigation of Stent Grafts in Aortic Dissection Trial. Circ Cardiovasc Interv (2013) 6(4), 407–416.

Patel R, Powell JT, Sweeting MJ et al. The UK EndoVascular Aneurysm Repair (EVAR) Randomised Controlled Trials: Long Term Follow-Up and Cost-Effectiveness Analysis. Health Technol Assess (2018) 22(5), 1–132

Powell JT, Brown LC, Forbes JF et al. Final 12-Year Follow-Up of Surgery versus Surveillance in the UK Small Aneurysm Trial. Br J Surg (2007) 94(6), 702–708.

Powell JT, Sweeting MJ, Thompson MM et al. Endovascular or Open Repair Strategy for Ruptured Abdominal Aortic Aneurysm: 30 Day Outcomes from IMPROVE Randomised Trial. BMJ (2014) 348, f7661.

Powell JT, Sweeting MJ, Ulug P et al. EVAR-1, DREAM, OVER and ACE Trialists. Meta-Analysis of Individual-Patient Data from EVAR-1, DREAM, OVER and ACE Trials Comparing Outcomes of Endovascular or Open Repair for Abdominal Aortic Aneurysm over 5 Years. Br J Surg (2017) 104(3), 166–178.

Rantner B, Kollerits B, Roubin GS et al (Carotid Stenosis Trialists' Collaboration). Early Endarterectomy Carries a Lower Procedural Risk Than Early Stenting in Patients with Symptomatic Stenosis of the Internal Carotid Artery: Results from 4 Randomized Controlled Trials. Stroke (2017) 48(6), 1580–1587.

Rerkasem A, Orrapin S, Howard DP, Rerkasem K. Carotid Endarterectomy for Symptomatic Carotid Stenosis. Cochrane Database Syst Rev (2020) 9(9), CD001081.

Rothwell PM, Gutnikov SA, Warlow CP (European Carotid Surgery Trialist's Collaboration). Reanalysis of the Final Results of the European Carotid Surgery Trial. Stroke (2003) 34(2), 514–523.

Sofat S, Chen X, Chowdhury MM & Coughlin PA. Effects of Statin Therapy and Dose on Cardiovascular and Limb Outcomes in Peripheral Arterial Disease: A Systematic Review and Meta-Analysis. Eur J Vasc Endovasc Surg (2021) 62(3), 450–461.

Thompson SG, Ashton HA, Gao L et al. Final Follow-Up of the Multicentre Aneurysm Screening Study (MASS) Randomized Trial of Abdominal Aortic Aneurysm Screening. Br J Surg (2012) 99(12), 1649–1656.

Thorbjørnsen K, Djavani Gidlund K, Björck M et al. Editor's Choice—Long Term Outcome after EndoVAC Hybrid Repair of Infected Vascular Reconstructions. Eur J Vasc Endovasc Surg (2016) 51(5), 724–32.

Vedantham S, Goldhaber SZ, Julian JA et al (ATTRACT Trial Investigators). Pharmacomechanical Catheter-Directed Thrombolysis for Deep-Vein Thrombosis. N Engl J Med (2017) 377(23), 2240–2252.

Veith FJ, Gupta SK, Ascer E et al. Six-Year Prospective Multicenter Randomized Comparison of Autologous Saphenous Vein and Expanded Polytetrafluoroethylene Grafts in Infrainguinal Arterial Reconstructions. J Vasc Surg (1986) 3(1), 104–114.

Valenti D, Mistry H, Stephenson M. A Novel Classification System for Autogenous Arteriovenous Fistula Aneurysms in Renal Access Patients. Vasc Endovascular Surg (2014) 48(7–8), 491–496

KEY BOOKS

Hirshberg A, Mattox K. Top Knife. 1st ed. Castle Hill Barns, Shrewsbury: TFM Publishing; 2014.

Khan M, McMonagle M. Trauma: Code Red. 1st ed. Milton: CRC Press; 2018.

Sidawy A, Perler B. Rutherford's Vascular Surgery and Endovascular Therapy. 9th ed. Philadelphia, PA: Elsevier; 2019.

PODCASTS

Behind the Knife: The Surgery Podcast. 2022. Big T Trauma Archives—Behind the Knife: The Surgery Podcast. [online] Available at: <https://behindtheknife.org/podcast-series/big-t-trauma/> [Accessed 21 January 2022].

Behind the Knife: The Surgery Podcast. 2022. The Premier Surgery Podcast | Surgical Education | Behind The Knife—Behind the Knife: The Surgery Podcast. [online] Available at: <https://behindtheknife.org/> [Accessed 21 January 2022].

Rasmussen, T., 2022. Vascular Trauma 1—Peripheral. [online] Audible Bleeding: The Vascular Surgery Podcast. Available at: <https://www.audiblebleeding.com/trauma-peripheral/> [Accessed 21 January 2022].

Index

Note: Locators in *italics* represent figures and **bold** indicate tables in the text.

A

AAA, *see* Abdominal aortic aneurysms
ABCDE approach, 101, 201, 226, 227, 235
Abdominal aortic aneurysms (AAAs)
  endovascular strategy *vs.* open repair
    EVAR-1, DREAM, OVER and ACE trials, 27
    meta-analysis of individual-patient data, 27–28
  juxtarenal, *see* Juxtarenal AAA
  MASS, 21
  non-ruptured infra-renal
    aortic necks and access for EVAR, 107–109, *108, 109*
    ESVS Guideline Recommendations, 104–107
    examination, 103
    history, 103
    management plan, 103–104
    overview, 104, *105*
  ruptured, *see* Ruptured AAA
  ruptured infra-renal
    definitive management, 110
    ESVS Guideline Recommendations, 111–112
    examination, 110
    history, 109–110
    immediate management, 110
Above ankle amputation, *see* Guillotine amputation (above ankle)
Above-knee amputation, 2, 188, 275, 307; *see also* Amputation
  intra-operatively, 304–305
  post-operatively, 305
  pre-operatively, 304
ACE trial, 27–28
Acute iliofemoral deep vein thrombosis, 36
Acute limb ischaemia, 77; *see also* Ischaemia
  bilateral lower limb ischaemia (case), 95–97
  lower limb
    examination, 77
    history, 77
    relevant ESVS guideline recommendations, 78–79, 80
  Rutherford 2A left arm ischaemia (case), 84–87
  Rutherford 2B acute left leg ischaemia (case), 87–90
  Rutherford 2B acute right leg ischaemia (case), 90–92, 93–95
  thrombolysis (case), 99–102

thrombosed popliteal aneurysm (case), 97–99
  upper limb
    diagnosis and immediate work-up, 81
    relevant ESVS guideline recommendations, 81, 82
ADSORB trial, 30, 146
  aortic remodelling, 30
Amlodipine, 54, 63, 65, 123, 126, 141, 257, 265, 268
Amputation
  above ankle, *see* Guillotine amputation (above ankle)
  above-knee, *see* Above-knee amputation
  BASIL trial, 4
  below-knee, *see* Below-knee amputation
  hallux, *see* Hallux amputation
  intermittent claudication undergoing early revascularisation, 1–3
  lower limb amputation in England, 4–5
  transmetatarsal, *see* Transmetatarsal amputation
Angioplasty
  balloon, *see* Balloon angioplasty
  CFA, 75
  iliac, 75–76
  PT, 64
  SFA, 73–75, 88
Ankle brachial pressure index (ABPI), 47, 51, 55, 69, 134, 191, 194
Antiplatelet therapy, 11, 72, 79, 106, 149, 151, 155, 162, 238
  Antithrombotic Trialists' Collaboration, 10
  for prevention of death, myocardial infarction, and stroke, 10
Aorto-bifemoral bypass, 1, 338
Aortoiliac aneurysms
  AAA, *see* Abdominal aortic aneurysms
  complex juxtarenal AAA (case), 126–127
  EVAR complications (case), 128–130
  infra-renal AAA and chronic renal failure (case), 119–122
  standard percutaneous EVAR (case), 122–125
  symptomatic 7.5-cm infra-renal AAA (case), 116–119
Apixaban, 65, 66, 110
Aspirin
  after infra-inguinal bypass surgery, 13
  CAPRIE trial, 10–11
  Dutch Bypass Oral Anticoagulants or Aspirin Study, 13
  rivaroxaban with or without aspirin, 11

349

ATLS protocol, 227, 230, 232, 234–236, 240, 245, 247, 251
Atorvastatin, 47, 53, 54, 56, 63, 70, 87, 120, 123, 125, 126, 155, 211, 257, 261, 265, 268, 283, 285, 288
ATTRACT trial, 36, 201

B

Balloon angioplasty, 3, 4, 91, 129, 171–174, 178, 179, 184, 205, 212, 213; *see also* Angioplasty
BASIL (Bypass *versus* Angioplasty in Severe Ischaemia of Leg) Trial
  analysis of amputation and overall survival, 4
  RCT evidence, 3–4
Below-knee amputation, 306; *see also* Amputation
  intra-operatively, 306–307
  JMF reflections, 307–308
  post-operatively, 307
  pre-operatively, 306
BEST-CLTI trial, 57
Best medical treatment (BMT), 30
Bilateral lower limb ischaemia, 95–97
Bisoprolol, 116
Bottle-top crepe bandage technique, 177
Brachial embolectomy
  intra-operatively, 293–294
  post-operatively, 294
  pre-operatively, 293
  special points, 294–295
Brachiocephalic fistula creation
  intra-operatively, 317–319
  post-operatively, 319
  pre-operatively, 317
Button-hole technique, 174

C

Calliper placement, 104
CAPRIE (Clopidogrel *versus* Aspirin in Patients at Risk of Ischaemic Events) trial, 10–11, 56
Carotid Artery Risk Score (CAR score), 151
Carotid artery stenosis (CAS), 16–17
Carotid endarterectomy (CEA), 151
  antiplatelet therapy, 155
  infected carotid endarterectomy patch (case), 256–261
  intra-operatively, 278–280
  post-operatively, 281
  pre-operatively, 278
  stroke after, 153
  for symptomatic carotid stenosis, 16–17, 154–162
  technical aspects of, 152–153
CASPAR (Randomised, Placebo-Controlled Clopidogrel and Acetylsalicylic Acid in Bypass Surgery for Peripheral Arterial Disease) trial, 13–14

Catheter-directed thrombolysis (CDT), 34, 35
CAVA trial, 201
CaVenT trial, 201
CDT, *see* Catheter-directed thrombolysis
CEA, *see* Carotid endarterectomy
CFA, *see* Common femoral artery
CFV, *see* Common femoral vein
Charcot foot deformity, 65
Chronic limb-threatening ischaemia (CLTI), 69; *see also* Ischaemia
  ESVS and NICE Guideline Recommendations, 69–70
  examination, 68–69
  following iliac angioplasty, 75–76
  history, 68
  multi-level SFA disease with tissue loss (case), 71–73
  right leg with tissue loss, failed previous SFA angioplasty (case), 73–75
  severe aortoiliac occlusive disease (case), 70–71
Chronic venous disease
  bilateral symptomatic varicose veins, 189–193
  deep venous obstruction (case), 196–198
  venous leg ulceration (case), 193–196
CIA, *see* Common iliac artery
CLASS (Randomised Trial of Treatments for Varicose Veins) trial, 30–31
Claudication
  calf, 153
  intermittent, *see* Intermittent claudication
  short distance, 54, 68, 70, 75, 77, 99, 100, 134
  venous, 197, 198
Clinical, Etiological, Anatomical, Pathophysiological (CEAP) classification, 30, 192, 194
Clopidogrel, 11–14, 51, 54, 56, 58, 68, 70, 71, 101, 103, 107, 120, 135, 150, 155, 156, 281
CLTI, *see* Chronic limb-threatening ischaemia
Cochrane review
  CEA for symptomatic carotid stenosis, 16–17
  thrombolytic strategies *vs.* standard anticoagulation for DVT, 36–37
Common femoral artery (CFA), 55, 57, 64, 70, 93, 104, 109, 122, 123, 134, 135, 187, 188, 205, 236–237, 237, 250, 284, 286, 289, 331
  angioplasty, 75
  distal CFA lumen, 94
  endarterectomy, 88–90, 109
  longitudinal arteriotomy, 94
Common femoral endarterectomy
  intra-operatively, 282–283
  post-operatively, 283
  pre-operatively, 282
Common femoral vein (CFV), 36, 75, 189, 190, 197, 201, 202, 204, 237, 312, 314

Common iliac artery (CIA), 90, 114–115, 123, 206, 221, 290
Compartment syndrome (lower limb)
 examination, 83
 history, 83
 relevant ESVS guideline recommendations, 83
COMPASS trial, 12, 56
Complex juxtarenal AAA, 126–127
Compression therapy, 32–34, 33, 194, 196
Computed tomography (CT), 23–24, 52, 76, 104, 111, 113, 117, 138, 155, 179
Computed tomography angiogram (CTA), 52, 78, 104, 111, 113
Confidence interval (CI), 11, 12, 14, 19, 24, 29, 32, 34, 35, 37
Coronary heart disease, 5
Cox proportional hazard models, 2
Cox regression analysis, 32
CPEX testing, 117–118, 120, 123, 127
Crawford classification, 131, 132, 133
CREST trial, 16

D

Deep-vein thrombosis (DVT)
 acute iliofemoral, 36
 of lower limb, standard anticoagulation for, 36–37
 pharmacomechanical catheter-directed thrombolysis for, 34–35
Deep venous obstruction, 196–198
Descending thoracic aortic aneurysm
 case study, 140–144
 incidental finding of asymptomatic 9 cm (case), 137–139
 ruptured (case), 139–140
Diabetes, 1, 5, 8, 47, 52, 54, 59, 63, 64, 87, 97, 104, 126, 153, 159, 160, 180, 208, 214, 219, 257, 265, 268
Diabetic foot disease
 fulminant diabetic foot sepsis (case), 65–67
 examination, 65
 FRCS question time, 66
 history, 65
 JMF reflections, 67
 Dutch Bypass Oral Anticoagulants or Aspirin Study, 13
 neuroischaemia 2 (case), 63–65
 JMF reflections, 58–59
 Relevant ESVS Guideline Recommendations, 57–58
 neuropathy 1 (case), 59–62
 JMF reflections, 62–63
Documentation
 clear, 41
 importance of, 40
 recommendations/principles, 40
Doppler waveforms, 134

DREAM trial, 27–28
DRIL (distal revascularisation interval ligation), 182, 183
Dutch Bypass Oral Anticoagulants, 13
DVT, see Deep-vein thrombosis

E

Early endarterectomy
 randomised controlled trials, 16
 symptomatic stenosis of internal carotid artery, 16
Early venous reflux ablation (EVRA) trial
 early endovenous ablation in venous ulceration, 33–34
 long term clinical and cost-effectiveness of, 34
 randomised trial of, 33–34
Echocardiogram, 70, 104, 120, 123, 127, 141, 186, 219, 232, 273, 290, 294
ECST trial, 15, 157
EIA, see External iliac artery
Endoleaks, 19
 risk of, 17
 type 2, 26–27, 129–130
 type 1A, 18, 107–108, 119, 128–129
 type 1B, 18
EndoVac technique, 260–261
Endovascular aneurysm repair (EVAR)
 Achilles heel, 17
 EVAR-1, 27–28
 EVAR-2, 25, 26
 for infrarenal AAA, 18–19
 long term follow-up and cost-effectiveness analysis, 25–27
Endovascular intervention, 1, 56, 59, 68, 69, 73, 78, 137, 157, 172, 173, 212, 213, 241, 295
Endovascular strategy vs. open surgical repair
 for abdominal aortic aneurysm
  EVAR-1, DREAM, OVER and ACE trials, 27–28
  meta-analysis of individual-patient data, 27–28
 of juxtarenal abdominal aortic aneurysms, 20–21
 for ruptured abdominal aortic aneurysm
  comparative clinical effectiveness and cost effectiveness of, 24–25
  randomised trial, 24–25
ESCHAR (compression therapy alone vs. compression plus surgery in chronic venous ulceration), 31–32
ESVS Guideline Recommendations, 69–70
European Carotid Surgery Trial, 15
EVA-3S trial, 16
Exercise
 programme, 1, 52–53, 326
 testing, 106, 117, 120, 273
 tolerance, 47, 54, 59, 123, 126, 141, 143, 211, 257, 261, 265, 268

External iliac artery (EIA), 70, 75, 90, 93, 102, 114–115, 187, 238, 271, 282–283

F

Femoral above-knee popliteal bypass (reversed ipsilateral GSV)
  intra-operatively, 284–285
  post-operatively, 285
  pre-operatively, 284
Femoral below-knee popliteal bypass (reversed ipsilateral GSV)
  intra-operatively, 286–287
  post-operatively, 287–288
  pre-operatively, 286
Femoral embolectomy
  intra-operatively, 289–290
  post-operatively, 290
  pre-operatively, 289
  special point, 290
Femoropopliteal artery of leg
  paclitaxel-coated balloons and stents in, 7–8
  risk of death following application of, 7–8
Femoropopliteal bypasses, 2, 7
FEVAR (fenestrated endovascular aneurysm repair) cohort, 20–21
Fishmouth incision method, 304
Fistula aneurysm, 169–171
Fistula planning assessment, 163–166
Foot debridement
  intra-operatively, 300
  post-operatively, 300–301
  pre-operatively, 300
FRCS exam, 1, 39, 43–44, 45, 68, 73, 86–87, 94, 103, 134, 153, 163, 177, 189, 223, 256, 345
Fulminant diabetic foot sepsis, 65–67
  examination, 65
  FRCS question time, 66
  history, 65
  JMF reflections, 67
Furosemide, 48, 63

G

Gangrene, 3, 6, 47, 51, 55, 68, 69, 71, 73, 180, 268
General Anaesthesia versus Local Anaesthesia for Carotid Surgery (GALA), 14–15
Good Medical Practice, 42
Good Surgical Practice, 42–43
GRADE methods, 37
Great saphenous vein (GSV)
  bilateral GSV distribution, 190
  endovenous ablation
    intra-operatively, 311–312
    post-operatively, 312
    pre-operatively, 311

reversed ipsilateral GSV, 284–288
stripping
  intra-operatively, 313–314
  post-operatively, 314
  pre-operatively, 313
GTN spray, 87, 261
Guillotine amputation (above ankle), 66; see also Amputation
  foot debridement, 66–67
  intra-operatively, 309–310
  post-operatively, 310
  pre-operatively, 309

H

Haematoma, 239–240
Hallux amputation, 298; see also Amputation
  intra-operatively, 298
  post-operatively, 298–299
  pre-operatively, 298
HALO effect, 312
Hazard ratio (HR), 11, 12, 14, 19, 23, 27, 29, 32, 34, 118
Home-based exercise programme, 1
Hospital Episode Statistics (HES) database, 4
Hypertension, 5, 47, 52, 53, 56, 58, 65, 87, 93, 97, 104, 112, 116, 123, 126, 139, 141, 146, 149, 153, 156, 157, 160, 161, 162, 180, 208, 211, 214, 219, 257, 261, 265, 268

I

ICSS trial, 16
Ileo-femoral DVT, 199–202
Iliac artery aneurysms
  background, 114
  basic management principles, 115
  clinical presentation, 114–115
  endovascular repair, 115
  ESVS Guideline Recommendations, 116
  open surgical repair, 115
  pelvic circulation, 116
IMPROVE (open vs. endovascular repair) trial, 23
Indices of Multiple Deprivation 2010 (IMD) score, 4
Infected carotid endarterectomy patch, 256–261
Infected prosthetic femoral-distal bypass, 268–272
Infrainguinal arterial reconstructions, 6–7
Infra-inguinal bypasses, 3, 6, 13, 58, 78
Infra-renal AAA and chronic renal failure, 119–122
Insulin, 49, 59, 63, 268; see also Diabetes
Intermittent claudication, 7, 12, 59, 63, 100, 211, 214, 331
  examination, 51
  history, 51
  management plan, 52–53
  management plan, NICE Guidelines 2021, 52
  revascularisation with intermittent claudication, 52

risk of amputation, 1–3
undergoing early revascularisation, 1–3
Internal carotid artery (ICA) stenosis, 16, 150, 153, 154, 156–158, 160, 242–244, 258, 259, 260, 279, 280
Internal iliac artery (IIA), 90, 114–116
Intravenous thrombolysis (IVT), 161
Investigation of Stent Grafts in Aortic Dissection (INSTEAD) trial
  INSTEAD-XL trial
    endovascular repair of type B aortic dissection, 29
    long term results of randomised, 29
  strategies for type B dissection, 28–29
Ischaemia
  acute limb, see Acute limb ischaemia
  CLTI, see Chronic limb-threatening ischaemia
  mesenteric, 19, 93, 145, 211
  severe limb, 3, 4
  spinal cord, 93, 138, 146, 163
  upper limb, 93, 145, 294–295
Isosorbide mononitrate, 261
IVDU groin
  after fact, 188
  definitive management, 186
  examination, 185
  final crucial points, 188
  history, 185
  immediate management (hosing groin), 185–187
  other technical considerations, 187–188

J

Juxtarenal AAA, 112; see also Abdominal aortic aneurysms
  basic management principles, 112
  defined, 112
  endovascular strategy vs. open repair for, 112–113
  ESVS Guideline Recommendations, 113
  FEVAR vs. OSR, 20–21

K

Kaplan–Meier analysis, 2, 12, 29

L

Lansoprazole, 59
Levothyroxine, 257
Losartan, 126
Lower-limb fasciotomy
  intra-operatively, 296–297
  post-operatively, 297
  pre-operatively, 296
Lower limb ischaemia, 6, 81, 88, 93, 145; see also Ischaemia
  bilateral, 95–97

Lower limb venous thromboembolism
  ileo-femoral DVT (case), 199–202
  May-Thurner syndrome (case), 205–207
  Phlegmasia Cerula Dolens (case), 202–205
  superficial venous thrombosis (case), 207–210

M

Machete attack, 227–230
Major adverse cardiovascular events (MACE), 9
May-Thurner syndrome, 205–207
MDT, see Multidisciplinary team
Mesenteric ischaemia, 19, 93, 145, 211; see also Ischaemia
  acute, 217–222
  chronic, 211–217
Metformin, 54, 59, 63, 65, 87, 126, 265, 268
MI, see Myocardial infarction
MILLER procedure, 184, 184
Mini-MDT, 155, 160, 216
MRC/BHF Heart Protection Study of Cholesterol, 8–9
Multicentre Aneurysm Screening Study (MASS)
  cost effectiveness analysis of screening for AAA, 21
  final follow-up of, 22
  randomised trial of AAA screening, 22
  sex differences after endovascular aneurysm repair for infrarenal, 18–19
Multidisciplinary team (MDT)
  aortic, 109, 114, 120, 121, 123–125, 127, 142
  mini-MDT, 155, 160, 216
  vascular, 69, 76, 100, 118, 157, 158, 161, 188, 197, 198, 201, 207, 212, 214, 258, 260, 266, 272
Multiple stab avulsions
  anaesthetic for, 312
  intra-operatively, 313–314
  post-operatively, 314
  pre-operatively, 313
Myocardial infarction (MI), 2, 9–15, 10, 47, 71, 116, 137, 156, 159, 238, 239, 263, 277

N

NASCET trial, 15, 157
Nellix stent graft system, 17–18
Neuroischaemia, 54–57
  JMF reflections, 58–59
  Relevant ESVS Guideline Recommendations, 57–58
Neuroischaemia 2, 63–65
Neuroischaemic heel ulceration, 63–64
Neuropathic diabetic foot sepsis, 60, 66
Neuropathy 1, 59–63
NICE Guidelines
  intermittent claudication, management plan, 52

Recommendations, 69–70
for varicose veins, 191–192
Non-ruptured infra-renal
aortic necks and access for EVAR, 107–109, *108*, *109*
ESVS Guideline Recommendations, 104–107
examination, 103
history, 103
management plan, 103–104
overview of, 104, *105*
Non-ST segment myocardial infarction
(NSTEMI), 238

O

Odds ratio (OR), 19, 24–26
Open AAA repair (elective, infra-renal); *see also*
Abdominal aortic aneurysms
intra-operatively, 273–276
post-operatively, 276
pre-operatively, 273
reflections on open aortic surgery, 276–277
Open surgical repair (OSR), 143, 250
EVAR with, 25, 27
FEVAR *vs.,* 20
iliac artery aneurysms, 115
of ruptured AAA, 111
TAAA, 132
OR, *see* Odds ratio
Oral anticoagulants, 13
OSR, *see* Open surgical repair
OVER trial, 27–28
Oxford Risk Score, 151, 157

P

Paclitaxel-coated balloons or stents, 7–8
PAD, *see* Peripheral arterial disease
PAI, *see* Proximalisation of arterial inflow
Parachute technique, 275, 280, 283
Patient counselling, 38–39
PCDT, 36
Peripheral arterial disease (PAD), 2, 52, 75, 88, 180,
193, 299, 301, 303, 305, 307
CASPAR trial, 13–14
dose on cardiovascular and limb outcomes, 9
effects of statin therapy, 9
management, 5
Peritoneal dialysis tube insertion (open)
intra-operatively, 320–321
post-operatively, 321
pre-operatively, 320
Peritoneal dialysis tube removal
intra-operatively, 322–323
JMF reflections, 323–324
post-operatively, 323
pre-operatively, 322

PFA, *see* Profunda femoris artery
Phlegmasia Cerula Dolens, 202–205
Polytetrafluoroethylene (PTFE), 6, 7, 74, 99, 176,
181, 221, 242, 270
Popliteal aneurysm
examination, 134
history, 134
investigations (acute), 135
investigations (non-acute), 134
management (acute), 136
management (non-acute), 135
stenting, 135–136
Popliteal embolectomy
intra-operatively, 291–292
post-operatively, 292
pre-operatively, 291
Post-thrombotic syndrome (PTS), 34–35
Profunda femoris artery (PFA), 188, 282–284, 286,
289–290
origin of, 94, 187
Prosthetic bypass, 4, 73, 100, 101, 177, 269, 270, 272
Proximalisation of arterial inflow (PAI), 182
PTFE, *see* Polytetrafluoroethylene
PTS, *see* Post-thrombotic syndrome
Pulmonary function tests, 70, 104, 106, 117, 123,
141–142, 273

Q

Quality Adjusted Life Year (QALYs), 25

R

Radiofrequency ablation, 33, 312
Ramipril, 48, 54, 63, 87, 116, 123, 141, 208, 261, 265
Rankin score, 150, 151, 161, 162
Renal infarction, 93
Revascularisation
with intermittent claudication, 1–3, 52
rivaroxaban in peripheral artery disease after, 12–13
Revised Venous Clinical Severity Score (r-VCSS),
189, 192
Rivaroxaban
with or without aspirin with stable peripheral or
carotid artery disease, 11
in PAD after revascularisation (VOYAGER trial),
12–13
Rope ladder technique, 177
RUDI (revision using distal inflow), 182, *183*
Ruptured AAA, 23; *see also* Abdominal aortic
aneurysms
comparative clinical effectiveness and cost
effectiveness of, 24–25
endovascular strategy *vs.* open repair for, 23–25, 111
randomised trial, 24–25

Ruptured infra-renal
  definitive management, 110
  ESVS Guideline Recommendations, 111–112
  examination, 110
  history, 109–110
  immediate management, 110
Rutherford 2A left arm ischaemia, 84–87
Rutherford 2B acute left leg ischaemia, 87–90
Rutherford 2B acute right leg ischaemia, 90–95

S

Saphenofemoral junction (SFJ), 190, 193, 284, 286,
    311–314
  ligation
    intra-operatively, 313–314
    post-operatively, 314
    pre-operatively, 313
Saphenous vein bypass, 4, 79
Severe limb ischaemia, 3, 4; see also Ischaemia
SFA, see Superficial femoral artery
SFJ, see Saphenofemoral junction
Short saphenous vein (SSV), 32, 66, 189, 193, 307, 309
Simvastatin, 8–9, 65, 116, 125
Smoking cessation, 1, 52, 69, 70, 73, 100, 104, 112,
    115, 131, 149, 214, 217, 331
Snorkel or chimney technique, 138
Society for Vascular Surgery Lower Extremity
    Threatened Limb Classification System, 5–6
SPACE trial, 16
Spinal cord ischaemia, 93, 138, 146, 163; see also
    Ischaemia
SSV, see Short saphenous vein
Standard percutaneous EVAR, 122–125
Statin therapy
  and dose on cardiovascular and limb outcomes
    in PAD, 9
  systematic review and meta-analysis, 9
STEAL syndrome
  banding/plication, 181, 182
  DRIL (distal revascularisation interval ligation),
    182, 183
  MILLER procedure, 184, 184
  overview of management for vascular access, 181
  PAI (proximalisation of arterial inflow), 182
  principles, 180–181
  radial artery ligation or embolisation, 183–184
  RUDI (revision using distal inflow), 182, 183
Stenosis
  carotid artery, see Carotid artery stenosis
  of ICA, see Internal carotid artery stenosis
  symptomatic carotid, 16–17, 153–162
Stroke, 10
  after carotid endarterectomy, 153
  antiplatelet therapy for, 10

ipsilateral ischaemic stroke, 17, 157
ischaemic stroke, 10–11, 13
risk of, 15–17
Superficial femoral artery (SFA), 1–2, 47, 49, 51,
    55, 70, 98, 122, 187, 188, 234–235, 282–286,
    289–290, 305
  angioplasty, 73–75, 88
  lesion, 89
  multi-level SFA disease with tissue loss, 71–73
  origin of, 94
  stenosis, 89, 90
Superficial venous thrombosis (SVT), 207–210
Supervised exercise programme, 1, 52, 53, 326
Surgery-first strategy, 3
SVT, see Superficial venous thrombosis
Symptomatic carotid artery disease
  broad management overview, 152
  decision-making around carotid intervention
    (from ESVS Guidelines), 151
  definitive management options, 151
  examination, 150
  history, 150
  initial management, 150–151
  other considerations, 151–152
  stroke after carotid endarterectomy, 153
  symptomatic carotid stenosis (case), 153–162
  technical aspects of carotid endarterectomy,
    152–153
Symptomatic 7.5-cm infra-renal AAA, 116–119

T

TAAA, see Thoracoabdominal aortic aneurysm
Temporal artery biopsy
  intra-operatively, 315
  JMF reflections, 316
  post-operatively, 316
  pre-operatively, 315
TEVAR (thoracic endovascular aneurysm repair),
    28–30, 138–140, 142–144, 146, 148, 149,
    261–263
  access options for insertion, 140
  infected thoracic aortic stent, 261–265
  as local anaesthetic percutaneous
    approach, 142
Thoracoabdominal aortic aneurysm (TAAA), 20;
    see also Abdominal aortic aneurysms
  background, 131
  basic management principles, 131
  Crawford classification, 132
  endovascular repair, 132
  JMF reflections, 133
  open surgical repair, 132
  Relevant ESVS Guideline Recommendations,
    132–133

Thrombolysis
  acute limb ischaemia, 99–102
  catheter-directed, *see* Catheter-directed
    thrombolysis
Thrombolysis, 99–102
Thrombosed graft, 171–174
Thrombosed popliteal aneurysm, 97–99
Thyroxine, 47, 59, 257
Ticagrelor, 63, 64, 238
TORPEDO trial, 201
Transmetatarsal amputation, 302; *see also* Amputation
  intra-operatively, 302–303
  post-operatively, 303
  pre-operatively, 302
Type B aortic dissection
  acute (case), 145–147
  chronic (case), 147–149

U

UK EVAR Randomised Controlled Trials, *see*
    Early Venous Reflux Ablation trial
UK small aneurysm trial
  follow-up of, 22–23
  surgery *vs.* surveillance in, 22–23
Upper limb ischaemia, 93, 145, 294–295; *see also*
    Ischaemia

V

Vacuum-assisted closure (VAC) technique, 62, 64,
    67, 112, 187, 260, 261
Varicose veins
  bilateral symptomatic varicose veins, 189–193
  CLASS trial, 30–31
  comparing treatments, 31
  outcomes of, 31
VASCP trial, 157
Vascular access
  early access complication (case), 166–169
  failure to mature (case), 178–180
  fistula planning assessment (case), 163–166
  late access complications (case), 174–177
    fistula aneurysm (case), 169–171
    thrombosed graft (case), 171–174
  STEAL syndrome, 180–184
Vascular death, 9–13, 13
Vascular graft and endograft infection
  infected abdominal aortic stent (EVAR) (case),
    265–268
  infected carotid endarterectomy patch (case),
    256–261
  infected prosthetic femoral-distal bypass (case),
    268–272

infected thoracic aortic stent (TEVAR) (case),
    261–265
  overall baseline ESVS guideline
    recommendations, 256
Vascular MDT, 69, 76, 100, 118, 157, 158, 161, 188,
    197, 198, 201, 207, 212, 214, 258, 260, 266, 272
Vascular patient
  general principles, 45
  introductory statements, 45–46
  presentations, 46–50
Vascular trauma
  aortic transection/pseudoaneurysm, 232–234
  brachial artery laceration, 225–227
  central line iatrogenic injury to right subclavian
    artery, 250–251
  femoral artery bleeding, 235–238
  final comments on, 255
  gunshot wound, 251–252
  haematoma, 239–240
  iatrogenic injury to radial artery, 238–239
  ischaemic limb, 234–235
  laparoscopic port injury, 223–225
  left supraclavicular fossa, haemodynamically
    unstable, 247–249
  machete attack, 227–230
  open femur fracture with superficial femoral
    artery injury, 234–235
  pain with hypotension, 244–247
  principles of operative management of vascular
    injuries, 240–244
  stab wound, 230–232
  trauma surgery on axillosubclavian artery
    complex, 252–255
Venous Clinical Severity Score, 30, 35
Venous leg ulceration, 193–196
Venous thromboembolism (VTE), 35, 125
  lower limb, *see* Lower limb venous
    thromboembolism
  prophylaxis, 283, 285, 287, 310, 313
  recurrent, 36
  risk assessment, 311, 312, 314
Villalta score, 35
VOYAGER trial, 12–13, 56, 76, 89, 283, 285, 288
VTE, *see* Venous thromboembolism

W

Wound, Ischaemia, and Foot Infection (WIfI)
  risk stratification based on, 5–6
  stage, 6, 47, 49, 55–58, 69–70, 73, 100

Y

Yorkshire Kidney Screening Trial, 119

Printed in the United States
by Baker & Taylor Publisher Services

Printed in the United States
by Baker & Taylor Publisher Services